# second edition

# Safety

## Alton L. Thygerson
*Brigham Young University*

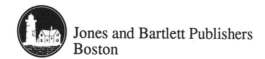
Jones and Bartlett Publishers
Boston

*Editorial, Sales, and Customer Service Offices*
Jones and Bartlett Publishers
20 Park Plaza
Boston, MA 02116

*Library of Congress Cataloging-in-Publication Data*

Not available at press time.

ISBN 0-86720-272-6

Printed in the United States of America
95 94 93 92 91          10 9 8 7 6 5 4 3

Dedicated to the most important people in my life — my family

# Contents

## 9

### MOTOR VEHICLE ACCIDENTS                                      94

## 10

### FALLS                                                        120

# 14

## POISONING                                                    171

# 15

## FIREARM ACCIDENTS                                            197

# 16

## COLD AND HEAT INJURIES                                       205

# 17

## ELECTRIC CURRENT INJURIES

224

# 18

## DISASTERS

233

# 19

## OCCUPATIONAL SAFETY

250

## 20

**SCHOOL SAFETY**

## 21

**SPORTS AND RECREATIONAL SAFETY**

## 22

**SAFETY INSTRUCTION**

# 23

## LEGAL ASPECTS OF ACCIDENTS 303

## INDEX 319

# Preface

The chief goal of this book is to present an account of the foundations of safety, which involves accident prevention and injury control, in such a way as to make it both understandable and interesting to readers with little or no previous knowledge of the subject.

Although there are many professional and lay opinions concerning the accident problem, the foundations for a science of accident prevention and injury control remain inadequate. This book is an attempt to present that needed foundation.

The book deals with terms such as "accident" and "safety." Other relevant content includes a chapter on risk-taking, another on determining causes of accidents, a third devoted to strategies for accident prevention and injury control, plus chapters on the main types of accidents (such as drowning, falls, and firearms). Examples of other concepts not extensively covered in most safety textbooks include: accident proneness, using accident data, and special safety instructional problems (e.g., scare tactics).

A special feature of this book is the use of anecdotal "boxes" providing pertinent world records, accounts of unusual accidents, historical background, and relevant quotes. Also, case studies of lawsuits with a brief explanation of court decisions are included.

A book of this kind has to reflect the author's experience. First, like many people, I have been exposed to many of the hazards discussed herein and have personally experienced several. In addition, I have spent over 20 years teaching safety education courses at public school, college, and university levels. I have enjoyed a close association with several professional safety organizations and a wide consulting experience in safety.

I have also drawn upon long hours of extensive library research over a period of many years. My many years of experience as author of a weekly newspaper column devoted to safety, a monthly journal feature in *Emergency: The Journal of Emergency Services*, and several other safety-related books have also enhanced this book.

Indebtedness to numerous persons is freely acknowledged. In some cases it has been possible to document this fact in specific citations and acknowledgments. The helpful cooperation of numerous publishers in giving permission to quote from their publications is gratefully acknowledged. Appreciation is also extended to those at Prentice-Hall who helped in the development and production of this book.

Alton L. Thygerson

# Safety

# 1

# Introduction

The safety of the American people has never been better. In this century we have witnessed a remarkable reduction in life-threatening accidents along with other public health problems (e.g., infectious and communicable diseases). Nevertheless, accidents rank as the most frequent cause of death for persons between the ages of one and thirty-eight. Moreover, trauma (accidental death and injury) is a seriously neglected public health problem in the United States.

It is the thesis of this book that further improvements in the safety of the American people can be achieved through a commitment to accident prevention and control.

Since 1912, the accidental death rate in the United States has been reduced from eighty-two per 100,000 persons to forty (a reduction of over 50 percent). The reduction in the overall rate during a period when the nation's population more than doubled has resulted in 2,400,000 fewer accidental deaths than would have been the case if the rate had not been reduced.[1]

Much of the credit for this must go to earlier efforts of prevention, based on new knowledge obtained through research. But some of the recent gains are due to measures by government to eliminate hazards and reduce their undesirable effects in the event of an accident. However, we have the scientific knowledge to decrease even further the trauma toll from accidents in which the loss of human life is great.

The message should be clear that much of today's accidental death and disability can be averted. Modest expenditures of dollars can yield high dividends in terms of both lives saved and an improvement in the quality of life.

The case for preventing accidents and controlling their effects has been established in part by a number of accomplishments. Some of the most successful examples are packaging poisonous agents in child resistant containers, equipping refrigerator doors to open easily from the inside, and banning thousands of unsafe toys.

Compared with many diseases of far less consequence, the prevention of death, injuries, and property damage due to accidents has received relatively little scientific attention. Moreover, the expenditure of money for research in the safety area is quite small when compared with the money spent on other public health problems (such as heart disease, cancer, etc.).

Although individual behavior is clearly important to accident causation, emphasis on personal responsibility ignores the important role of the social, political, economic, and physical environments that largely determine behavior. Often pleas for safer lifestyles are likely to be ineffective. Efforts to modify individual behavior will continue, but other successful approaches should be utilized that give automatic protection without requiring any special action on the part of these being protected.

## WHAT IS AN ACCIDENT?

The definition of an "accident" is complicated and not easily understood. Though all of us have had an accident and assume that we know what an accident is, it is more difficult to define than you may think.

Read through each of the statements in Table 1-1 and place a check mark in the blank space if you believe that the statement represents an accident as the term is used within the field of safety.

There are two major attributes of accidents—unintended "causes" and undesirable "effects." These two factors seem to constitute the major elements of most definitions of the term "accident." For example, in the United States the most widely accepted definition of an accident is the one used by the National Safety Council: "that occurrence in a sequence of events which usually produces unintended injury, death, or property damage."[2] Two subfactors essential in the definition of an accident are: (1) the suddenness of the event (in seconds or minutes) and (2) the damage resulting from one of the forms of physical energy (e.g., mechanical, thermal, chemical, etc.).

### Unintended Causes

What is meant by an "unintended cause"? The so-called "act of God," such as being hit by lightning or drowning in a flood, is generally considered an unintended cause. At the other end of the scale is an "act of man," where it is clear that the cause was due to some human behavior.

Most people experience daily unintended events that are called accidents (e.g.,

**TABLE 1-1.  Which Are Accidents?**

Directions: Check the items which you consider to be an accident.

_____  1.  A depressed woman died from an overdose of Valium.

_____  2.  An animal trainer was bitten to death by a tiger.

_____  3.  A woman fell off a trolley car with no apparent injuries but then sued on the claim that she became a nymphomaniac because of the fall.

_____  4.  While hurrying to meet a manuscript deadline, a secretary made a typing mistake.

_____  5.  A college student became very angered when a professor forgot an appointment.

_____  6.  Two people were trampled to death by irate soccer fans rioting over a referee's decision.

_____  7.  A professional golfer received minor injuries after being struck by lightning.

_____  8.  A driver was angered when another vehicle barely missed him.

_____  9.  A college student caught a cold from his girl friend.

_____  10.  During a bank robbery, a security guard was shot and killed.

_____  11.  Residents of St. George, Utah, show high cancer death rates after receiving excessive amounts of radiation fallout from nuclear bomb testing in Nevada during the 1950s.

_____  12.  The family car's right fender was bent while a teenager family member was backing the car out of the garage.

_____  13.  Due to twenty-five years of jarring while operating a bulldozer, the operator developed a lumbar (low back) disc pain.

_____  14.  A two-year-old child died after swallowing aspirin obtained from his mother's purse.

_____  15.  An elderly couple died from hypothermia after being stranded in their car during a winter blizzard.

These statements should have been checked: 2, 7, 12, 14, and 15. These situations meet the criteria for an accident as defined in the field of safety.

mistakes in typing, forgetting an appointment) but are not physically injurious. Usually only those events resulting in physical injury, death, and/or property damage are labeled as accidents in the field of safety.

BOX 1-1

Whatever can go wrong, will.

*—Murphy's Law*

It is important to differentiate between events that are intentional and those that are unintentional.[3] Unintentional events include accidents (drowings, falls, etc.) and disasters (tornadoes, earthquakes, etc.). Intentional acts include crime (homicide, theft, assault, arson, etc.), suicide, wars, and riots. Therefore, if intent can be shown to precede the injury, the occurrence becomes a criminal act, not an accident. The focus of the field of safety is upon unintentional causes which have resulted in undesirable effects (death, injury, and/or property damage).

It is also important to note that the term "unintended" covers only damage from one of the forms of physical energy in the environment (e.g., mechanical, thermal, chemical, electrical, or ionizing radiation). Thus, if a person inadvertently swallows poison and is damaged, the event is called an accident. However, if that same person swallows a polio virus and is injured, the result is called a disease and is rarely considered accidental.

Edward Suchman[4] indicates that the term "accident" is more likely to be used when the event manifests the following three major characteristics:

1. Degree of expectedness—the less the event could have been anticipated, the more likely it is to be labeled an accident.
2. Degree of avoidability—the less the event could have been avoided, the more likely it is to be labeled an accident.
3. Degree of intention—the less the event was the result of a deliberate action, the more likely it is to be labeled an accident.

These characteristics could include many daily activities such as losing things or forgetting appointments, but within the context of the safety field, physical injury, death, and/or property damage must result. In other words, an injury indicates that an accident happened. The injury also occurs over a relatively short period of time (seconds or minutes).

### Undesirable Effects

What is meant by "undesirable effects"? Physical injury in the medical sense can range from minor cuts to death. At any rate, the term "injury" usually refers to damage resulting from sudden exposure to physical or chemical agents, while the result of long-term exposure is usually classified as disease.

Death, injury, and/or property damage—undesirable effects of an unintentional event—do *not* in themselves constitute the accident, but are the results of it. In other words, injury, death, and/or property damage only indicate that an accident has occurred if they result from a sudden or short-term exposure to physical and/or chemical agents.

BOX 1-2

---

Whatever can happen to one man can happen to every man.

*—Seneca*

---

For example, if a driver falls asleep at the wheel but awakes in time to avoid a collision, the event involves no physical injury or damage and is not considered an accident.

An injury could be psychological in nature. Examples include anger, fear, and embarrassment. Such result would not ordinarily be classified as an accident.

BOX 1-3 *UNUSUAL BUT TRUE*

> Bob Aubrey of Ottawa, Ontario had been blind for eight years, tripped over his guide dog and banged his head on the floor. His sight was instantly restored.
>
> —National Safety Council, *Family Safety*

All consequences of accidents need not be entirely negative or undesirable. For example, though a child is burned by touching a hot pan or pot, he learns very quickly that pans and pots can be hot and can cause pain. Thus, this child avoids future contact with hot pans and pots (or possibly even any hot object) and is not burned again. This child's experience, though temporarily painful, has a long-term positive effect. See Table 1-2.

BOX 1-4 *UNUSUAL BUT TRUE*

> Edwin Robinson, legally blind and partially deaf, was standing under a poplar tree near his Falmouth, Maine, home during an electrical storm. A bolt of lightning struck him, restoring his sight and hearing.
>
> —National Safety Council, *Family Safety*

Another example is the after effects of a disaster. Though human life may be taken, survivors learn that living in certain river bottoms in the spring of the year or being near a beach during a hurricane or tsunami should be avoided.

It is not suggested that everyone try to experience things in order to determine consequences. Rather, all people should gain from others' experiences. This is the basis for all instruction and education—a shortcut to experience, but also an avoidance of hazards which may have undesirable effects.

**TABLE 1-2. Accidental Scientific Discoveries**

| DISCOVERY | DISCOVERER | YEAR |
|---|---|---|
| Electrical current | Luigi Galvani of Italy | 1781 |
| Practical photography | Louis Daguerre of France | 1837 |
| Vulcanized rubber | Charles Goodyear of the United States | 1839 |
| X-rays | Wilhelm Roentgen of Germany | 1895 |
| Radioactivity | Henri Becquerel of France | 1896 |
| "Popsicle" (trade name) | Frank Epperson of the United States | 1923 |
| "Teflon" (trade name) | Roy J. Plunkett | 1938 |

Some safety experts question whether injuries or damages should be included in a definition of the term "accident" since a resulting injury is the outcome and does not constitute the accident. Why a person is injured is a separate question from why he was involved in an accident.

The two attributes found in most definitions of an accident (unintentional causes and undesirable effects) are independent of each other. It is, for example, possible for a person to fall down the stairs (the unintended event) without hurting himself (the injury). The two factors can assist in determining the appropriate countermeasures to be used in combating the accident problem. "Accident prevention" pertains to the efforts (such as education, prohibitions, licensing) to deal with the unintentional causes of accidents. "Injury control" pertains to the mitigation (rescue, safety belts, emergency medical care, helmets) of injury, death, and/or property damage.

"Accident prevention" has been criticized on the basis that it is not effective enough and does not convey the idea of the basic problem (injuries) and of the desired end (reducing losses due to injuries). Some experts show evidence that countermeasures to the injury problem should not be limited to prevention, but should include any stage of the injury-producing process. The term suggested is "injury control" rather than "accident prevention." this may appear to be an improvement, but it makes no distinction between accidental (unintentional) injury and intentional injury. It would appear that property damage is not clearly identified either, since "injury" usually refers in most cases only to physical human body damage.

Preventing accidents and their undesirable effects requires a clear concept of what an accident is. Unfortunately, even safety experts disagree on its definition. In fact, the many definitions of an accident complicate accident prevention and ininjury control. Moreover, the common definition and fatalistic connotation of the word "accident" appear to be an obstacle since the word implies, to many people, that something unexpected and unpleasant has occurred, but it:

- couldn't be helped, it was an accident.
- was inevitable and would have happened to anyone.
- was unforeseen, and therefore, uncontrollable.
- is not our fault, and therefore we shouldn't be blamed.

Nevertheless, the word is too deeply entrenched in the language to go out of use. In summary, the word "accident," as commonly used in the field of safety, refers to a sudden unintended event which results in death, injury, and/or property damage from one of the forms of physical energy.

## WHAT IS SAFETY?

There seems to be no general acceptance of what is implied or denoted in the term "safety." Kenneth Licht[5] has identified five distinct ways in which the word "safety" is used:

I. Examples of Safety or Its Derivative Used in a Health Context
   A. Visitors to exotic lands are cautioned that the public drinking supply may not be *safe*.
   B. Air pollution was so bad last winter that it was *unsafe* for elderly people and those with respiratory problems to go outside.
   C. Many persons still consider it *unsafe* to store canned foods in their original containers.
   D. Even persons with sensitive skin may use this product with complete *safety*.

II. Examples of Safety or Its Derivative Used in a "Security Context
   A. Always carry your credit cards in a *safe* place.
   B. We guarantee the highest interest rates with complete *safety*.
   C. Our recently expanded campus police force has made this the *safest* campus in the state.
   D. Ladies, for your personal *safety*, learn self-defense techniques at our health club.

III. Examples of Safety or Its Derivative Used in a "Special" or "Technical" Context
   A. Don't be half-*safe;* use . . . . . . . deodorant.
   B. The *safety* we scored in the final quarter beat State and made our homecoming a complete success.
   C. Be sure the *safety* is on until you're ready to fire.
   D. It is *safe* to assume that most people prefer comfort to distress.

IV. Examples of Safety or Its Derivative Used in an "Accident Prevention" Context
   A. It's a good practice to have your car *safety*-checked before your vacation trip.
   B. The right way is the *safe* way.
   C. Worn tires are more *unsafe* at today's expressway speeds than they were when average speeds were lower.
   D. Platform shoes may be stylish, but they're certainly *unsafe*.

V. Examples of Safety or Its Derivative Used in an "Accident Mitigation" Context (Note: This category deals with efforts to reduce (mitigate) the consequences of accidents. It takes up where accident prevention leaves off. Hard hats, for example, have little to do with accident prevention, but everything to do with accident mitigation. A closer examination of the concept of accidents and accident mitigation will follow.)
   A. *Safety* rules require hard hats be worn on this job.
   B. More than half the states now have *safety* regulations requiring eye-protection articles be worn in all shops and labs.
   C. Energy-absorbing steering columns, padded dashes and corner posts, recessed handles, knobs, and other hostile projections have made the new cars much *safer*.
   D. A first-aid course is essential to anyone interested in a career in *safety*.

In his book, *Of Acceptable Risk*, William Lowrance[6] explores the meaning of safety. A thing is safe, according to Lowrance, if its risks are judged to be acceptable; and judging the acceptability of that risk (judging safety) is a matter of personal and social value judgment. Safety can change from time to time and be judged differently in different contexts.

Lowrance points out that the term "safety" is vague as used in the past and has long been misused. He contends that risks, not safety, are measured. A thing is safe if its attendant risks are judged to be acceptable.

Lowrance differentiates by saying that:

Measuring Risk—a measure of the probability of harm—described as a scientific activity.
Measuring Safety—a judgment of the acceptability of risks—described as a value-judging activity.

We all face varying degrees of risks. An example of an "acceptable risk" would be an act almost every one of us performs many times a week: opening our mail. Have you ever gotten a paper cut while tearing open the flap of an envelope? That is an injury associated with a very common item, a paper envelope. Yet we do not consider a paper envelope hazardous. The risk of injury involved in tearing open an envelope is acceptable.

Objects with sharp edges present an interesting example of "unacceptable risks" which also can be considered "acceptable" depending on the circumstance. Anything with a sharp edge is hazardous. But we simply accept the risk whenever we use a knife, and we use it carefully to minimize the hazard. However, very young children do not understand these concepts of *risk* and *hazard*, and they certainly cannot exercise the same kind of care as adults. So while a sharp edge on a kitchen knife constitutes an acceptable risk to an adult, the risk becomes unacceptable for children. Similarly, a sharp edge on a child's toy presents an unacceptable risk.

Remember, Lowrance defines *risk* as something we can *measure* and *safety* as something we must *judge*. Take the matter of the paper envelope. We can measure the severity of the cuts and the probability or the frequency with which they occur. This gives us a measure of the *risk* involved in opening a paper envelope. Next, we judge whether this risk is worth taking. Yes, we say, it is. We judge that paper envelopes are *safe*.

In our example of the knives, we can measure the risk of a cut. We judge that knives are safe for adults, who can handle them carefully, but are unsafe for children, who cannot. On a child's toy, a sharp edge produces such a high probability of harm, poses such a high risk, that we judge it unsafe. See page 43 for more information on how to judge what is safe.

## WHY STUDY ABOUT ACCIDENTS AND SAFETY?

### Awareness

Individuals should be aware of the main accident problems. Have you ever visited a place and then been surprised at how often you heard or read about that place afterward? The place had been mentioned just as frequently before you visited it, but you never noticed these comments until you were acquainted with it; thereafter, you found meaning in each reference because it related to something that had become familiar. Similarly, if we are aware of a particular accident problem, we notice each reference to it in the newspaper, possibly take time to read a magazine article about it, or become more attentive when it comes up in conversation. In this way we constantly increase our knowledge of a problem and the validity of our judgments about it.

### Factual Knowledge

An intelligent analysis must rest upon facts. It makes little sense to discuss an accident problem unless someone in the group knows what he or she is talking about. Although fact gathering will not solve any problem automatically, it is impossible to analyze a problem until the facts have been collected, organized, and interpreted.

Misconceptions about safety, accidents, and injuries exist because all the facts may not be known or presented. Unfortunately, these misconceptions and myths persist yet, in spite of educational efforts. (See Figures 1-1 and 1-2.) As a self-check for misconceptions, see how well you perform on the test in Table 1-3.

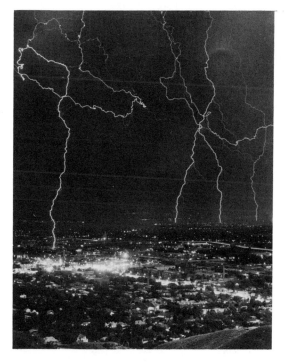

**FIGURE 1-1**
Does lightning ever strike twice in the same place? Photo courtesy of the *Deseret News.*

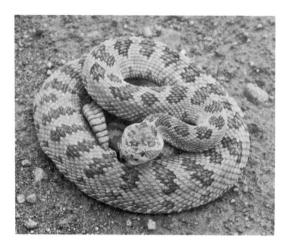

**FIGURE 1-2**
Myths exist about the rattlesnake. The venom of bees, wasps, and hornets causes more deaths in the United States each year than are caused by the venom of rattlesnakes. Photo courtesy of the Utah Division of Natural Resources.

## The Science of Accident Prevention and Injury Control

*It is valuable that we have a general understanding of how and why accidents occur, how people are affected by accidents, and how we can deal with them.* This provides a frame of reference within which we can catalog data and study specific problems. If we have a thorough understanding of the science of accident prevention and injury control we can intelligently organize and analyze data on any particular accident. In addition, this understanding enables us to interpret new data

**TABLE 1-3    Test on Safety Misconceptions**

Directions: Place a check mark in front of the statement if you believe it to be true.

_____    1.    A person hit by lightning usually dies instantly.

_____    2.    Lightning never strikes twice in the same place.

_____    3.    Red is the hunter's best clothing color.

_____    4.    A rattlesnake gives warning before striking.

_____    5.    It is impossible to stay afloat in water for long with clothes on.

_____    6.    If a boat overturns, you should swim to shore.

_____    7.    A drowning person always comes up for air three times.

_____    8.    Coffee will help sober up a drunk.

_____    9.    Smaller vehicles can stop in less time and distance than larger ones.

_____    10.    Pumping the brakes helps stop a car more quickly on icy roads.

_____    11.    A rattlesnake has to be coiled up to strike.

_____    12.    Sharks won't attack close to shore.

_____    13.    Moss always grows on the north side of a tree trunk.

_____    14.    There is a difference between "flammable" and "inflammable."

_____    15.    The only way you can get poison ivy is to touch the plant.

Number 10 should have been checked as true. All the other statements are false.

correctly and to keep up to date. Accident data often become obsolete and accident problems may change considerably within a few years. For example, there is a change in concern about motorcycle and snowmobile death and injury statistics and a decrease in concern about abandoned refrigerators and ultrathin plastic clothing covers as potential hazards. Yet, if the individual understands the science of accident prevention, he or she will not find it hard to interpret new data and understand new accident trends.

Our attitudes and values determine the meanings we find in the facts we observe. A study of some widespread fallacious attitudes toward accidents may help show why people react to facts so differently. Such a study may also help show why we may always have accident problems.

Listed below are some fallacious beliefs presented by authors Richardson, Hein, and Farnsworth:

1. The "other fellow" concept, whereby it is assumed that accidents happen to other people but won't happen to you.
2. The "your number's up" concept, whereby it is assumed that "when your number is up," you will get hurt and there is nothing you can do about it.
3. The "law of averages" concept, whereby accidents and injuries are shrugged off as due to inevitable statistical laws.
4. The "price of progress" concept, whereby accidents are rationalized as the inevitable price of scientific advancement.
5. The "spirit of '76" concept, whereby living dangerously is glorified and safety measures are regarded as sissy.
6. The "act of God" concept, whereby accidents are seen as divinely caused—for punishment or for some purpose unknown to us.[7]

### A Sense of Perspective

Some people find the study of accidents upsetting. Just as people are frightened by all the diseases they find listed in a medical textbook, some individuals are disturbed by the great amount of expressed or implied criticism of our society that they find in a safety course. For others, awareness of imperfections which result in accidents may become an obsession. They are so distressed with the tragedy, suffering, and waste caused by an accident-plagued society that they fail to see more encouraging aspects of the total picture. We need a sense of perspective if we are to see without exaggeration or distortion.

### Appreciation of the Proper Role of the Expert

Opinions are not equally valuable. If we want a useful opinion on why our head throbs or our car stalls, we ask the appropriate experts. However, as we ponder accidents, we hesitate to ask the safety expert and confidently announce our own opinions, perhaps after discussing the questions with others who know no more than we.

This contradiction stems from our failure to distinguish between *questions of knowledge* and *questions of value.* In questions of knowledge there are right and wrong answers, whereas in questions of value there are differences of opinion. The layman and the expert are equally qualified to answer questions of value, but they are not equally qualified to answer questions of knowledge. For instance, the question of whether leisure time should be used in viewing operas or football games is a matter of value. But the question of whether a four-phase driver education program is more or less effective than a two-phase driver education program requires expert knowledge to answer.

Stated in simple terms, *the role of the expert is not to tell people what they should want, but to tell them how they may best get what they want.* Even experts are not infallible; all may be wrong on a given issue. When experts disagree, no one answer should be considered positive or final. Experts in safety agree that accidents are caused and do not "just happen"; the layman who feels an accident was an event which could not have been avoided reveals his ignorance.

In the field of safety, the function of the expert is to provide accurate descriptions and analyses of accidents and to show laymen what consequences may follow each countermeasure proposal. However, experts have met with limited success when they have attempted to tell people what would be best for them in a given situation. It usually takes a near-accident, an accident, or even a tragedy before people become sufficiently concerned and motivated to take overt action. Recall from page 8 that experts measure risk, while safety is unusually determined by personal and social value judgments.

The task of the individual is to learn how to recognize an expert and guide his own thinking by expert knowledge rather than by guesswork.

## NOTES

1. National Safety Council, *Accident Facts* (Chicago: National Safety Council, 1984), p. 10.
2. ____., p. 97.
3. Kenneth F. Licht, "Safety: What Is It?" *School Safety World Newsletter*, 1, no. 3 (Summer 1973), 3.
4. Edward A. Suchman, "A Conceptual Analysis of the Accident Phenomenon," in William Haddon, Jr., Edward A. Suchman, and David Klein, eds., *Accident Research* (New York: Harper & Row, Publishers, Inc., 1964), p. 276.
5. Kenneth F. Licht, "Safety and Accidents—A Brief Conceptual Analysis and a Point of View," *Journal of School Health,* XLV, no. 9 (November 1975), 530–31.
6. William W. Lowrance, *Of Acceptable Risk* (Los Altos, Calif.: William Kaufmann, Inc., 1976), p. 8.
7. Charles E. Richardson, Fred V. Hein, and Dana L. Farnsworth, *Living* (Glenview, Ill.: Scott, Foresman & Company, 1975), pp. 339–40.

# 2

# Magnitude of the Accident Problem

## EXTENT OF ACCIDENT OCCURRENCE

Reading statistics can be quite dull. Reading accident statistics may be repulsive as well. However, accident statistics of any kind tell us only where and how accidents happened, but not why. Let us consider some general accident statistics.

Every year in this country approximately one hundred thousand accidental deaths are reported by the National Safety Council. This averages out to one death every five minutes.[1] About nine million disabling injuries are reported annually. Disabling injuries are not reported on a nationwide basis, therefore the total numbers of injuries are estimates and should not be compared from year to year. Death accounts are more accurate than data on nonfatal injuries, which are often under-reported and under-estimated; for many types of accidents records are almost nonexistent.

Table 2-1 ranks accidents with other major causes of death. The tragedy of the high accidental death loss is that trauma kills thousands who otherwise could expect to live long and productive lives, whereas those afflicted with heart disease, cancer, stroke, and many chronic diseases usually die late in life.

The human suffering and financial loss from preventable accidental death constitute a public health problem second only to the ravages of ancient plagues or world wars. In making comparisons of fatal accidents with war, it must be kept in

13

TABLE 2-1   Accidents and Other Causes of Death

| RANK | CAUSE OF DEATH |
|------|----------------|
| 1 | Heart disease |
| 2 | Cancer |
| 3 | Stroke (cerebrovascular disease) |
| 4 | Accidents |
|   |     Motor vehicle |
|   |     Falls |
|   |     Drowning |
|   |     Fires, burns |
|   |     Suffocation — ingested object |
|   |     Poisoning by solids and liquids |
|   |     Firearms |
|   |     Poisoning by gases and vapors |
| 5 | Pneumonia |
| 6 | Diabetes mellitus |
| 7 | Chronic liver disease, cirrhosis |
| 8 | Atherosclerosis |
| 9 | Suicide |
| 10 | Homicide |
| 11 | Certain conditions originating in perinatal period |
| 12 | Nephritis and nephrosis |

Source: National Safety Council, *Accident Facts*, 1984, p. 8.

mind that nearly everyone is exposed to accidents, but relatively few are exposed to war deaths. The point is that we are very much concerned about war and its effects, but to be unconcerned about a domestic problem which causes as much or even more damage betrays a paradox in human thought and values.

One in four Americans is annually injured badly enough to require medical attention or activity restriction for at least one day. Accidents cause more deaths each year than all infectious diseases combined. Although accidental deaths were reduced by over 50 percent during the past seventy-five years, trauma from accidents still poses a major problem.

The accident picture in the United States is grim; yet it is fair to assume that without organized safety efforts and safety education, America's accident record would be even more shocking than it is. Following heart disease, cancer, and stroke, accidents are the fourth principal cause of death in the United States. Accidents are the leading cause of death among those persons aged one to 38 years.[2]

We often think of accidents only when they are catastrophes because these events make newspaper headlines. From a statistical point of view, a catastrophe is an accident in which five or more lives are lost.[3] It is significant that a very small percentage of accident catastrophes occur as a result of natural forces such as floods, hurricanes, tornadoes, and earthquakes (see Figure 2-1). Rather, the majority of newspaper headline catastrophes are caused by some kind of human failure which results in airplane crashes, mine cave-ins, explosions, and the like. However, the

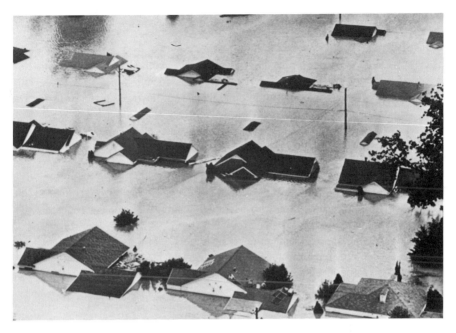

**FIGURE 2-1** Disasters occur in all parts of the world. That they will come is certain. Photo courtesy of the American National Red Cross.

record of natural catastrophes reveals that relatively few lives are lost in this way when contrasted with the total number of deaths resulting from other types of unspectacular, unpublished accidents.

## SURVEYS OF ACCIDENTS AMONG THE GENERAL PUBLIC

The National Health Survey, conducted by the National Center for Health Statistics, is a survey of households to collect information on the number of injuries sustained by household members during the two weeks prior to the survey interview. (It should be noted that other health information is also surveyed.) The total number of injuries is then estimated for the entire United States based upon these findings from approximately 40,000 households. We realize that differences in definition produce different injury totals when we compare the results of the National Health Survey with the totals presented by the National Safety Council.

An examination of accident injury data gathered from the general population suggests the following conclusions:

1. Estimates of the number of accidents based solely on the data of deaths or reported injuries are incomplete.

2. Data derived from these sources point out the need for a standard accident definition and reporting system.

The question of definition—and *who does the defining*—is a crucial one. For example, one may never detect or report the housewife who burns her fingers. This type of incident occurs commonly in daily living and illustrates how large numbers of accidents remain unknown.

## ESTIMATES OF THE COST OF ACCIDENTS

Reliable estimates of the overall cost per annum of accidents in the United States are difficult to make, and those who have investigated the problem conclude that even approximate figures would be inaccurate.

We can compare accident costs to an iceberg—only a small portion that we can actually see and measure appears above water. The indirect and hidden costs form the rest of the iceberg, the part below water that is not easily measured. Examples of costs are listed in Table 2-2.

**TABLE 2-2  Some Social and Economic Consequences of Accidents**

| | SOCIAL | | ECONOMIC |
|---|---|---|---|
| 1 | Grief over the loss of loved ones | 1 | Costs of rescue equipment required |
| 2 | Loss of public confidence | 2 | Accident investigation and reporting |
| 3 | Loss of prestige | 3 | Fees for legal actions |
| 4 | Deterioration of morale | 4 | Time of personnel involved in rescue |
| 5 | Denial of education | 5 | Medical fees (doctors, hospitals, etc.) |
| 6 | Lack of guidance for children | 6 | Disability costs of personnel badly injured |
| 7 | Psychological effects of a change in standard of living | 7 | Replacement cost of property damaged or lost |
| 8 | Psychic damages affecting behavior | 8 | Slowdown in operations while accident causes are determined and corrective actions taken |
| 9 | Embarrassment | 9 | Loss of income |
| 10 | Lost pride | 10 | Loss of earning capability |
| 11 | Inconvenience | 11 | Rehabilitation costs for those who have lost limbs, mental abilities, or physical skills |
| 12 | Adversely affected interpersonal relationships (anger, resentment, etc.) | 12 | Funeral expenses for those killed |
| | | 13 | Pensions for injured persons or for dependents of those killed |
| | | 14 | Training costs and lower output of replacements |
| | | 15 | Production loss for employer |

## GEOGRAPHICAL DISTRIBUTION OF ACCIDENTS IN THE UNITED STATES

### Regional Accident Rates

Rates of reported accidents vary widely from one region to another. In accidental death rates, the Middle Atlantic region ranks lowest. The Rocky Mountain and Southern States regions have the highest rates of accidental deaths. Various explanations could be offered for these wide variations, but they would probably still not account for all the variations found.

### Rural-Urban Variations

Accident death rates tend consistently to decrease with greater density of population. The difference in rates between the most densely populated and the least densely populated communities is sizable.

## GENERAL CHARACTERISTICS OF THE ACCIDENT VICTIM

The "typical" accident victim exists only as a vague abstraction created from statistical figures. Nevertheless, statistics enable us to say:

1. Most accident victims are males. After the first year of life, males have more accidents than females, at all age levels.
2. Most accident victims are young. Accidents are the leading cause of death for persons aged one to thirty-eight years; however, the rate for accidental deaths is highest for those over seventy years of age, with the fifteen to twenty-four year age group next highest.
3. Accidental death rates are highest in rural areas. The Rocky Mountain and Southern regions of the United States have the highest accident rates.
4. Most accidental deaths occur in a motor vehicle, but most injuries occur in the home. This is explained by the high speeds involved in motor-vehicle accidents resulting in death; whereas, the home is not as lethal, but because of time spent there accounts for the most injuries.
5. Most accidents happen to the victim in a cyclical manner, reaching peaks in frequency on certain days and at a particular time of the year. Weekends and the summer months of June, July, and August have the highest rates.

As will be discussed in Chapter 3, accurately assessing facts presents a real problem.

## SOCIAL AND ECONOMIC CONSEQUENCES OF ACCIDENTS

Accidents produce consequences of grave importance in terms of death, injury, and property damage. Table 2-2 presents in brief form some social and economic implications of accidents.

TABLE 2-3   Years of Potential Life Lost by Causes of Death

| CAUSE OF DEATH | YEARS OF POTENTIAL LIFE LOST BEFORE AGE 65 BY PERSONS DYING IN 1982 | ESTIMATED NUMBER OF PHYSICIAN CONTACTS DECEMBER 1981 |
|---|---|---|
| ALL CAUSES (includes data not shown separately) | 9,429,000 | 84,586,000 |
| Accidents | 2,367,000 | 4,610,000 |
| Malignant neoplasms | 1,809,000 | 1,403,000 |
| Diseases of heart | 1,566,000 | 4,956,000 |
| Suicides, homicides | 1,314,000 | — |
| Cerebrovascular diseases | 256,000 | 557,000 |
| Chronic liver diseases and cirrhosis | 252,000 | 86,000 |
| Pneumonia and influenza | 118,000 | 1,067,000 |
| Chronic obstructive pulmonary diseases and allied conditions | 114,000 | 2,025,000 |
| Diabetes mellitus | 106,000 | 2,312,000 |

Source: Centers for Disease Controls.

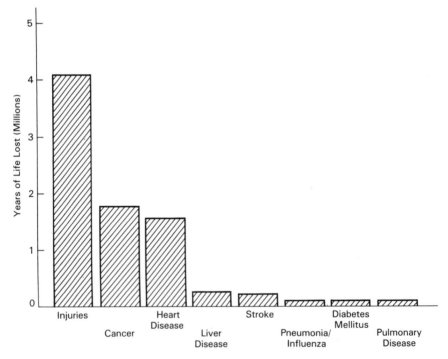

FIGURE 2-2 Potential Years of Life Lost Prior to Age 70 from Eight Leading Causes of Death. From *The Injury Fact Book* by Susan P. Baker, Brian O'Neill, and Ronald S. Karpf (Lexington, Mass.: Lexington Books, D.C. Heath and Company, Copyright 1984, D.C. Heath and Company).

We should consider the serious consequences of accidents in terms of their disruptive effects on the home, on the family, and on employment. The notions of "life years lost" and "working years lost" are helpful in gauging the magnitude of the accident problem. Table 2-3 and Figure 2-2 show us that accidental deaths are responsible for a greater number of years of potential life lost than are deaths from any other cause.[4]

## NOTES

1.  National Safety Council, *Accident Facts*, 1983, p. 11.
2.  All statistical data in this book are from the National Safety Council, *Accident Facts*, 1984, unless otherwise noted.
3.  Metropolitan Life Insurance Company, *Statistical Bulletin* (January 1975), p. 6.
4.  Nelson S. Hartunian, Charles N. Smart, and Mark S. Thompson, *The Incidence and Economic Costs of Major Health Impairments* (Lexington, Mass.: D.C. Heath and Company, 1982).

# 3

# Using Accident Data

The first decennial census was taken in the United States in 1790. However, it was not until after the turn of the twentieth century that accident data were collected systematically.

## ACCIDENT FACTS

Issued annually by the National Safety Council, *Accident Facts* now constitutes a most reliable source of nationwide frequency for all types of accidents reported in the United States.[1] In addition to presenting annual reports on the four principal classes of accidents, *Accident Facts* presents data on rates and trends; hence this compendium is an available source for evaluating the relative efficiency of accident-prevention attempts. The National Safety Council has been aided in the collection and interpretation of accident data by many organizations, companies, and individuals.

## OTHER SOURCES OF ACCIDENT STATISTICS

Except for statistical studies made by individual investigators which are usually limited to small samples of accident victims, the large-scale gathering of statistical data is necessarily a task of the government. At present, there are several sources available for accident statistics:

*National Center for Vital Statistics.*  This government agency summarizes death certificates. Details are brief. Reports often state "victim fell," or "victim poisoned"—and little else.

*National Center for Health Statistics.*  This federal agency conducts the National Health Survey annually. This survey of about forty thousand households is primarily concerned with health problems. Accidents are included, but are a relatively small portion of the survey. Its weakness is that it does not get enough information. Although forty thousand households are contacted annually, the interviewer asks for accident experience of household members during only the previous two-week period. This totals about eight thousand person-years of exposure annually. Thus, if a type of accident occurs only twenty-five thousand times a year, we can expect to find only one case in the National Health Survey for that year. From the survey, then, one gets overall totals—a broad perspective of what is going on; but one does not get the details needed. Numerical differences between National Health Survey totals and the National Safety Council totals occur and are due mainly to differences in the injury definitions used.

*National Electronic Injury Surveillance System (NEISS).*  This is a national data system used to determine the magnitude and scope of consumer product-related injuries. NEISS gathers data daily through a computer system located throughout the United States. Certain accident cases are assigned for follow-up interviews to collect detailed information. The details, available through on-site visits so that photographs can be taken, the product examined or collected, and measurements made or done by telephone interviews, establish the relationship between the victim, the consumer product, and the environment.

NEISS enables the identification of hazards. NEISS data are supplemented by death certificate records for fatalities throughout the United States and by newspaper accounts.

*National Center for Statistics and Analysis.*  This center is under the jurisdiction of the National Highway Traffic Safety Administration and operates data collection and analysis programs to support motor vehicle and highway safety efforts.

The Center's major data collection systems include:

*Fatal Accident Reporting System (FARS)* Which is a census of every fatal motor vehicle accident in the United States, containing information obtained from state records.

*National Accident Sampling System (NASS)* which is a nationally representative sample of all police-reported traffic accidents and contains detailed information beyond what is available in state record systems. Data are collected by trained accident investigatiors under contract to NHTSA.

*State Agencies.* Organizations such as state departments of vital statistics, highway departments, and safety councils frequently collect, analyze, and distribute information on the incidence of accidents in their particular geographical area and special interest and responsibility.

*Research Reports.* Excellent sources of information on specific accident problems are available through the safety literature. (See Table 4-1.) Many of the research reports are located in public and university libraries.

## NEED FOR ACCIDENT DATA

Why do we need accident data? Such data provide evidence that an accident and injury problem exists, and that it is important to know of its existence. Actually, severe accidents are rare events in the life of most individuals and few persons can get any clear understanding of their importance as a social and economic problem solely from their own experience. A second reason for having accident data is the need to evaluate the effectiveness of accident prevention and injury control countermeasures.

Data usually comes in statistical form, and statistics are of two types:

1. *Descriptive statistics* provide methods of organizing, summarizing, and communicating data. Most of the accident and injury statistics are descriptive in nature. Total sums, ratios, averages, and percentages are examples of descriptive statistics.
2. *Inferential statistics* provide methods for making inferences from the descriptive data. Research reports usually use inferential statistics. Examples of such statistics include statistics indicating differences between groups and statistics showing relationships. A college course in statistics is needed to properly understand and interpret the use of inferential statistics.

## PROBLEMS OF STATISTICAL ANALYSIS

Statistics play an important role in accident prevention. The reasons statistics are not used more is probably because of what some call a "statistical neurosis."

An early statistician coined a phrase that has since been repeated to generations: "It's not that the figures lie—it's that the liars figure." Although deceptive figures do appear in accident statistics, it is probable that the largest number of statistical studies are compiled by those desiring to inform rather than misinform. Nevertheless, a statistic that misleads through honest error can be just as confusing as one that is deliberately constructed to misrepresent. In the following paragraphs we will discuss several sources of error found in accident statistics; these may be divided into the following groups: sources of error in *collection, presentation,* and *interpretation.*

### Sources of Error in the Collection
### of Accident Statistics

*Deliberate suppression.*   There are several forms of suppression. One can be attributed to administrative self-protection rather than to darker motives. Keeping the accident rate down is a perennial concern of administrators. Frequently, a slightly injured worker is immediately returned to the job to keep the factory record spotless, even if the injured worker should be home after the accident resting from the shock and caring for his injury.

Only a few accident statistic errors in collection result from distortions introduced deliberately or negligently. The following sources of error are highly difficult or impossible to eradicate.

*Failure to complain.*   Since an accident is not known until someone reports it, any statistic that purports to represent the total number of any type of accident that has taken place is necessarily an informed guess based on the addition of an estimated number of *unreported* accidents of the same category. Certain types of accidents tend to be reported with much greater accuracy than others. For example, deaths resulting from motor-vehicle accidents are usually reported quite accurately because there are legal requirements to make such reports and great value is placed upon human life. However, motor-vehicle accidents causing less than one hundred dollars worth of damage may go unnoticed and even unreported as a result of legal stipulations and one hundred dollar deductible insurance coverage which may not require the reporting of small accidents. Even reports of damage costs may be totally in error since most estimated costs are quite subjective in nature.

*Geographical variations in the definition of certain accidents.*   There is one obstacle hindering a uniform system of accident reporting which will not be overcome until all jurisdictions employ similar definitions for classifying accidents. For example, different definitions yield different statistics. In Belgium and Italy a person is considered a highway fatality only if he dies at the accident scene. In France an interval between injury and death that would still permit such a classification is three days, twenty-four hours in Spain, thirty days in Britain, and a year in the United States and Canada.

*Differences in the reporting of accidents within the same area.*   An administrator has his biases. If a relative or a person with high status has an accident, the administrator may never report it in order to keep a record clear of any blemish that might hinder future promotions and advancements for that person. Another example was given by William E. Tarrants at a National Safety Congress:

A mid-western manufacturing plant with a fairly stable injury frequency rate decided to hire a full-time safety engineer to see if this rate could be cut down. Within a short time after the safety engineer was hired, the injury frequency rate nearly doubled. Should we conclude that the safety engineer caused these accidents and quickly fire him? A closer look revealed that the safety engineer instituted a new accident investigation and reporting system which produced more reports of disabling injuries, thus increasing the frequency rate.[2]

*Lack of uniformity in collecting and recording techniques.* Tallying the number of known accidents is a considerably more complicated process than it would seem to be. A motor-vehicle accident is usually witnessed, whereas there may be no witnesses to a home accident involving minor cuts or burns, making accurate reporting more difficult.

### Sources of Error in the Presentation of Accident Statistics

When we consider statistical data there is probably no assertion more misleading than the frequently heard statement: "The figures speak for themselves." Because long columns of figures convey an impression of factuality, it is essential to discuss the more common misunderstandings that arise from faulty presentation of data.

*Misleading use of simple sums rather than rates.* The fact that Town *A* records fifty motor vehicle deaths as compared with one hundred reported by Town *B* does not necessarily mean that Town *B* is twice as accident-ridden as Town *A*. If Town *B* has four times the population of Town *A* the reverse is true. Total accident figures do not become meaningful until they are transformed into *rates* (ratios or percentages) based on the total population under consideration. Similarly, this principle applies to changes in the incidence of accidents. Town *C*, in 1990, may report twice as many accidents as it did in 1970—yet its population may have doubled during this period. If this is true, then the accident rate remains the same.

*Misleading use of averages and percentages.* The precaution of translating simple sums into averages and percentages does not assure the proper presentation of data; these measures can be misleading as the raw totals. Consider the following statement: "The average number of accidents per family in the Lakeview residential area is three per year." This statement gives the impression that each family living in the Lakeview residential area has about the same number of accidents each year. This assumption may not be correct at all. A count reveals that five families live in the area. Three households report one accident, whereas the fourth family reports two accidents that year. The fifth family has a total of ten among its members. Thus the "average" figure obtained by adding the total number of accidents and dividing by five is mathematically accurate but misleading.

As the illustration demonstrates, an *average* is meaningless without information about the variation of the measures that compose it.

*Pitfalls of graphic presentations.*    For some readers, long columns of figures are not only impressive but downright intimidating. For this reason statisticians and publicists often present their findings graphically or pictorially. Although this method presents material in quick, easy-to-comprehend form, it can also mislead the reader.

### Sources of Error in the Interpretation of Accident Statistics

*The "self-evident" conclusion.*    Mark Twain observed that there are three kinds of lies—plain lies, damned lies, and statistics. This humorous statement implies that statistics can be manipulated to support any point of view. The use of statistics, however, should not be completely dismissed, for statistics mislead and confuse only when one does not know how to interpret them. There are elaborate formulas for determining the significance and reliability of a statistic. This text offers some simple tests which the reader can apply.

There are some basic criteria which should be applied in analyzing or interpreting accident information and data:

1. Who compiled and reported the information (e.g., background, reputation, and experience of the individual or group)?
2. Why is the information provided (e.g., to inform the public, sell a product, or other motives)?
3. When was the information compiled (e.g., recently or long ago)?
4. How is the information presented?
5. Where did the information come from (e.g., research findings or personal opinion)?
6. Is the information accurate and reliable (e.g., sound conclusions or questionable data)?
7. What of it (e.g., important or insignificant)?

The problems with many of the sources of accident data are: (1) information incomplete, (2) reporting on only severe types, (3) information not easily available or not made public, (4) inaccuracies, and (5) variations in definition of accident and/or injury.

The statement that "four times more fatalities occur on the highways at 7 P.M. than at 7 A.M." can be misleading. People fail to realize that more people are killed in the evening than in the morning simply because more people are on the highways at that hour to be killed. An amusing example of nonsense statistics is found in Table 3-1.

**TABLE 3-1    Pickles Will Kill You**

Pickles will kill you: Every pickle you eat brings you nearer to death. Amazingly the "thinking man" has failed to grasp the terrifying significance of the term "in a pickle." Although leading horticulturists have long known that Cucumis sativus possesses an indehiscent pepo, the pickle industry continues to expand.

Pickles are associated with all the major diseases of the body. Eating them breeds wars and communism. They can be related to most airline tragedies. Auto accidents are caused by pickles. There exists a positive relationship between crime waves and consumption of this fruit of the cucurbit family. For example:

Nearly all sick people have eaten pickles. The effects are obviously cumulative.

99.9% of all people who die from cancer have eaten pickles.

100% of all soldiers have eaten pickles.

96.8% of all communist sympathizers have eaten pickles.

99.9% of all the people involved in air and auto accidents ate pickles within 14 days preceding the accident.

93.1% of juvenile delinquents come from homes where pickles are served frequently.

Evidence points to the long-term effects of pickle eating:

Of the people born in 1839 who later dined on pickles, there has been a 100% mortality.

All pickle-eaters born between 1849 and 1859 have wrinkled skin, have lost most of their teeth, have brittle bones and failing eyesight—if the ills of eating pickles haven't already caused their death.

Even more convincing is the report of a noted team of medical experts: rats force-fed with 20 pounds of pickles per day for 30 days developed bulging abdomens. Their appetites for WHOLESOME FOOD were destroyed.

In spite of all the evidence, pickle-growers and packers continue to spread their evil. More than 120,000 acres of fertile soil are devoted to growing pickles. Our per capita yearly consumption is nearly four pounds.

Eat orchid petal soup. Practically no one has as many problems from eating orchid petal soup as they do from eating pickles.

The field of safety and accident prevention is replete with figures, statistics, numbers, and ratios. However, there is little literature available regarding the proper use of accident statistics. William Tarrants, at a National Safety Congress, presented information which he felt was pertinent:

During World War II about 375 thousand people were killed in the United States by accidents and about 408 thousand were killed in the armed forces. From these figures, it has been argued that it was not much more dangerous to be overseas in the armed forces than to be at home. A more meaningful comparison, however, would consider rates of the same age groups. This comparison would reflect adversely on the safety of the armed forces during the war—in fact, the armed forces death rate (about 12 per thousand men per year) was 15 to 20 times as high, per person per year, as the over-all civilian death rate from accidents (about 0.7 per thousand per year).

The same fallacy is noted in the widely publicized statistical appraisal which states that "Sometime during the Korean War we passed a grim milestone. One day an American soldier fell in battle. He was the millionth American soldier to die in our wars since the nation was born. A few months later the 1,000,000th American perished in a modern highway traffic accident. [*Author's note:* The two millionth traffic fatality occurred in 1974. Based on projections, the toll will reach three million in 1990.] Our wars go back to 1776. The traffic figure starts with 1900." The article concludes that "war is dangerous business but getting from one place to another by automobile is even more dangerous." Again, we should consider rates, not numbers, and comparisons should also consider the same age groups.

Peacetime versions of the same fallacy are also common. We often hear that "off-the-job activities are more dangerous than places of work, since more accidents occur off-the-job" or that "The bedroom is the most hazardous room in the home since more injuries occur in the bedroom than any other room." Here again the originators fail to consider differences in quantity of exposure, type of exposure, age, and other influencing factors.[3]

*The confusion of correlation with cause.* In Chapter 7 "causes" of accidents will be discussed in detail. A favorite method of searching for "causes" is to hunt for statistical associations. It is often claimed, without real justification, that there are associations and correlations between contributing factors and accidents. Individuals often have difficulty contrasting the association of these factors with the total situation; illustrations are given in Table 3-2 to help them overcome this difficulty. The central point is that a genuine association exists *only* when two things appear together *either more frequently or less frequently than would normally be expected.*

Whenever two factors are associated, there are at least four possibilities as to why:

1. A causes B (epileptic seizure causes auto accident).
2. B causes A (auto accident causes seizure due to head injury).
3. Both A and B are caused by C (both seizure and auto accident are caused by flickering roadside lights).
4. A and B are independent and the "association" is by chance.

TABLE 3-2  When Does a Percentage Indicate a Statistical Association?

| IF: | WE NEED TO KNOW: | BEFORE TRYING TO DECIDE: |
|---|---|---|
| 50% of fatal accidents involve drinking drivers. | What percent of all driving is done by drinking drivers? | Whether drinking drivers contribute more or less than their share of fatal accidents. |
| 50% of injuries to boys in the first three school grades are due to lack of safety knowledge. | What percent of all boys of similar age lack safety knowledge? | Whether lack of safety knowledge is associated with school injuries to boys. |
| 30% of fatal accidents involve vehicles being driven too fast. | What percent of all driving is done beyond the speed limit? | Whether driving too fast is correlated with fatal accidents. |
| 300% as many deaths occur off the job as on the job. | What percent of time is spent both on the job and off the job? | Whether a worker is safer at work than elsewhere. |

The above shows how a statistical association never identifies the cause; it merely states that two factors move together, without indicating why. To explain what causes what, inferential statistics must be used, and this requires specialized training.

Sometimes an association or correlation is highly significant, even though the question of causes remains unanswered. For example, several insurance companies found that boys making good grades had fewer motor vehicle accidents than students making low grades. The company did not need to know the cause of this association, this fact alone was enough to permit them to cut premiums for boys who could show an average of "B" or better.

## NOTES

1. *Accident Facts* may be obtained from the National Safety Council, 444 North Michigan Avenue, Chicago, Illinois 60611. Large public libraries may have copies for use.
2. William E. Tarrants, "Removing the Blind Spot in Safety Education Teacher Preparation," *School and College Safety*, National Safety Congress Transactions (Chicago: National Safety Council, 1965), p. 107.
3. *Ibid.*, pp. 107–8.

# 4

# The Safety Movement

## THE SAFETY TREND

Accidents have always plagued mankind. One of the earliest accounts of a concern for safety occurs in the eighth verse of the twenty-second chapter of Deuteronomy: "When thou buildest a new house, then thou shalt make a battlement for thy roof, that thou bring not blood upon thine house, if any man fall from thence." From this early admonition until the Industrial Revolution of the 1880s, accidents were the concern of the individual. The Industrial Revolution brought many changes—new hazards and new responsibilities which affected more people.

Factory inspections were introduced in England as early as 1833 and were designed to alleviate some of the worst hazards. But not until the twentieth century was any really effective attack made upon industrial hazards. Governmental regulations and controls were gradually formulated by most states in this country.

Effective labor legislation was passed between 1910 and 1915 and consisted of workmen's compensation laws. These laws required that the employer contribute to the costs of any work injury, whether or not a worker had been negligent.

Increased interest in safety also resulted in the formation of the National Safety Council in 1912. Initially formed out of concern for industrial safety, this agency was later expanded to include all aspects of safety and accident prevention.

We can see how effective the safety movement has been by examining accident rates for the past several decades. In general, statistics available for accidents indicate a definite decrease. However, the accident problem remains a significant one. There is still much room for improvement.

The National Safety Council reports that from its formation in 1912 to the present, accidental deaths per hundred thousand population have decreased over 50 percent, and if the rate had not decreased, nearly 2.5 million more people would have died as a result of accidents.[1] Of course, the success of death prevention is a result of the efforts of many organizations and individuals to alleviate accidental death.

We should be proud of the progress since 1912, but comparisons should be made for the past decade. Original concern focused on physical conditions. Since the 1930s, unsafe acts have been emphasized. Even with the progress shown in the total accident picture, we still need to reexamine our techniques for further success.

## ORGANIZATIONS AND AGENCIES

Consistent and organized safety efforts have reduced the toll of accidents and their undesirable effects. Even so, they are still a major public health problem. Various organizations and agencies have emphasized to varying degrees accident prevention and injury control.

Since there are several hundred national organizations with the word safety in their title, the list below is by no means comprehensive in identifying those organizations and agencies with a specific interest in safety. In most cases the title of the organization identifies its main focus and interests. Anyone interested in a professional career in safety would do well to contact these and other safety organizations and agencies, remembering that the private sector of industry and business also employs thousands of safety specialists.

**Government Agencies**

U.S. Consumer Product Safety
  Commission (CPSC)
Washington, D.C. 20207

National Injury Information
  Clearinghouse
5401 Westbard Avenue – Room 625
Washington, D.C. 20207

National Highway Traffic Safety
  Administration (NHTSA)
400 7th St., N.W.
Washington, D.C. 20590

Federal Aviation Administration (FAA)
800 Independence Ave., S.W.
Washington, D.C. 20591

U.S. Coast Guard
Office of Boating Safety
Washington, D.C. 20590

Occupational Safety and Health
  Administration (OSHA)
200 Constitution Ave., N.W.
Washington, D.C. 20210

Clearinghouse for Occupational Safety
  and Health Information
4676 Columbia Parkway
Cincinnati, Ohio 45226

Division of Poison Control
Food and Drug Administration
5600 Fishers Lane; Room 18B-31
Rockville, Maryland 20857

Federal Emergency Management
  Agency (FEMA)
Washington, D.C. 20472

U.S. Fire Administration
16825 South Seton Ave.
Emmitsburg, Maryland 21727

Mine Safety and Health Administration
  (MSHA)
4015 Wilson Boulevard
Arlington, Virginia 22203

**Professional Organizations**

American Association for Health,
  Physical Education, Recreation, and
  Dance (AAHPERD)
1900 Association Drive
Reston, Virginia 22091

American Society of Safety Engineers
  (ASSE)
850 Busse Highway
Park Ridge, Illinois 60068

American Academy of Safety Education
  (AASE)
c/o Jack N. Green, Sr.
Safety and Driver Education
North Carolina A & T State University
Greensboro, North Carolina 27411

American Driver and Traffic Safety
  Education Association (ADTSEA)
123 North Pitt St.
Alexandria, Virginia 22314

**Other Organizations**

National Safety Council (NSC)
444 North Michigan Ave.
Chicago, Illinois 60611

Insurance Institute for Highway
  Safety (IIHS)
Watergate 600; Suite 300
Washington, D.C. 20037

National Fire Protection Association
  (NFPA)
Batterymarch Park
Quincy, Massachusetts 02269

American National Red Cross
17th and D Streets, N.W.
Washington, D.C. 20006
or contact local chapter

American Automobile Association
  (AAA)
8111 Gatehouse Road
Falls Church, Virginia 22042

National Rifle Association (NRA)
1600 Rhode Island Ave., N.W.
Washington, D.C. 20036

Motorcycle Safety Foundation (MSF)
P.O. Box 120
Chadds Ford, Pennsylvania 19317

American Trauma Society
P.O. Box 13526
Baltimore, Maryland 21201

To keep well informed and up to date on safety information and developments, referring or subscribing to the safety periodicals in Table 4-1 is recommended.

## DISASTERS

Chapter 2 dealt briefly with the number of deaths resulting from disasters. As you will recall, the number of deaths from disasters is proportionately small when compared with other causes of accidental death; yet events called disasters receive front-page coverage in newspapers and news magazines.

The loss of life from disasters has decidedly influenced attempts to prevent needless death and injury. Table 4-2 presents a list of disasters with their respective death tolls and, more important, includes efforts made for reducing deaths and injuries following these disasters.

**TABLE 4-1**  Safety Periodicals

| TITLE OF PERIODICAL | ISSUED | PUBLISHER | EMPHASIS |
|---|---|---|---|
| Professional Safety | monthly | American Society of Safety Engineers | occupational safety |
| Journal of Traffic Safety Education | quarterly | California Safety Association | driver education |
| Family Safety | quarterly | National Safety Council | all accident types |
| National Safety News | monthly | National Safety Council | occupational safety |
| Traffic Safety | bi-monthly | National Safety Council | traffic/motor vehicle safety |
| Journal of Safety Research | quarterly | National Safety Council and Pergamon Press | all accident types but primarily traffic safety |
| Accident Analysis and Prevention | bi-monthly | Pergamon Press | traffic/motor vehicle safety |

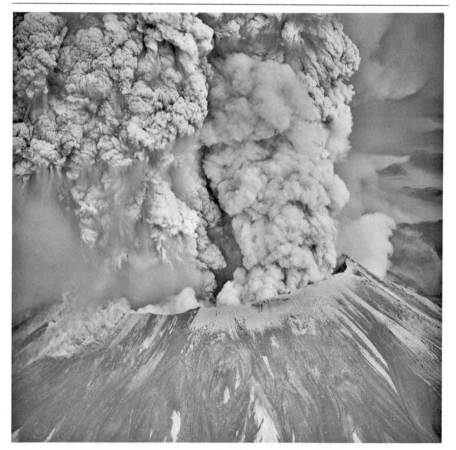

**FIGURE 4-1**  Mount St. Helens Volcano. Photo courtesy of FEMA.

TABLE 4-2 Disasters and Their Effects on Safety Measures

| TYPE | LOCATION AND DATE | TOTAL DEATHS* | RESULTS |
|---|---|---|---|
| Fire | City of Chicago, Illinois October 9, 1871 | 250 | Building codes prohibiting wooden structures; water reserve |
| Flood | Johnstown, Pennsylvania May 31, 1889 | 2209 | Inspections |
| Tidal wave | Galveston, Texas September 8, 1900 | 6000 | Sea wall built |
| Fire | Iroquois Theatre, Chicago, Ill. December 30, 1903 | 575 | Stricter theater safety standards |
| Marine | "General Slocum" burned East River, New York June 15, 1904 | 1021 | Stricter ship inspections; revision of statutes (life preservers, experienced crew, fire extinguishers) |
| Earthquake and fire | San Francisco, California April 18, 1906 | 452 | Widened streets; limited heights of buildings; steel frame and fire-resistant buildings |
| Mine | Monongah, West Virginia December 6, 1907 | 361 | Creation of Federal Bureau of Mines; stiffened mine inspections |
| Fire | North Collinwood School Cleveland, Ohio March 8, 1908 | 176 | Need realized for fire drills and planning of school structures |
| Fire | Triangle Shirt Waist Co. New York March 25, 1911 | 145 | Strengthening of laws concerning alarm signals, sprinklers, fire escapes, fire drills |
| Marine | *Titanic* struck iceberg Atlantic Ocean April 15, 1912 | 1517 | Regulation regarding number of lifeboats; all passenger ships equipped for around-the-clock radio watch; International Ice Patrol |
| Explosion | New London School, Texas March 18, 1937 | 294 | Odorants put in natural gas |
| Fire | "Cocoanut Grove," Boston, Mass. November 28, 1942 | 492 | Ordinances regulating aisle space, electrical wiring, flameproofing of decorations, overcrowding, signs indicating the maximum number of occupants; administration of blood plasma to prevent shock and the use of penicillin |
| Plane | Two-plane air collision over Grand Canyon, Arizona June 30, 1956 | 128 | Controlled airspace expanded; use of infrared as a warning indicator |

*Source: Based upon information from *Accident Facts* (1984), by permission of the National Safety Council.

The Galveston tidal wave of September 8, 1900, in which approximately six thousand lives were lost, was the most devastating disaster on record in the United States. A cyclone and tidal wave on November 12, 1970, struck East Pakistan, resulting in a disaster of proportions unprecedented in this century. The cost in lives from this natural disaster will never be reckoned accurately—a loss of more than half a million lives has been estimated.

The world's worst disaster on record (other than the Biblical account of Noah and the flood) occurred in 1887; a flood took 900,000 lives along the Hwang Ho River in China's Hunan Province.

## TECHNOLOGY

We become aware of the impact of technology on safety and accident loss reduction by looking at various innovations. Whether the innovation be safety lenses (eyeglasses), safety belts (lap and harness types in automobiles), safety hats (steel or other hard material), safety shoes (steel-toed), or safety guards (on electrical saws)—all of which are widely accepted today—we can be sure that formerly they were viewed as quite unacceptable and met with widespread resistance.

## LEGISLATION

Laws and regulations have resulted in a substantial reduction of injuries and fatalities. Examples can be given in air travel, railroads, boating, and mining, among others.

The case of motorcycle helmet laws in the United States portrays the effects of a law aimed at the reduction of death and injury. From 1960 to 1969 in order to qualify for safety program and highway funds, forty states enacted laws requiring motorcyclists to wear helmets. The law resulted in helmet use by more than 99 percent of motorcyclists. The law also had a dramatic effect on motorcyclists' fatalities. A study of eight states that adopted the law, compared to eight contiguous states without the law during the same period, found that motorcyclist deaths declined an average 30 percent following enactment of the law but did not change in the other states.

By 1975 all but three states had helmet-use laws that met the federal standard, but these three states did not lose any federal funds. Within three years, twenty-seven states changed their laws to allow most motorcyclists to ride without helmets. Comparison of helmet use and motorcyclist deaths before and after the repeal of the laws found use declined by more than half, on average, and deaths increased to rates that prevailed prior to the original enactment of the helmet-use laws.

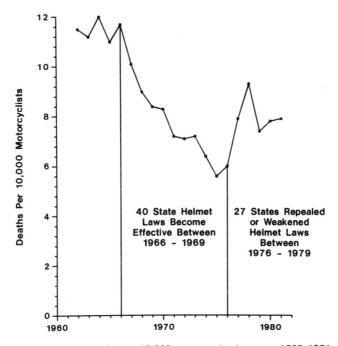

**FIGURE 4-2** Motorcyclist deaths per 10,000 motorcycles by year, 1962-1981. From *The Injury Fact Book* by Susan P. Baker, Brian O'Neill, and Ronald S. Karpf (Lexington, Mass.: Lexington Books, D.C. Heath and Company, Copyright 1984, D.C. Heath and Company).

### Major Safety Legislation

Despite tremendous gains in averting accidents and reducing death, injury, and property damage, the associated costs and losses to society still exist. Therefore, as an effort to combat specific accident types and injury losses, the federal government has passed several major safety laws. These laws include:

1. *The Highway Safety Act* was enacted to reduce motor vehicle injuries and fatalities by establishing a national highway safety program. This program required the establishment of uniform highway safety program standards upon which states and communities could organize their programs. Examples of standard areas include: periodic motor vehicle inspection, motorcycle safety, driver education, driver licensing, emergency medical services, pedestrian safety, and pupil transportation safety.
2. *The Occupational Safety and Health Act* was passed to assure, as far as possible, every working man and woman in the nation safe and healthful conditions and to preserve human resources. Thus, employers are required to provide a workplace free from hazards that are likely to cause death or injury to employees.

3. *The Consumer Product Safety Act* was created with the aim of protecting consumers against unreasonable risk of injury from hazardous products.

4. *The Federal Boat Safety Act* applies to all vessels used primarily for non-commercial purposes with the intention of creating a comprehensive boating safety program.

5. *The Federal Fire Prevention and Control Act* was enacted to reduce human and property loss through better fire prevention and control.

6. *The Federal Coal Mine Health and Safety Act* and the *Federal Metal and Nonmetallic Mine Safety Act* both regulate safety and health standards in the mining industry.

7. *Federal Hazardous Substances Act* was designed to require the labeling of hazardous products. A warning of the hazardous nature of a product in addition to any other pertinent safety information is to be presented on the container. Removal of products from sale that are hazardous and cannot be handled adequately through labeling is another feature of the law.

8. *Flammable Fabrics Act* was designed to ban the manufacture and sale of highly flammable fabrics used in clothing and interior home furnishings.

9. *Poison Prevention Packaging Act* was aimed at protecting people, especially small children, from various poisonous substances found around the house. A number of toxic and dangerous products are required to be sold in child-resistant packaging (e.g., aspirin, prescription drugs).

10. *Refrigerator Safety Act* was designed to protect against an individual's being trapped and suffocating inside a refrigerator by having it equipped with a device enabling the door to be opened easily from the inside.

### Laws Directed at Individuals

There is a widespread use of laws and regulations which attempt to reduce accidents and their undesirable effects, and the imposition of new laws or regulations or changes in old laws or regulations often result in strenuous debate. The debate often focuses upon the right of the government to impose and enforce a law over the rights of individual freedom.

Although there are gaps in knowledge about the effects of laws and regulations directed at individual behavior, the evidence suggests some emerging principles regarding what works and what does not. H. Laurence Ross,[2] writing about deterring the alcohol-impaired driver, points out that laws have three basic components that separately and jointly can influence their effectiveness:

1. Likelihood of apprehension must be perceived to be high.
2. Swiftness of administering penalty must be assured.
3. Severity of penalty need not be extreme.

Most efforts aimed at influencing human behavior aim at making the law "tougher" by focusing on the severity of the punishment with little attention paid to the other two components. Ross points out that severe penalties by themselves do not deter offenders.

## ECONOMIC COSTS

Only in recent years has the economic cost of accident prevention and injury control efforts been considered. Before, the cost of countermeasures seldom was an issue. In fact, some felt that a man's life was expendable. For example, when the Railway Safety Act was being considered in 1893, a railroad executive said that it would cost less to bury a man killed in an accident than to put air brakes on a railroad car.[3]

The struggle to eliminate or reduce the number of accidents and their undesirable consequences is based chiefly on two aspects: (1) cost and (2) regard for human life and well-being. It has been found that safety programs are good for business. Moreover, the first concern of almost everyone is for his or her health and safety. If these are safeguarded in one's everyday activities, the person is more productive and effective.

It has been estimated that the losses from accidental death, injury, and property damage are probably between $100 billion and $200 billion per year. A reduction in accident losses could therefore save billions of dollars annually.

Unfortunately, accident prevention and injury control programs are often undertaken because of compulsion or force from the government rather than for economic or moral reasons.

In recent years cost-benefit analysis has been a major consideration before implementing accident prevention and injury control countermeasures. The premise of cost-benefit analysis is that the benefits should equal or exceed the costs. Thus, there is concern when a countermeasure costs more than the social benefits.

The choice between two accident countermeasures that cost about the same but have different effectiveness is easy to make, as is the choice between countermeasures that have widely different costs but similar effectiveness. Unfortunately, safety decisions are usually not that simple.

## MASS MEDIA

In their effects upon the daily lives of people, the mass media has probably changed more in the last fifty years than in all the preceding history of mankind. At the turn of the century, radio and television were unknown, the motion picture was a curiosity. Books were rarely available for other than the upper-middle and upper classes.

Since then, the mass media has become one of the most powerful influences on people's behavior and opinions. For example, though it is very difficult to document, television shows depicting car chases and crashes in which people seldom get injured could have a definite effect on people's driving habits. Television heroes rarely buckle safety belts, and magazine ads glamorize alcohol consumption. Such daily influences do not tend to promote a safer lifestyle.

Positive influences have resulted from the mass media as well, such as the showing of disaster films depicting the need for high-rise building evacuation plans or the acquisition of swimming skills. Books can also be powerful influences for change. For example, Ralph Nader's book, *Unsafe At Any Speed*, drew such national attention to a certain automobile model that the manufacturer made major modifications in the car's suspension system only to have the public already so acutely aware of the car's defects that sales dropped dramatically, resulting in the elimination of the car from production.

## VALUES

How to spend one's life is answered only by one's choices among values. To this most important of all questions, science has no complete answer. Values are matters of preference, not matters of factual knowledge. Any attempt to say which values people ought to hold makes one a philosopher, not a scientist.

Nevertheless, almost all societies and cultures stress the value of human life and the preservation of self, family, and friends. Because this concept is almost universal, it is a major influence for emphasizing safety.

## NOTES

1. National Safety Council, *Accident Facts* (Chicago: National Safety Council, 1984), p. 10.
2. H. Laurence Ross, *Deterring the Drinking Driver* (Lexington, Mass.: D.C. Heath and Company, 1982), pp. 102–4.
3. Willie Hammer, *Occupational Safety Management and Engineering* (Englewood Cliffs, N.J.: Prentice-Hall, Inc., 1981), p. 1.

# 5

# Hazards, Risks, and Risk-Taking

The world seems to be a very hazardous place. Every day newspapers, radio, and television announce that some catastrophic accident has taken place. Everyone seems to be constantly subjected to an array of hazards.

The term "hazard" refers to a condition with the potential of causing death, injury, or property damage. Most hazards become dangerous only when humans interact with them. The term "danger" expresses a relative exposure to a hazard. A hazard may be present, but there may be little danger because of the precautions taken. Hazards must be identified before they can be controlled.

Hazards have always existed. Not all hazards are man-made. Technology does not always deserve the blame. Man has always had to contend with natural catastrophes, poisoning from plants, fire, and hypothermia. Although many of the old scourges have been conquered and in many ways we are better off than ever before, we still are confronted by new hazards such as radiation, electrocution, and automobile and airplane crashes.

The term "risk" refers to possible loss or the chance of a loss. Risk-takers often willingly expose themselves to hazards to obtain some possible gain, especially when in their personal evaluation, the possible gains outweigh the possible losses. Among the possible "rewards" or gains for successful risk-taking are: saving time, gaining status, experiencing a thrill, eliminating a hazard, meeting a dare or a challenge, and receiving a monetary reward.

Risk is a natural occurrence in human life. From an optimistic point of view, life is an adventure and man is continually pushing into new endeavors which are frequently dangerous. If there were no adventures nor excitement, no suffering or opposition, there would be no choice in life. Life itself would be rather monotonous. Without risk in our lives, no distinctively human kind of life would exist. Risk-taking in the sense of deciding to do one thing or another, is a critical and important part of being a human being.

From the moment we are born we are subject to hazards of all kinds. We continually run the risk of becoming injured or becoming a fatality in an accident. For each act of behavior, such as crossing a street or driving a car, there is an element of risk. The degree of risk may vary with time and situation; some risks are personal, some involve other people.

## VOLUNTARY AND INVOLUNTARY RISKS

Risks can be subdivided in a variety of ways. One useful method separates voluntary and involuntary risks, although these terms have caused some confusion as to their meaning. In general, voluntary risk-taking involves some motivation for gain or benefit by the risk-taker. Involuntary risk-taking refers to the fact that the risk-taker does not have the opportunity to assess the benefits or options of his actions.

Someone who climbs mountains does so by choice and accepts whatever risk may be associated with the activity, whereas the risks arising from natural disasters, such as earthquakes or floods, cannot readily be avoided. The risk from mountain climbing is voluntary, while the natural disaster risks are involuntary. The distinction is not, however, always clear—guiding mountain climbers may be the only occupation open to a particular individual, so that the voluntary nature of his or her choice is qualified. Similarly, in principle at least, it is possible to move away from an area where the risk of floods or earthquakes is high. Nevertheless, the point is one to be kept in mind when considering the acceptability of risk.

## INDIVIDUAL TENDENCIES TO TAKE RISKS

Any person who is directly faced with a dangerous situation makes his own judgments on risk-taking. When an individual feels he cannot, by himself, make a voluntary risk decision, the help of experts is often sought. Such experts might include physicians, safety professionals, or athletic trainers, who are especially competent to aid people because of their experiences and training. The degree to which the risk-taker considers the "expert" a "true" expert and the extent to which the advice is acceptable to the risk-taker determines how fully the advice is accepted. For example, if an ophthalmologist advised a worker to wear safety goggles to protect his eyes, the worker would tend to accept that opinion. But if a fellow worker suggested the same thing, the advice would have a lesser likelihood of being acceptable.

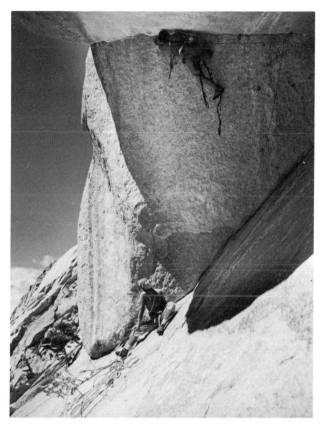

**FIGURE 5-1** Mountain climbers accept whatever risks they encounter. Photo courtesy of Gerald Peterson, UDOT.

The degree of knowledge about hazards and risks falls into four classifications: (1) risk completely known to the risk-taker; (2) risk is hidden from the risk-taker; (3) risk information is easily available, but the risk-taker makes no attempt to use or acquire this information; and (4) risks are uncertain and undefined to all; no information is available.

An opinion about undesirable effects can change risk-taking behaviors. For example, an automobile driver may believe that an accident will seldom happen to him; then, immediately after witnessing a serious automobile accident, his opinion may change radically and he will seek to avoid an automobile accident by driving more cautiously than before, at least for a short time. Being too familiar with a hazard can lead to another view about the danger of a hazard. For example, most people try to avoid high tension power lines, but electrical linesmen tend to become less concerned by the danger as they daily work around the lines. Familiarity can generate a less cautious attitude.

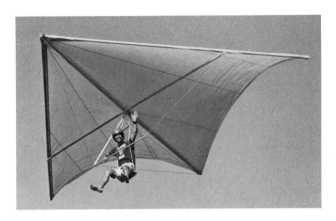

**FIGURE 5-2** Risk-takers make their own judgments about danger. Photo courtesy of Dan Poynter.

## EXPRESSING RISK

There are three general methods of expressing risk: (1) those which apply relative methods; (2) those which use probabilities of occurrences of accidents; and (3) those which show a relation to exposure.

The relative method is simpler than the others, has many different forms, and is more widely used. The hazard is rated according to a standard. A rating scale may be adopted (1 to 10, 1 to 6, etc.) by which the risk level is assessed. For example, a liquid that has a flash point of 225°F may be more fire-safe than one that has a flash point of 150°F.

Probabilities of future occurrences of a specific type of accident can frequently be estimated from past experience if the experience has been over a long period of time, for a large population, and if the events to be assessed will occur under conditions similar to those under which the experience data were derived. The National Safety Council may predict that a certain number of persons will die in traffic accidents during a specific holiday. If the weather or the availability of gasoline should be different from that when the experience data were derived or from any assumptions the National Safety Council made, the actual number of fatalities will differ from the predicted number.

Table 5-1 gives a list of probabilities of an individual's having a fatal accident in the course of a year in certain types of accidents. The values shown were derived by dividing the total number of fatalities in the United States in a single year for a specific accident type into the total population that same year. This expresses the overall risk to society; the risk to any particular individual obviously depends on his exposure and a host of other factors.

Risks often are expressed in relation to exposure so that different risks can be compared. For example, in looking at different modes of transportation for passengers one might make comparisons in terms of fatality rates per passenger miles

**TABLE 5-1  Probability of Having a Fatal Accident**

| ACCIDENT TYPE | NUMBER OF DEATHS* | CHANCE OF DEATH** |
|---|---|---|
| All accidents | 105,000 | 1 in 2,157 |
| Motor vehicle | 52,600 | 1 in 4,300 |
| Falls | 12,300 | 1 in 18,400 |
| Drowning | 7,000 | 1 in 32,357 |
| Fires, burns, and deaths associated with fires | 5,500 | 1 in 41,181 |
| Suffocation—ingested object | 2,900 | 1 in 73,064 |
| Poisoning by solids and liquids | 2,800 | 1 in 80,892 |
| Firearms | 1,800 | 1 in 125,833 |
| Poisoning by gases and vapors | 1,500 | 1 in 151,000 |
| All other types | 18,400 | 1 in 125,833 |

*Source: National Safety Council, *Accident Facts,* 1981 (covers 1980 accidental deaths).
**Based on United States 1980 population of 226.5 million.

traveled. Thus, in a recent year the death rate per hundred million passenger miles was: for automobiles, 1.2 deaths; for commercial airplanes, 0.4 deaths; for passenger trains, .05 deaths; for public buses .04 deaths.

## JUDGING SAFETY[1]

Safety is not measured; risks are measured. A thing is safe if its risks are judged to be acceptable. In other words, safety is the degree to which risks are judged acceptable.

The dictionary defines "safe" as "free from risk." Nothing can be absolutely free of risk. Everything thought to be safe, under some circumstances, can cause harm. Because nothing can be absolutely free of risk, nothing can be said to be absolutely safe. There are degrees of risk, and consequently there are degrees of safety.

Notice that this definition emphasizes the relativity and judgmental nature of the concept of safety. It also implies that two activities are required for determining how safe things are: (1) measuring risk and (2) judging the acceptability of that risk (judging safety), which is a matter of personal and social value judgment.

A false expectation is that safety experts can measure whether something is safe. They cannot because they can assess only the probabilities and consequences of events, not their value to people. Safety experts are prepared mainly to measure risks. Deciding whether people should be willing to take risks is a value judgment that the experts are little better qualified to make than anyone else.

Safety can change from time to time and be judged differently. Knowledge of risks evolves, and so do our personal and social standards of acceptability. For example, our decision whether to cross a street is different in different situations, depending on whether we are out in the rain, are carrying a heavy load of groceries,

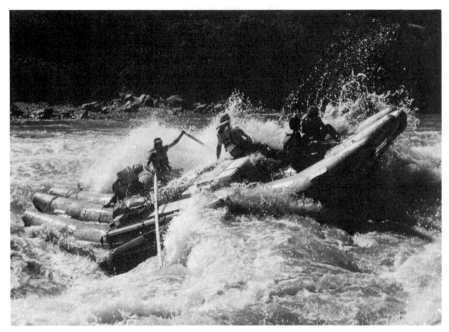

**FIGURE 5-3** Knowledge of risks evolves, and so do our personal and social standards of acceptability. Photo courtesy of Gerald Petersen, UDOT.

or are already late for an appointment. A power saw that is safe for an adult may not be safe in the hands of a child.

A risk estimate can assess the overall chance that a fatal accident will occur, but cannot predict any specific event. From past experience we can determine how many falls in the home will occur, but we cannot predict who, when, or exactly where the fall will occur.

Recall that determining safety involves two different kinds of activities: (1) risk-measuring—measuring the probability and severity of harm (a scientific activity); and (2) safety-judging—judging the acceptability of risks (a value activity).

The following table illustrates risk-measuring activities in the left-hand column, and corresponding safety-judging in the right column:

| RISK-MEASURING | SAFETY-JUDGING |
| --- | --- |
| 1. Bicycles rank first as a consumer product hazard (expressed by comparing). | 1. Mandatory bicycle safety standards (i.e., reflectors, wheels, brakes, chains, etc.) have been issued by the U.S. Consumer Product Safety Commission. |
| 2. Each American has one chance in 232 of being dog bitten each year (expressed by probability of occurrence). | 2. Most communities have regulations about dogs being licensed and leashed, under verbal command, or confined. |

3. Each American has one chance in 5,000 of being a traffic fatality (expressed by probability of occurrence).

3. The federal government has established standards in areas of traffic safety (i.e., alcohol control, driver education, enforcement, etc.)

How safe is safe enough is a value judgment. Scientists are not any more equipped to make value judgments about how safe things ought to be than any other person. It is dangerous to assume that those with technical or scientific expertise are especially qualified to make such judgments. Decisions, however, are often made by the experts because nobody else is prepared or willing to make them.

## COPING WITH HAZARDS

When a risk-taker sees a new hazard, he has three options: fight, flee, or accept the imposed risk.

A risk-taker may seek to reduce his chances of injury by fighting the manner in which the hazard is imposed. For example, if an irrigation canal is scheduled to be constructed near a residential area and it poses the potential problem of having

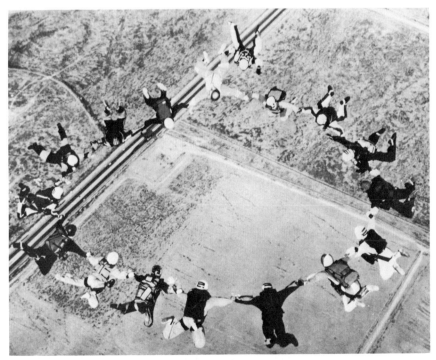

**FIGURE 5-4**  Those engaged in risk-taking activities often spend many hours learning ways to minimize the hazards. Photo courtesy of the *Deseret News*.

young children drown in the canal, then residents of the area can attempt to have the canal redirected away from the homes or to have the canal fenced or covered.

A risk-taker may seek to reduce the chances of injury or death by removing himself from the hazard. For example, using the same problem cited above, a home owner could elect to sell his house and move to another location.

The third way of coping with a new hazard is to do nothing and accept the risk and hope that an injury will not occur.

## PERSONAL GUIDELINES FOR RISK-TAKING

Risk is a relative thing. What may be risky to one person may be an everyday event to another. The margin of danger varies from person to person and even changes for the same person in different situations. In some risk-taking activities the margin of danger is the same for all. For example, in sky diving or mountain climbing, risk is obviously relative to the skill and experience of the participant—less skill increases the risk. However, in Russian roulette with a six-chamber revolver and only one bullet, the margin of danger is the same for all participants—there is no skill involved.

Most societies have their high risk-takers. Whether they be Vikings or astronauts, they have received a hero's reward. Sports such as bullfighting, football, snow skiing, and sky diving all involve risk. Today's heroes in these sports have spent many hours learning ways to minimize the hazards. Here are guidelines to consider when personally taking risks:

- Never risk more than you can afford to lose.
- Do not risk a lot for a little. Control emotions in a dangerous situation. Carefully identify what is the risk—a loss or a gain. Avoid risks merely because of a dare or for reasons of principle.
- Consider the odds and your intuition. There is a difference between taking a chance where there is no control and a situation where you are a major factor.

## HAZARDS CONTROLLED BY TECHNOLOGY

As technology develops, new methods to control hazards are being found. These controls come in two forms: (1) hazards before considered uncontrollable can now be controlled to various degrees, and (2) more effective controls are found for hazards that are already controllable. An example of the first case is the research in progress on means of controlling tornadoes, either through cloud seeding or explosive disruption of the funnel. The degree of success of such controls is not yet established, but they are being tested. In the second case, new developments in building design (i.e., automatic sprinklers) are resulting in changes in building codes and, it is hoped, in better control of serious fires.

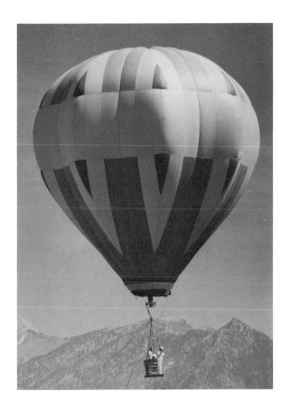

**FIGURE 5-5**
What may be risky for some may not be risky for others. Photo courtesy of Gerald Petersen, UDOT.

## FEAR TO RISK

Even though few people are killed in commercial aviation in the United States, there are twenty-five to thirty million Americans who are afraid to fly. These same people think nothing at all of driving their own cars without safety belts fastened, in spite of the fact that fifty thousand people will die in automobile crashes in a year's time.

There are three principles that govern perception of risk:

1. *Feeling in control.* People who drive "in control" or ski "in control" take risks, while a passenger on a plane feels little control over the situation.
2. *Size of the event.* Single big events (e.g., natural and human-caused disasters) are feared excessively and such events are often exaggerated by the media. One or two people dying in an automobile crash does not sound nearly as bad as forty-five dying in a plane crash.
3. *Familiarity.* It is hard to fear the familiar and hard not to fear the unfamiliar. For example, it is easy to fear elevators if you stay out of them; it is hard to fear them if you ride elevators several times every day.

**TABLE 5-2  Risk-Taking**

STEP #1:    Rate your participation in the following behaviors.
            1 = frequently    2 = sometimes    3 = never

| STEP #1 COLUMN | | | STEP #2 COLUMN | STEP #3 COLUMN |
|---|---|---|---|---|
| _____ | 1. | flying in a small private plane | _____ | _____ |
| _____ | 2. | flying in a commercial airliner | _____ | _____ |
| _____ | 3. | swimming alone | _____ | _____ |
| _____ | 4. | driving without safety belts on | _____ | _____ |
| _____ | 5. | living on an active earthquake fault | _____ | _____ |
| _____ | 6. | living in a "tornado belt" state | _____ | _____ |
| _____ | 7. | working in an underground coal mine | _____ | _____ |
| _____ | 8. | jay-walking across a street | _____ | _____ |
| _____ | 9. | exceeding the 55 mph speed limit | _____ | _____ |
| _____ | 10. | waving away or swatting at a bee | _____ | _____ |
| _____ | 11. | tubing on a bumpy downhill course | _____ | _____ |
| _____ | 12. | riding double on a bicycle | _____ | _____ |
| _____ | 13. | petting or feeding a large stray dog | _____ | _____ |
| _____ | 14. | keeping guns and ammunition together | _____ | _____ |
| _____ | 15. | sleeping in a house without a smoke detector | _____ | _____ |
| _____ | 16. | driving a small compact car | _____ | _____ |
| _____ | 17. | taking pills or medicine in the dark | _____ | _____ |
| _____ | 18. | talking with food in your mouth | _____ | _____ |
| _____ | 19. | stopping incompletely at stop signs | _____ | _____ |
| _____ | 20. | driving/riding a motorcycle | _____ | _____ |

STEP #2:    For those statements that you marked as 1, try to identify one or more of the following reasons that explains why you participate.

    a.  save time
    b.  seek a thrill
    c.  gain money
    d.  meet a dare
    e.  perform a necessary function
    f.  gain recognition, status, attention
    g.  eliminate a hazard
    h.  other reason

STEP #3:    For those statements that you marked as 2 or 3 in Step #1, try to identify one or more of the following reasons that explains why you do not participate.

    1.  It is not economical for me. It might cost me more than the personal benefits derived.
    2.  It is too inconvenient. The time and hassle are not worth the benefits.
    3.  It is too dangerous. An injury could happen.
    4.  It does not provide enough psychological reward (i.e., thrill, recognition, etc.)
    5.  I do not have enough skill to participate.

**NOTES**

1. The definition of safety and the concepts in this section are based on and are adapted from William W. Lowrance, *Of Acceptable Risk*.

# 6

# Philosophical Implications

## BASIC ASSUMPTIONS OF SAFETY

There are certain assumptions existing which aid in the understanding of our situation relating to safety in the world in which we live. These assumptions include:

- Hazards exist with the potential for causing death, injury, and property damage. Most hazards become dangerous only when humans interact with them.
- Basic laws and order of the physical world exist. We do not live in a chance world, but one governed by laws. For example, the solar system moves in mathematically correct orbits, enabling us to land a man on the moon. The earth's gravitational pull determines that what we throw into the air is pulled back to the earth; this always happens—even though the object might be a car that plunges off a mountain road taking the occupants to their deaths. Likewise, we know what will happen if we fall into a vat of boiling steel or come in contact with high tension electric power lines.
- Every law has both a punishment and a reward to it. There are opposites in all things. If not, the life known by humans would be mundane and monotonous.
- We are free agents, but we are prevented from doing what we want by limits set upon us by the environment in which we live, as well as by various social circumstances and limitations of the physical body. Being a free agent means that we can do what we please, but we will suffer the consequences of our actions—good or bad.
- Even though we are free to choose our course of action, we are not free to choose the consequences of our actions. Disobedience to law results in a

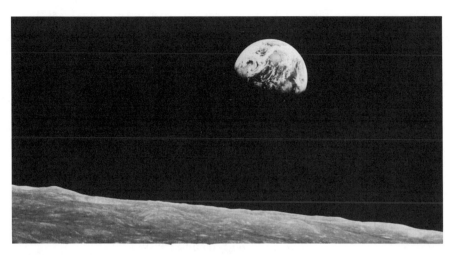

FIGURE 6-1 We live in a world governed by laws, not by chance. Exploration of the solar system and other accomplishments are possible when the laws are known. Photo courtesy of the National Aeronautics and Space Administration.

punishment. For example, if we touch a hot flame, we are burned. Obedience to law provides a reward. If we drive properly around a curve in the road, for example, we stay on the road.

- A knowledge of the basic laws can be acquired vicariously or through actual experience. It is important to realize that it is not necessary to break a law to learn what to avoid.

- To be adventurous is a natural aspect of human behavior and such adventure enriches life. In fact, progress depends on the adventurous urge (e.g., exploration which results in new discoveries).

- Because we are able to choose, we are responsible for our actions. "Responsibility" is here defined as the ability to fulfill our needs, and to do so in a way that does not deprive others of the ability to fulfill their needs. Acquiring responsibility is a complicated, lifelong process. Responsibility is learned through involvements with responsible fellow human beings.

- Because human lives are intermingled, what one person does may vitally affect someone else. When automobile accident insurance premiums rise, the owner of a car with an accident-free record becomes alarmed. After all, he or she is paying for others' accidents. Thus, other people's behavior affects us. When an automobile crosses through the freeway median guardrail and crashes into another car, killing its occupants, a stranger's actions have had a tragic effect on innocent people.

## WORTH OF A HUMAN LIFE

What value is to be placed on a human life? How can we determine its worth? Two things will give some indication of the value of human life: (1) what these lives have cost up to this point—the labor, material, and struggle that has gone into their creation and development; and (2) the effective use to which they can be put—the benefits that result from productivity and contribution to society.

How much is a human life worth? All people have worth. Almost everyone recognizes a moral obligation to minimize the loss of life—most religions and philosophies are based upon the tenets that human life has worth and life is worth living.

The value of life often is measured in terms of money—how much is a company or a parent willing to pay to protect those under their stewardship from accidental death. For example, a parent may place a great deal of emphasis on safety by purchasing and using child restraints for their automobile, smoke detectors for the home, and appliances with UL ratings. Another parent may take none of these precautions.

There have been numerous ways in which the worth of a human life has been determined:

1. *Legal limitations.* Several states have set limits on the amount a victim's dependents can collect if someone else is held liable for his death in an accident. Other states have no limitations. Internationally, liabilities are sometimes limited by agreement among countries whose citizens could be involved.

Another aspect is that the life of a person who has no dependents usually has little or no legal value. Awards by courts are computed in a variety of ways. For example, a common method predicts the victim's total income had he lived to normal life expectancy, less his cost of living, and calculated on the basis of accrual of interest.

2. *Replacement method.* Replacing a productive, contributing life is costly. The military services have identified for the various military ranks the worth (in dollars) of individuals.

Another example is the replacement cost of housework of a woman who cares for her family full-time. Several methods have been used for such determinations, but suffice it to say, the calculations usually amount to a sizable amount of money.

Still another example is the loss to society by the premature impairment or death of persons with great talents and abilities (see Table 6-1). It is impossible to measure the intangible potential that was never realized because of an accidental death. Certainly the world would gain by increasing the length of life of talented people. In fact, the period of greatest achievement for artists, authors, scientists, and scholars occurs during mid-life according to several experts. Much depends, however, on such factors as the field of endeavor and the age at which creative work is begun. Most creative people maintain a high level of productivity throughout their lives. For example, the career of Thomas Edison reveals that, while the inventor's highest peak of discovery came at the age of thirty-five, he remained active and creative into his eighties.

3. *Insurance aspects.* The amount of insurance collected in the event of a death is another consideration.

4. *Accumulated assets.* Often appearing in the news media are listings of the richest people in the United States or in the world. Income tax collecting agencies (federal, state) appraise the worth of individual holdings at various times (e.g., probate court, bankruptcy, real estate values, etc.).

**TABLE 6-1 Contributions Lost Due to Accidental Death**

| NAME | CONTRIBUTION(S) | TYPE OF ACCIDENT | AGE AT DEATH |
|------|-----------------|------------------|--------------|
| Queen Astrid | Ruler of Belgium | Automobile crash | 30 |
| Albert Camus | French author and Nobel Prize winner for Literature | Automobile crash | 47 |
| Philippe Cousteau | Photographer, author, deep-sea diver and son of famous oceanographer | Seaplane crash | 37 |
| Pierre Curie | French Nobel Prize winner for Physics | Struck by truck while walking | 47 |
| James Dean | American movie star | Automobile crash | 24 |
| Princess Grace | Wife of Prince Rainier III of Monaco; former American movie actress, known as Grace Kelly | Automobile crash | 52 |
| Audie Murphy | American war hero; movie star | Small plane crash | 46 |
| Knute Rockne | Famous Notre Dame head football coach | Small plane crash | 34 |
| Will Rogers | American humorist, political analyst, movie star | Small plane crash | 58 |
| Percy Bysshe Shelley | English poet | Drowned while sailing during a storm | 29 |
| Natalie Wood | American movie actress | Drowned after falling from private boat | 43 |

NOTE: Some gained fame that their names are instantly recognizable. Others are included because of noteworthy activities or achievements in their lifetime, even though their names are less well known.

BOX 6-1 *THREE FAMOUS PEOPLE WHO SURVIVED CRITICAL ACCIDENTS TO ACHIEVE SUCCESS*

1. Ben Hogan, golfer

   In 1949 he survived a near-fatal auto accident. After months of rehabilitation, he began playing golf again and the following year won the National Open.

2. Glenn Cunningham, track star

   As a youngster his legs were horribly burned in a fire. Doctors feared he would not walk again. However, he not only walked, but was the top miler in the world for many years.

3. Conrad Adenauer, German leader

   Almost killed in 1917 when he fell asleep while driving and crashed into a streetcar. He went through the windshield head first and his face was slashed beyond recognition. He survived, though his face was terribly scarred, and became chancellor of Germany after World War II.

5. *Value of the human body's chemicals.* Most people have heard that the human body is worth a few dollars on the basis of its minerals. However, the biologic chemicals found in human blood and tissue have an astronomical market value. Refer to Table 6-2 for examples of several compounds and their value.

6. *Social status.* Symbols of achievement and status are often used to place or determine someone's worth. Location of one's home, clothing labels, size and make of automobiles, type of employment, number of people at social functions (e.g., weddings, parties, funerals) all are examples of criteria used to determine one's worth.

Too often, we wrongly judge and evaluate a person's worth by material possessions rather than other standards such as contributions to society through service or creativeness.

**TABLE 6-2   Value of the Human Body's Compounds**

Using a chemical supply catalog, Daniel A. Sadoff, a University of Washington animal researcher, recently calculated the value of every marketable substance in a normal 150 pound body. Some of his findings appear below. Totaling the market values, Sadoff estimates we are each worth a million dollars.

| COMPOUND | AMOUNT IN BODY (150 LB.) | VALUE |
|---|---|---|
| Cholesterol | 140 g | $       525.00 |
| Fibrinogen | 10.2 g | $       739.50 |
| Hemoglobin | 510 g | $   2,550.00 |
| Albumin | 153 g | $   4,819.50 |
| Prothrombin | 10,200 U | $ 30,600.00 |
| IgG | 34 g | $ 30,600.00 |
| Myoglobin | 40 g | $100,000.00 |

## DEATH

One of the most universal and solemn experiences shared by the human race is the inescapable fact of death. In fact, most of us hope for a long life and a quick death, but only a minority of the population has this wish fulfilled.

Two possibilities confront us: either we can die young and bring sorrow to family and friends, or we can live and feel sorrow as family and friends die. Such a statement is not pessimistic; it is simply true. For, sooner or later, in one way or another, all must die. How we as human beings act and react in the face of death has always been one of the principal concerns in life.

BOX 6-2

"I'm not afraid to die. I just don't want to be there when it happens."

— *Woody Allen*

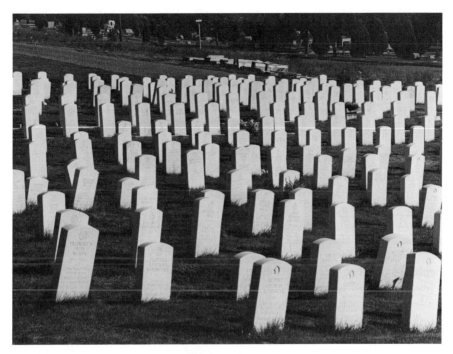

**FIGURE 6-2** A universal experience which comes to everyone is death. Photo courtesy of the *Deseret News*.

There seems to be an almost universal desire among men to continue to live. The desire for prolonging our lives is so strong, not only in human beings, but also in other forms of life, that the first law of nature is termed "the law of self-preservation." So deeply is the desire to live implanted in mankind that a human being will go to almost any length in order to preserve his own life.

BOX 6-3

> To everything there is a season . . . a time to be born, and a time to die . . .
> — *Ecclesiastes 3:1-2*

We seldom come in contact with the dead since few people die at home or in public places. Death takes place primarily in a hospital. However, some time in our lives we will be directly confronted by death.

It has been demonstrated that one's attitudes toward death can be improved (e.g., you can learn to accept death as a reality of living and be more comfortable with it).

Our attitudes toward our individual deaths affect not only the way we view death, but also the way in which we live our lives. For example, if one views his or her own death with horror, one may have considerable difficulty in mustering the courage necessary to cross a street in heavy traffic. If, on the other hand, death is conceived as a pleasurable and exciting experience, one may not hesitate to go over Niagara Falls in a barrel. Thus, an examination of death may provide clues as to our risk-taking behavior. The amount of risk-taking we are willing to do may be a function of our conception of death.

We can learn from death. To learn what is cold, we must learn what is hot. Likewise, is it not also logical that to learn about life, we must be aware of what death is?

## SAFETY VALUES

Values are the things that people hold to be important. They are the things that people want or care about. Values are the guides that tend to give direction and purpose to live. Values represent a way of life.

In this book we are concerned with a particular value—the prevention of accidents and the control of death, injury, and property damage. We do make judgments about what is safe or unsafe. These judgments are value judgments.

The early slogan "Safety First," which made safety sound unattractive because it seemed to put safety ahead of every other consideration, came from an unfortunate circumstance. At the turn of the century, a man named Henry C. Frick, president of the Henry C. Frick Coke Company, inaugurated the country's first industry-wide safety campaign with the slogan, "Safety First, Quality Second, Cost Third." "Safety First" was lifted out of context and widely used by other companies. No longer was safety "first" only to quality and cost; the slogan seemed to put it ahead of everything.

We do *not* advocate safety as the main objective in life. We should not live by a timid and faint-hearted value. Safety is a positive concept, not a negative one. It is not meant to be a "thou-shalt-not" approach to life that holds people back.

If a person is to realize a useful and full life, the perception of safety as a positive value working with other individual and social values is essential. Safety as a value at times competes with time, status, personality shortcomings, bravery, adventure, and other values. Safety enables us to choose between experiences that are unproductive, absurd, and even stupid, and those that enrich our life, make it interesting and worthwhile. Safety is a means to an end—adventure, achievement of goals, progress (safety *for* as opposed to safety *from*).

Safety *for* enjoyment; safety *for* an effective life; safety *for* good health. These are some of the positive aspects of safety. The negative aspect, safety *from* death, injury, and property damage, should be discarded in favor of the positive approach. The safety *from* concept is only used with the very young, mentally deficient, and the senile elderly, since they are unable to understand the reason behind correct and safe procedures.

Safety *for* philosophy recommends activities with as much risk reduced as possible. Do not abandon snowmobiling, skiing, motorcycling, or any other activity simply because it has more risk than other activities—life then would become boring and unrewarding.

## ISSUES IN SAFETY

Since safety is determined by the judgments or evaluation of people, a natural result is that people will not always agree about how safe they want to be. Refer to pages 6 and 43 for further elaboration on how safety is determined.

Since there are differing points of view with regard to various accident and injury problems, these differences are called issues. These issues should be studied because they:

1. Need resolving or answering.
2. Can and do affect people and property.
3. Are interesting and provocative.

Listed below are some controversial issues relating to accidental death and injury:

1. Mandatory use of safety devices such as automobile safety belts and motorcycle helmets.
2. Driver education's effectiveness in reducing accidents.
3. Handgun control.
4. Football and other contact sports in high schools.
5. Types of insulation used in housing.
6. Small vs. large cars for safeness in the event of an accident.
7. Efforts to control drunk drivers.
8. Boxing.

# 7

# Determining Causes

## MULTIPLE CAUSE CONCEPT

Accidents generally result from a combination of closely interwoven factors. This is known as the multiple cause concept.

Each of the circumstances which contributes to an accident is *a* cause, while *the* cause is the combination of these factors, each of which is necessary but none of which is by itself sufficient.

A *circumstance* is any condition or action accompanying an accident whether it contributes to the accident or not. A contributing *cause* is a circumstance without which the accident would not have happened. A cause is always a circumstance, but a circumstance is not always a cause. Each cause, if it truly contributes to an accident, is of equal importance in that accident. Too often the event directly preceding an accident is labeled the cause. The multiple cause concept refutes this.

We may "get away with" violations for years because all the other essential ingredients for the accident are not present. On the other hand, an accident could occur the first time the violation is committed.

One example of an attempt to show the multifactorial background of accidents is the chart shown in Figure 7-1 developed by the National Safety Council.

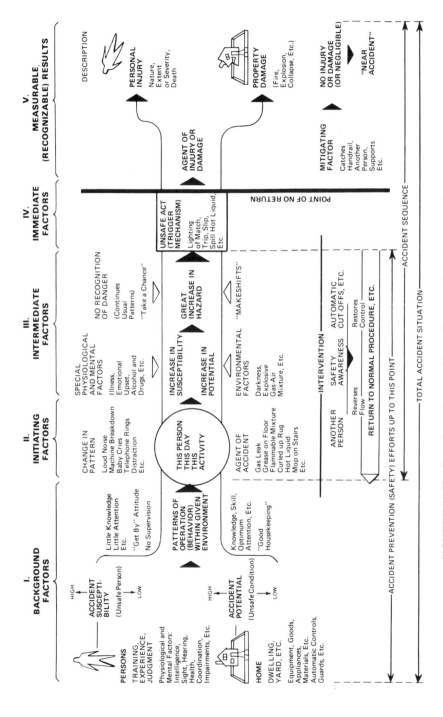

**FIGURE 7-1** The dynamics of home accidents. Courtesy of the National Safety Council.

## EPIDEMIOLOGY OF ACCIDENTS

"Epidemic" literally means "in or among people" and thus "common to, or affecting at the same time, many in a community." Formerly, epidemiology was defined as the medical science dealing with epidemics. It was most often found in public health programs that dealt with infectious and communicable diseases. However, heart disease, cancer, and accidents have also been studied by the epidemiological method. In relation to accidents, epidemiology is the study of why some get injured and some do not. John Gordon[1] (probably the first to use the epidemiological approach to the accident problem) and others emphasized the importance of viewing accidents as a public health problem because they play an increasingly significant role as a cause of death. They also stressed the fact that accident problems should be treated in the same way, with the same methods used in the epidemiological approach to other public health problems.

The epidemiological model includes the interaction of hosts, agents, and environmental factors. The *host* is the person killed or injured. The *agents* of injury are the various forms of energy in excessive amounts.[2] Mechanical energy is the usual agent for injuries involving motor vehicle crashes, falls, and gunshots. Thermal energy is the agent of burns. Chemical, electrical, and ionizing radiation are other forms of energy accounting for injuries. The lack of oxidation is the agent for drowning, choking, and other types of suffocation.

In epidemiological usage,[3] the term *vehicle* refers to any inanimate (nonliving) carrier that conveys damaging agents. The term *vector* is used to refer to animate (living) carriers. Most of the carriers of excessive energy are vehicles (e.g., cars, guns, etc.). A few are vectors (e.g., dogs, poison ivy, etc.).

No medical tool was more important than epidemiology in eliminating from Western civilization the old scourges of typhus, typhoid fever, cholera, plague, and many other diseases. Such can be the case for traumatic death and injury.

Precise knowledge is the only sound base for the implementation of accidental death and injury countermeasures. Safety programs based on sound epidemiological data must replace "hit-or-miss" safety programs. The fact that accidental death and injury are not often considered a public health problem is one of the reasons that they are indeed a public health problem.

## DESCRIPTIVE EPIDEMIOLOGY

Descriptive epidemiology is by far the most common form of epidemiology utilized today. It provides statistical ways by which we can measure the accidental death and injury problem. By use of various sources of information (household interviews, report forms from hospital emergency departments, police reports, state and local health departments, insurance records, etc.) the injury problem is described in terms of frequency rates and characterized as to host, agent, and environmental factors.

The National Safety Council, the National Center for Health Statistics, the National Electronic Injury Surveillance System, and the National Highway Traffic Safety Administration operate systems for reporting the accident data obtained by their descriptive epidemiology efforts.

At first glance the goal of describing death and injury occurrence in this way may seem trivial. However, such studies are of importance and can serve the following purposes:

1. Focus attention on a particular accidental death and injury problem;
2. Measure long-range trends;
3. Serve as a basis for further studies and research;
4. Identify clues to accident causation;
5. Provide data to determine priorities for action;
6. Provide data to determine effectiveness of countermeasure programs.

### Human

Human factors constitute a great concern in the descriptive epidemiology of accidents. Characteristics studied include age, sex, marital status, socioeconomic status, and physical condition.

*Age.* Age is one of the most important factors in accident occurrence. Some accidents occur almost exclusively in one particular age group, such as home fall fatalities. Other accidents occur over a much wider age span but tend to be more prevalent at certain ages than others.

The time of life at which an accident predominates is influenced by such factors as the degree of exposure to the agent at various ages and variations in susceptibility with age. The influence of age-related exposure is illustrated by lead poisoning, which is most prevalent in children.

Many injuries, such as in fatally injured adult pedestrians, show a progressive increase in prevalence with increasing age. It is tempting to regard an accident with this age pattern as being due merely to aging itself.

*Current Age Tabulations.* The tabulation of death rates in relation to age at one particular time, as in Table 7-1, is known as a current, or cross-sectional, presentation. This shows death rates as they are occurring simultaneously in different age groups; thus, different people are involved in each age group.

*Sex.* Some injuries occur more frequently in males, others more frequently in females. A sex difference in injury incidence initially brings to mind the possibility of hormonal or reproductive factors that either predispose or protect. For example, premenstrual syndrome (PMS) is a significant factor affecting women's susceptibility to accidents.

But men and women differ in many other ways, including habits, social relationships, environmental exposures, and other aspects of day-to-day living. The

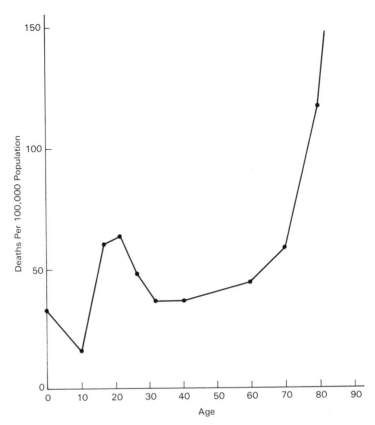

**FIGURE 7-2** Injury Death Rates by Age. From *The Injury Fact Book* by Susan P. Baker, Brian O'Neill, and Ronald S. Karpf (Lexington, Mass.: Lexington Books, D.C. Heath and Company, Copyright 1984, D.C. Heath and Company).

**TABLE 7-1  Accidental Death Rates by Age**

| AGE GROUPS | DEATH RATES* |
|---|---|
| All ages | 38.9 |
| Under 5 years | 22.4 |
| 5 to 14 years | 13.9 |
| 15 to 24 years | 48.4 |
| 25 to 44 years | 35.4 |
| 45 to 64 years | 34.3 |
| 65 to 74 years | 47.1 |
| 75 years and over | 135.2 |

*Deaths per 100,000 population in each age group. Rates are averages for age groups, not individual ages.

Source: Deaths are for 1983, latest official figures from National Center for Health Statistics.

higher male prevalence of traffic fatalities is at least partly related to the fact that, on the average, men drive automobiles more than women.

Sex differences in injury occurrence are important descriptive findings and often suggest avenues for further research. Such differences need explaining. See Table 7-2 and Figure 7-3 for a comparison between males and females.

TABLE 7-2  Male: Female Ratios of Death Rates by Cause, 1977-1979

| RATIO | UNINTENTIONAL INJURY | SUICIDE | HOMICIDE |
|---|---|---|---|
| 52:1 | | | Firearm (legal intervention) |
| 29:1 | Electricity (non-home) | | |
| 22:1 | Fall from ladder/scaffold | | |
| 19:1 | Machinery | | |
| 17:1 | Struck by falling object | | |
| 12:1 | Drowning (boat) | | |
| 10:1 | Motorcyclist | | |
| 7:1 | Fall from structure | | |
| | Explosion | | |
| | Lightning | | |
| | Firearm | | |
| 6:1 | Pedestrian (train) | Domestic gas | |
| | | Firearm | |
| 5:1 | Drowning (non-boat) | | Firearm |
| | Airplane crash | | Beating |
| | Cutting/piercing | | |
| | Electricity (home) | | |
| | Bicyclist | | |
| 4:1 | Opiate poisoning | Hanging | Cutting/stabbing |
| | Suffocation | Cutting/piercing | |
| | Motor vehicle exhaust | | |
| 3:1 | Alcohol poisoning | | |
| | Excessive cold | | |
| | Motor vehicle occupant | | |
| | Pedestrian | | |
| | Fall from other level | | |
| | Excessive heat | Motor vehicle exhaust | |
| 2:1 | Pedestrian (non-traffic) | Jumping | |
| | Exposure | | |
| | Housefire | | |
| | Aspiration (food) | | |
| | Natural disaster | | |
| | Aspiration (non-food) | | |
| | Fall on stairs | | |
| | Hot substance | Drowning | |
| 1:1 | Fall on level ———————————————————————————————————— | | |
| | Barbiturate poisoning | Barbiturate poisoning | |
| | | Psychotherapeutic drugs | |
| 1:2 | | | Strangulation |

Source: Susan P. Baker et al., *Injury Fact Book* (Lexington, MA: Lexington Books, 1984).

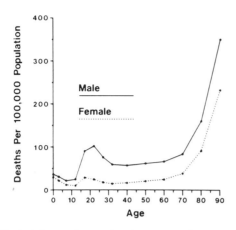

FIGURE 7-3 Death Rates from Unintentional Injury, by Age and Sex. From *The Injury Fact Book* by Susan P. Baker, Brian O'Neill, and Ronald S. Karpf (Lexington Books, D.C. Heath and Company, Copyright 1984, D.C. Heath and Company).

*Marital Status* is another important descriptive variable. Married persons have lower fatality rates than single persons. The unmarried have been shown to be more often involved in fatal traffic accidents than the married, and ski injuries are overwhelmingly found among the unmarried.

*Socioeconomic Status.* Some epidemiologists categorize socioeconomic status as an environmental factor. This factor can be and usually is measured by the occupation or income of the family head, by his or her educational level, or by residence, in terms of the value of the home or dwelling unit.

Low socioeconomic status appears to be related to lead poisoning, snowmobile injuries, and adult pedestrian deaths. On the other hand, drownings involving power boats and yachts, injuries or deaths related to private airplane crashes, and ski injuries are most often found among the high socioeconomic status groups.

*Physical Condition.* Although alcohol is among the most important human factors known to be related to severe injury and death, other drugs are becoming more frequently involved. The intoxicated have difficulty in escaping from a hazard (fire or submerged automobile), or intoxication becomes an obstruction that impedes those giving medical attention and treatment. Chronic health problems such as diabetes, epilepsy, and heart disease may also induce an accident. Overexertion and fatigue reduce the attention, sensory acuity, and reaction time of any individual.

### Place

Where accidental injuries occur is a matter of great importance. Comparison of injury and death rates in different places may provide clues to causation or serve as a stimulus to further fruitful investigation. See Table 7-3 for a comparison between rural and urban death rates. Examples of descriptive findings presented are international comparisons, comparisons of regions within the United States, and comparisons of areas within a city.

**TABLE 7-3 Rural: Urban Ratios of Injury Death Rates by Cause, 1977–1979**

| RATIO | UNINTENTIONAL INJURY | SUICIDE | HOMICIDE |
|-------|----------------------|---------|----------|
| 10:1 | Lightning; exposure | | |
| 9:1 | Machinery; natural disaster | | |
| 7:1 | Firearm | | |
| | Struck by falling object | | |
| 6:1 | Pedestrian (non-traffic) | | |
| | Excessive cold | | |
| | Drowning (boat) | | |
| 5:1 | Suffocation | | |
| | Motor vehicle occupant | | |
| 4:1 | Electricity (non-home) | | |
| | Explosion | | |
| 3:1 | Fall on level | | |
| | Clothing ignition | | |
| | Airplane crash | | |
| | Aspiration (non-food) | Firearm | |
| 2:1 | Alcohol poisoning | | |
| | Electricity (home) | | |
| | Motor vehicle exhaust | | Beating |
| | Drowning (non-boat) | | |
| | Cutting/piercing | | |
| | Motorcyclist | | |
| | Aspiration (food) | | |
| | Fall from ladder/scaffold | | |
| | Housefire | | |
| | Bicyclist | Motor vehicle exhaust | |
| 1:1 | | | |
| | Hot substance | | |
| | Excessive heat | | |
| | Pedestrian | | |
| | Pedestrian (train) | Drowning | |
| | Fall on stairs | Hanging | |
| 1:2 | Fall from structure | Psychotherapeutic drugs | Firearm (legal |
| | | Cutting/piercing | intervention) |
| | | Domestic gas | |
| 1:3 | | | Firearm |
| 1:4 | Barbiturate poisoning | | |
| 1:5 | | Barbiturate poisoning | |
| 1:6 | | | |
| 1:7 | | | Cutting/stabbing |
| 1:10 | | | Strangulation |
| 1:20 | | Jumping | |
| 1:29 | Opiate poisoning | | |

Source: Susan P. Baker et al., *Injury Fact Book* (Lexington, MA: Lexington Books, 1984).

*International Comparisons.* Because of the problems regarding the validity of fatality statistics (attributable to definition problems), it is difficult to take seriously small differences among nations in accident fatality rates. However, it is also difficult to explain away very large differences (e.g., where the death rate is in one country two or three times as large as the death rate in another). Large differences are impressive when both countries are known to have reasonably good vital statistics systems.

*Comparisons of Regions Within the United States.*   The availability of fatality statistics for states in the United States has permitted the discovery of interesting place-to-place variations in accidental death occurrence. Differences in fatality rates between urban and rural areas are a common finding. The higher fatality rate from traffic accidents in rural than in urban areas is consistent with the fact that faster driving occurs in rural areas, and it is the speed of the vehicle which is a major factor in death causation.

Geographic variation within the United States is quite distinctive, which suggests that climate or other factors may be involved (see Figure 7-4). For example, there is the finding in the United States of generally higher fatality rates for accidents in the mountain region. While hypotheses abound, to date no one has convincingly explained this geographic distribution of fatal accidents.

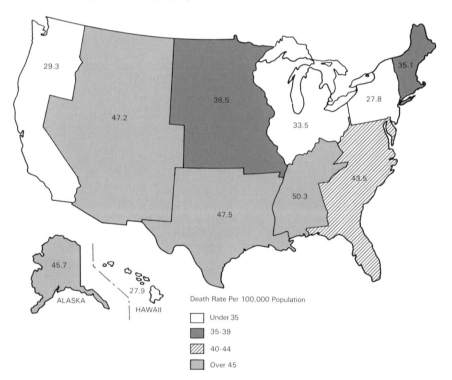

**FIGURE 7-4** Accidental mortality by geographic division, United States. Adapted from the National Safety Council, *Accident Facts*, 1984.

*Areas Within a City.*    When studying accidental injuries within a city, it is often desirable to plot the occurrence of such injuries in each census tract, since information about other characteristics of persons in each tract is available.

Lead poisoning, fire, and traffic accidents in cities have been mapped according to location with results showing definite geographic distribution.

### Time

The pattern of injury occurrence in time is often an extremely informative descriptive characteristic. A great variety of time trends may be found in the accident data; these involve simple increases or decreases of injury incidence, or more complex combinations of these changes in time.

*Short-Term Increases and Decreases in Injury Incidence.*    Short-term changes are those increases or decreases in injury incidence that are measured in hours, days, weeks, or months. For example, two-thirds of all drownings occur in the afternoon or early evening, and about 40 percent occur on Saturdays and Sundays. July is the peak month, with more than half occurring in the summer months, June through August.

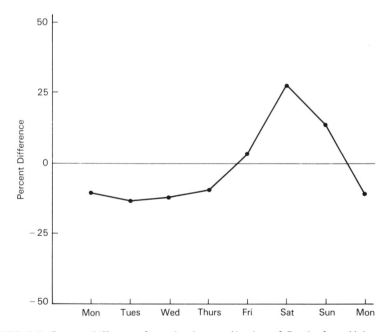

**FIGURE 7-5** Percent Difference from the Average Number of Deaths from Unintentional Injury, by Day of Week. From *The Injury Fact Book* by Susan P. Baker, Brian O'Neill, and Ronald S. Karpf (Lexington, Mass.: Lexington Books, D.C. Heath and Company, Copyright 1984, D.C. Heath and Company).

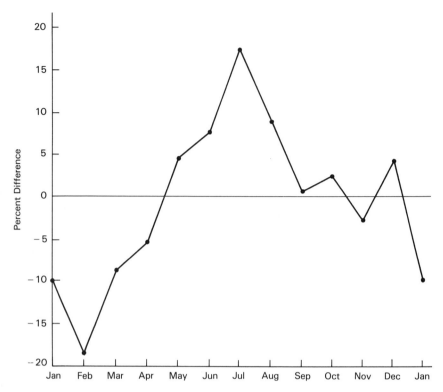

**FIGURE 7-6** Percent Difference from the Average Number of Deaths from Unintentional Injury, by Month. From *The Injury Fact Book* by Susan P. Baker, Brian O'Neill, and Ronald S. Karpf (Lexington, Mass.: Lexington Books, D.C. Heath and Company, Copyright 1984, D.C. Heath and Company).

*Epidemics.* An epidemic, or outbreak, is the occurrence of an injury type in members of a defined population clearly in excess of the number of cases normally found in that population. Thus, the spectacular, short-term increases (some lasting several years) of injuries associated with backyard trampolines, skateboards, water ski kites, abandoned refrigerators, and ultrathin plastic bags were suddenly major, nationwide accidental death problems.

*Recurrent or Periodic Time Trends.* The incidence of certain accidental injuries shows regular recurring increases and decreases. This regular pattern exhibits cycles. Many cycles occur annually and represent variation in injury occurrence. Seasonal variation is a well-known characteristic for drownings, which occur mainly during the summer months, whereas carbon monoxide poisoning is most prevalent during the winter months when people are spending large amounts of time enclosed in automobiles and buildings.

Shorter-term periodic variations have also been observed. For example, death rates from automobile accidents show weekly cycles with the highest rates occurring on weekends, especially Saturdays. To date there are no available statistics on the number of passenger-miles driven on each day of the week. Thus, it is not possible to state whether the weekend increase in deaths is due merely to an increased exposure of the population to the moving automobile or whether the risk of death per passenger-mile actually increases, possibly because of such factors as more reckless driving or more alcohol consumption on weekends.

*Long-Term Trends.*    Some accidental deaths exhibit a progressive increase or decrease in occurrence that is manifested over years or decades.

Figure 7-7 shows the death rates of accidents from 1910 to 1980. A marked decrease in fatalities from all accidents has occurred, representing about a 50 percent decrease. This decrease is believed to be due largely to a greater concern for safety. Rather than going back to 1910, it is suggested that only the past ten years should be considered.

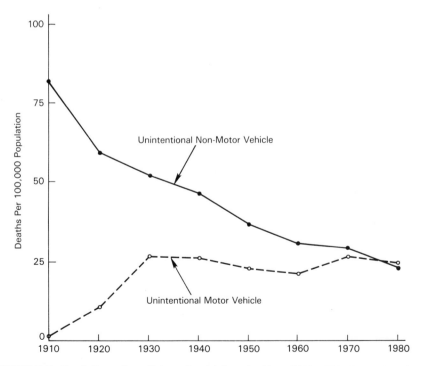

**FIGURE 7-7**  Death Rates from Unintentional Injury, by Year, 1910–1980. From *The Injury Fact Book* by Susan P. Baker, Brian O'Neill, and Ronald S. Karpf (Lexington, Mass.: Lexington Books, D.C. Heath and Company, Copyright 1984, D.C. Heath and Company).

## INVESTIGATIVE EPIDEMIOLOGY

Investigative epidemiology is used to develop specific data related to the causes of the injury which would then point to feasible countermeasures. Whereas descriptive epidemiology identifies the accident problem and information regarding who, when, and where, investigative epidemiology gives the specifics on causation.

Complex interactions among the human, the environment, and the agent are disclosed. The investigations are conducted by a team of experts. These "multidisciplinary teams" involve a variety of professionals: medical/paramedical, social/behavioral, and physical/environmental personnel, engineers, statisticians, and clerks. Nurses, pathologists, toxicologists, psychologists, sociologists, and physical therapists have provided the types of skills needed. The effort is a teamwork approach, which overcomes the failings of an individual specialist.

Such investigations include: (1) studies of a single type of injury where a small number of cases can provide clues, (2) on-site investigations, and (3) in-depth evaluations.

Marland of the U.S. Public Health Service says this about the value of investigative epidemiology:

> The most important characteristic of investigative epidemiologic data is its specificity. When provided with the specific facts of injury-producing events, those persons responsible for injury control can develop an equally specific countermeasure. By the same token, those responsible for implementing the countermeasure are confident in their actions—be it redesign of a product, a local building code, a state law or an educational program. These programs became successful because their specificity is related to the injury just as surely as a cause and effect.[4]

It must be stressed that all accident investigations should seek causes for the injuries as well as causes for the accident, looking into all phases—before, during, and after—and all aspects of the scene—human, agent, and environment.

Present efforts by investigative epidemiology teams are small. Examples of such teams in operation include: Federal Aviation Administration (FAA) investigations of airplane crashes, Consumer Product Safety Commission teams interested in product safety, National Highway Traffic Safety Administration (NHTSA) team investigating motor vehicle accidents.

### Obstacles to Acquiring Data

The multidisciplinary accident investigation teams have been encountering serious problems in obtaining information from people in the accidents they investigate. Witnesses or parties to the accident are often reluctant to divulge information. Despite the stated intention of the investigators to develop the data for research purposes only, parties confuse investigators with those seeking to bring legal actions against them or to involve them in such actions, both civil and criminal. As a result, people refuse access to information because they fear they will be harmed or embarrassed in some later legal action.

## HUMAN CAUSATION MODEL

Many safety experts strongly believe that human error or behavior is the basic cause behind all accidents, and that safety is primarily a human problem. Furthermore, they believe that successes in reducing accident death and injury rates will come from controlling human behavior.

A number of writers have discussed and attempted to classify types of human errors, and a great deal has also been written about causes of human behavior. While some of these writers and theorists have psychology and management backgrounds, most come from the technical areas of systems engineering, systems safety, and human factors engineering.

Robert Mager and Peter Pipe[5] have identified human behavior problems. Using the flowchart in Figure 7-8, we start out by citing an unsafe behavior such as "Joe doesn't wear his safety belt," or "Tom is not storing his lawn mower's gasoline in a safe can."

The second step is to ask the question, "Is it dangerous?" The main idea here is whether the alleged unsafe behavior is really a problem.

Then, assuming the unsafe behavior is dangerous, we go to the next step, which is the determination of whether the unsafe behavior is due to a deficiency of safety knowledge and/or skills. In essence, is the person in danger because the person *does not know how* to be safe?

If the answer is "yes" we might determine whether the person ever knew how to perform safely. If there is a genuine lack of safety knowledge and/or skills, then the main remedy would be either to change the safety knowledge and/or skill level (e.g., teach the person how to be safe) or remove the person from the dangerous situation.

If, on the other hand, the answer is "no"—the person is able to behave safely but does not, the solution lies in something other than in enhancing safety knowledge and/or skills. "Teaching" someone to do what the person already knows how to do is going to change neither safety knowledge and/or skills nor safe behavior.

Here is an illustration: A plant manager complains that every year two million dollars are lost because of accidents. He believes the employees can recognize a hazard when they see one, but that they do not report hazards. The manager tried putting safety posters on the walls and had employees watch safety films regularly. Nothing happened to the accident rate because this is a case where people know how to be safe but are not. No amount of information or exhortation will change this situation. What is needed is a change in the conditions or the consequences surrounding employees' unsafe behavior.

Determining whether lack of safety knowledge and/or skills is due to a lack of training is one of the more important decisions in the anlysis of unsafe behavior,

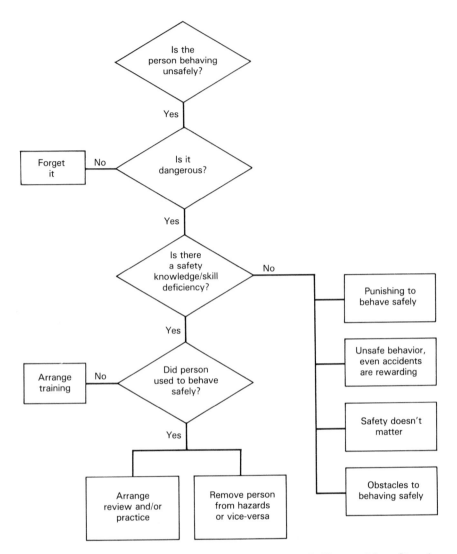

**FIGURE 7-8** Human Causation Model. Adapted from Robert F. Mager and Peter Pipe, *Analyzing Performance Problems* (Belmont, Cal.: David S. Lake Publishers, 1984).

and is often neglected. If safety knowledge and/or skills never existed, training would be useful. But if safe behavior once existed and now is discarded, training from the beginning would be overdoing it.

When safe behavior fades or disappears and accident rates increase, periodic review programs should be considered. Such programs can include occasional review sessions of safety knowledge and/or skills or feedback about safe behavior from others.

To this point, several solutions have been suggested pertaining to the person who does not exhibit safe behavior due to deficiencies of safety knowledge and/or skills.

When a person could behave safely if he really had to but does not, something other than safety instruction is needed. There are four general causes of such unsafe behavior:

1. It is punishing to behave safely.
2. It is rewarding not to be safe, or it is even rewarding to have accidents.
3. Safety does not matter.
4. There are obstacles to being safe.

When it appears that someone knows how to be safe but does not act that way, find out whether safe behavior has been leading to unpleasant results. Some examples of how it is punishing to act safely include: (1) It is time consuming or a waste of time; (2) it is inconvenient; (3) it is uncomfortable (e.g., helmets and goggles are hot); (4) an attitude to not "rock the boat" by reporting hazards exists; (5) it is considered unmanly ("sissies" use goggles or a guard); (6) it is difficult to use equipment because of guards, etc. If so, the remedy is to find ways to reduce or eliminate the negative effects and to create, or increase, positive or desirable consequences.

Secondly, there are cases where the consequences of unsafe behavior are more favorable than those that follow safe behavior. Examples of how unsafe behaviors are rewarded include: (1) injured victims gain attention and (2) those having been injured get to rest, get time off, etc. If so, the remedy is to find ways to reward those who are practicing safety.

Thirdly, sometimes unsafe behavior continues to exist not because the person does not know how to perform or because the person is not motivated, but because it simply does not matter whether the person behaves safely. Nothing happens if he is safe; nothing happens if he is unsafe. In a case where a person could be safe if he had to or wanted to, one of the things to look for is the consequence or benefit of being safe. If there is none then it may be necessary to arrange one. When you want someone to behave safely, one rule is to "make it matter."

Lastly, if a person knows how to be safe but does not behave that way, look for obstacles. Look for things that might be getting in the way of his safe behavior. Look for lack of time, lack of authority. Look for poorly placed or labeled equipment. Look for bad lighting and uncomfortable surroundings. Most people want to avoid accidents. When they do not, it is often because of an obstacle in the environment around them.

Once the reason is found for unsafe behavior, it is worth determining a worthwhile remedy or solution. Select from several solutions the most practical, economical, and easiest to use—the one most likely to give the most result for the least effort. This is cost effectiveness.

## SYSTEMS SAFETY APPROACH

The engineering techniques of systems analysis have also been proposed for the solution of safety problems. In its emphasis on the interaction of humans, machines, and environment, this approach is quite similar to the epidemiological one.

Too many well-written explanations of the systems safety approach have been published for this writer to elaborate further. Suffice it to define systems safety for the uninitiated with the hope that he or she will investigate further. Systems safety analysis is a logical, step-by-step method of examining situations with accident potential. It helps identify causes that could be overlooked if a less detailed method were used. Human, mechanical, and environmental factors are placed in an orderly, related schematic, inducing a logical thought process which leaves little to chance. It is a challenging and satisfying creative brain-storming approach.

While the systems safety approach has been highly successful in regard to the safe operations of some very complex systems, many problems yet remain in quantifying the influence of the human as an element in the system.

A system is an orderly arrangement of components which are interrelated and which act and interact to perform some task or function in a particular environment. The main points to keep in mind are that a system is defined in terms of a task or function, and that the components of a system are interrelated, that is, each part affects the others. Examples of systems are aircraft, production lines, and transportation.

No matter which method of analysis is used, it is important to have a model of the system. Most models take the form of a diagram showing all the components. This makes it easier to grasp the interrelationships and simplifies tracing the effects of malfunctions.

The systems approach to safety can help to change safety from an art to a science by classifying much of our knowledge. It can change the application of safety from piecemeal problem solving to a safety-designed operation. We can apply the question "What can happen if this component fails?" to the various elements of the systems and come up with adequate safety answers before the accident occurs, instead of after the damage has been done.

## OTHER HUMAN FACTORS

### Accident Proneness

Some people do have more accidents and injuries than others. In fact, a mere look around at friends and neighbors will usually identify several who have had more than their share of injuries.

Accident proneness refers to the existence of an enduring or stable personality characteristic that predisposes an individual toward having accidents. Critical words in this definition are the adjectives *enduring* and *stable*.

The concept of accident proneness has had a long and controversial history. English researchers were responsible for the early work (1919) which *created* the concept, which then *grew* in popularity through the 1920s, reaching its *peak* in the

BOX 7-1

> He is so unlucky that he runs into accidents which started out to happen to somebody else.
>
> *— Don Marquis*

late 1930s. Accident proneness was *questioned* in the 1950s and *rejected* in the 1960s. Since then, it made somewhat of a *comeback* in the 1970s. Needless to say, the accident proneness concept has been plagued with argument, debate, and confusion. This has largely resulted because the concept of accident proneness means different things to different people.

Misconceptions which have been associated with accident proneness include:

*Most accidents are caused by a few people.* This point of view has been represented by "20 percent of the people who have 80 percent of the accidents." The 20 percent were identified as being accident prone.

The major flaw in this concept is the fact that people who have accidents in one period of time are not necessarily those who have accidents in the next. That is, 20 percent of a population may indeed have 80 percent of the accidents during a two-year period, but during the next two years the 20 percent of the population involved in accidents does not include all of the original individuals. Thus, uneven accident involvement may best be explained on the basis of chance alone, and there is no reason to predict that an individual in the "20 percent group" will continue to be heavily involved in accidents.

*Accident proneness as a single personality trait.* Confusion arises because some authorities consider accident proneness as a single trait, while others will include in the accident prone definition a variety of psychological traits.

There is little agreement on what traits distinguish the accident prone personality. In fact, the descriptions often conflict. For example, one study found the accident prone to be passive and repressed, while another described him as impulsive and action oriented.

*Accident proneness as an influence found in all environments.* This view is depicted by the well-known quote, "a man drives as he lives," indicating that an "accident prone" person would be susceptible not only for a traffic accident but an accident in other surroundings as well (i.e., work, home, etc.).

*Accident proneness as an innate and unmodifiable trait.* Such a belief stigmatizes an individual and would be contrary to the popular idea that behavior can be modified. There are no known psychological traits that predict the probability of an accident with any accuracy.

People do change. Maturing with age and becoming married are examples of experiences which have influenced and even changed an individual's behavior and character.

*Accident repeaters are accident prone.*  Accident repetitiveness refers to the *descriptive* truth that some individuals have more accidents than others. Accident proneness is a theory and is offered as the *explanation* of why some people have more accidents than others. Evidence indicates that repeaters are not necessarily prone and that exposure to hazards may account for many of those having more than their share of accidents.

One of the reasons for the failure of the accident proneness theory has been the lack of agreement over its meaning. Accident proneness means different things to different people.

The bulk of evidence indicates that there is no such thing as a single type of "safe" or "unsafe" person. Rather, each individual has a range of behavior—some safe, others unsafe, depending on the environmental hazards to which he is exposed. Thus, instead of a single type of accident prone individual, there are many reasons why some individuals have more accidents than others.

For example, individuals vary considerably in their: (1) exposure to hazards, (2) ability to recognize and make judgments concerning hazards, (3) experience and training, (4) physical attributes (i.e., visual acuity, reflexes, etc.), and (5) exposure to social and environmental stresses.

The idea of accident proneness must be viewed as only one explanation for individual variations in accidents. There are other explanations which must always be considered.

Criticism of the accident proneness concept should not be taken to mean that personal factors do not play an important role in accidents. Categorization of human factors involved in accidents may be divided on a short-term and long-term basis.

BOX 7-2

> My only solution for the problem of habitual accidents . . . is for everybody to stay in bed all day. Even then, there is always the chance that you will fall out.
>
> *— Robert Benchley*

### Type I—Short-Term

*Emotional.*  This person is under stress. The stressful period can last anywhere from several weeks to several months and it may occur only a few times in a life-time or several times during a year. During this period, the individual is likely to show forgetfulness, inattention, unusual irritability, and other symptoms. Once the crisis is resolved, the individual goes back to his previous state of good adjustment.

*Physical.*  A person ill or recovering from an illness, fatigue, using alcohol or other drugs may be involved in a period of susceptibility for an accident.

### Type II—Long-Term

*Emotional.* In this category are individuals with "negative character traits" such as untrustworthiness, rudeness, and aggressiveness. This category reflects the usual definition of accident proneness—that of having a personality trait enduring over time, perhaps a lifetime. However, a person may change his character as the result of becoming more mature with age, education, the need to be approved, marriage, responsibility, or simply "slowing down" from old age.

*Physical.* People who are suffering physical conditions which may impair their ability to perform safely, such as failing eyesight, senility, untreated diabetes, seizures not under drug control, and a host of other physical conditions, may account for accident susceptibility. However, many people with known chronic ailments compensate for their condition and do perform safely, and, in fact, may even have better accident records than those who are healthier.

### Lack of Knowledge and Skills

With all the new inventions coming forth on a daily basis, no single individual can keep up with all the new innovations. If the innovation happens to be hazardous, people will get hurt in many cases merely because they did not know how to handle the new contraption. Examples of hazardous products later deemed unsafe include hot water vaporizers capable of severely burning when tipped over, electrical toy ovens with the potential of high-level temperatures, and power lawn mowers capable of ejecting foreign objects.

Another problem exists when a person could use a potentially hazardous object safely yet because he or she does so infrequently, the person endangers himself or herself.

### Imitation

People are strongly influenced by imitation. "Do as I say and not as I do" is a recognition of the fact that people sometimes learn more from imitation than we would like. Children acquire much of their behavior by watching parents and peers. Often they imitate behavior new to them following only brief exposure to it. Research confirms the fact that when you teach one thing and then do something else, the teaching is less effective than if you practice what you teach. Safe driving and use of safety belts are both examples of imitation's effects. We tell parents, "do not take medications in front of your children." The reason: fear that they will imitate the parent and become poisoned.

### Attitudes

It would be difficult to overemphasize the importance of attitudes relating to accidents. As is evident to most people, attitudes are of major significance in determining how safe a person might be.

An attitude is an internal state which affects an individual's choice of action toward some object, person, or event. The choice an individual makes is of a personal nature. For example, a person may choose to drive faster than the speed limit or use a power saw without a guard—the choice indicates his or her attitude.

Accidents may even affect attitudes. Certain beneficial attitudes may come from accidents. An involvement in an accident or witnessing an accident may foster greater respect for laws, social responsibility, and moral obligation. Thoughtfulness, courtesy, sportsmanship, and other qualities may sometimes result from accidents (e.g., an individual who causes an injury to another may become more thoughtful of others in similar future situations). There may also be negative attitudes resulting from accidents. Emotional disturbance, nervousness, anxiety, and other psychological problems may result from accidents. Fear, anger, hatred, and antisocial behavior may be also produced as a result of being involved in an accident.

Attitudes are a fundamental factor in safety. Attitudes stem from observation, learning, and experiences of an individual. It is often difficult to modify or change attitudes since they usually have been developed over a long period of time; nevertheless, attitudes can be altered toward a safer lifestyle.

### Alcohol and Other Drugs

Alcohol and drug abuse are behaviors with major implications in all areas of safety. More than half of the fatal motor vehicle accidents and up to 40 percent of adults dying in non-motor vehicle accidents (e.g., poisoning, falls, burns) had used alcohol. Reports indicate that almost half of all adults who drowned had consumed alcohol.

Drugs other than alcohol have not been shown to play a substantial role in accidents, although abuse of amphetamines, marijuana, or other drugs can seriously impair performance. Multiple drug use, especially the combination of alcohol with one or more other drug, creates additional problems.

### Emotions

Little information in this area is available. However, the likelihood of accidents increases when people are emotionally upset. An emotional state (e.g., anger) can carry over the manner of driving or other behavior which involves hazards.

BOX 7-3  *UNUSUAL BUT TRUE*

NEW ORLEANS (AP)—Mourners gathered Friday for Michael Scaglione, 26, who was killed after he threw a golf club and the clubhead rebounded and stabbed him in the throat, severing the jugular vein.

Police said Scaglione made a bad shot and threw his club against a golf cart. When the shaft broke and the head rebounded, he was struck in the throat.

Other members of the foursome said Scaglione staggered back, gasped, "I stabbed myself," and pulled the piece of golf club from the wound.

Surgeons said if Scaglione had not done that he might have lived, since the metal might have reduced the gush of blood. Rushed to a hospital, he was revived temporarily, but died later.

Nearly all people have periods in which they experience emotional stress. During these periods they will tend to be less alert and less attentive to what they are doing, and there will be a tendency to have accidents.

Various types of emotions may contribute to accidents. Extreme fear, anger, nervousness, or anxiety are examples.

### Fatigue

Evidence shows that as persons become tired they are more likely to experience accidents. The true magnitude of the fatigue problem is not known; however, it is a larger problem than accident data indicates in all areas of safety—motor vehicle, school, work, etc.

There are basically two types of fatigue: "task or skill induced" fatigue and fatigue from other factors, of which sleep deprivation is the most common. "Task or skill-induced" fatigue results from long hours of doing essentially the same thing resulting in loss of alertness and difficulty in responding properly to hazards.

### Stress

The old concept of "accident proneness" (e.g., a lifelong personality trait) has been largely abandoned today as an explanation of accident causation and involvement. Instead we should be looking at the acute situational factors which may precipitate an accident. In fact, accident involvement often can be explained by personal stresses which cause a person to perform in such a manner as to increase his or her accident chances.

Everyone has experienced stress; moreover, we have some degree of stress all of the time. Everyone has a different level of stress tolerance, which means each individual is capable of handling different amounts and kinds of stress. However, everyone has his or her limits.

### Society's Values

The American values taught in homes and schools include:

- Competitiveness in an aggressive style is acceptable.
- Masculinity implies toughness and aggressiveness.
- Excitement and challenges should be sought, and risk-taking is justified in seeking them.

These are the values exemplified by our historical heroes. These beliefs and others have allowed the United States to excel in all areas (e.g., sports, finance, technology, etc.). All of this is relevant to accidents because these values suggest that exposure to hazards in a certain type of lifestyle is the ideal. Such a lifestyle lends itself to involvement in accidents.

### Biorhythm

The biorhythm theory proposes that many accidents occur on certain critical days, which are calculated from a person's birth date.

The biorhythm concept was developed in the early 1900s by Wilhelm Fliess, a Berlin physician, and Herman Swoboda, a Viennese psychologist. Working separately they concluded that each of us has a 23-day physical cycle and a 28-day emotional cycle. Late in the 1920s, Alfred Telscher, an Austrian engineer and teacher, added a 33-day intellectual cycle after observing his students' academic performance. The work of these three men forms the basis of today's biorhythm theory.

The use of biorhythm appears to be widely exaggerated—at least in the United States. Only a few organizations will admit using the theory, and mostly to promote safety awareness, not to predict accidents.

The biorhythm cycles are usually depicted as curves, with a positive phase, a negative phase, and a zero or "critical point," when the lines cross the axis from positive to negative, or vice versa. Although negative days are regarded as less favorable than positive days, it is the critical days—occurring about six times a month—that are considered most upsetting.

Opinions on the validity of biorhythms vary. Some claim the theory has been successfully used in accident prevention programs by companies in the United States, Japan, and Europe, while others say the research results are inconclusive.

There are other types of biological cycles. For example, the strongest cycle is the 24-hour circadian rhythm. Various body functions that move in a 24-hour pattern are impressive: temperature, blood pressure, respiration, blood sugar, urine volume, coordination, and many others.

When the circadian rhythm is upset, problems can result. Everyone is familiar with the fatigue and disorientation that results from a long period without sleep. Other examples of upsetting the rhythm include "jet lag" in travelers flying long distances across several time zones, and shift work on jobs.

### Physical and Medical Conditions

Medical conditions and physical defects are frequently associated with accidents. The following items are not all-inclusive list, but they have been indicted as causes of accidents: circulatory problems, diabetes, narcolepsy, premenstrual syndrome, epilepsy, vision and hearing defects, among many others.

### NOTES

1. John E. Gordon, "The Epidemiology of Accidents," *American Journal of Public Health*, XXXIX (April 1949), 504–15.
2. William Haddon, Jr. "Advances in the Epidemiology of Injuries as a Basis for Public Policy," *Public Health Reports* 95, no. 5 (September-October 1980), 412–13.
3. *Ibid.*, p. 413.
4. Richard E. Marland, "Injury Epidemiology," *Journal of Safety Research*, (September 1969), p. 102.
5. Robert F. Mager and Peter Pipe, *Analyzing Performance Problems* (Belmont, Calif.: Fearon-Pitman Publishers, Inc., 1970).

# 8

# Strategies for Accident Prevention and Injury Control

**CHOOSING COUNTERMEASURES**

Measures to prevent accidents and reduce injuries have been in existence since ancient times (for example, shoes to protect against sharp stones). Many worked so well (such as evacuation in times of floods and volcanic eruptions) that they are still in use.

Traditional, often ineffective, approaches to safety have been based largely on piecemeal, unsystematic perceptions of accident causes and countermeasure options. Utilization of the criteria listed below will aid in determining countermeasures:

1. Priority should be given to countermeasures that will be the most effective in reducing injury losses and need not be based on causes which contributed to the accident. Some examples of this would be: using a net for an acrobat rather than urging him or her to "perform safely" and not to fall; placing thermal insulation on the handles of cooking pots, pans, and electric irons rather than telling users never to touch them with their bare hands; putting shoes on children rather than cautioning them not to stub their toes.
2. A mixture of countermeasures is best since a single measure will rarely solve the problem.
3. Quickness in obtaining positive results from a particular countermeasure is important.

4. Economic factors should play a major role in the choice of options. The often-heard statement that "it's worth it, if it saves just one life" is not true if, for the same amount of money or other resources, more than one life can be saved. Cost-effectiveness compares the cost of alternative ways of meeting a particular goal, whereas cost-benefit analyses assess the net financial gain or loss to society of implementing a particular safety program. Cost-effectiveness and cost-benefit analyses are often misapplied and misunderstood in decisions concerning safety programs.

   Cost-effective designs should be chosen to minimize societal costs. Because of difficulties in determining the value of life and limb, cost-benefit studies would be appropriate only in the evelution of countermeasures intended to reduce property damage, but not save lives and reduce injuries.

5. In most cases, the less that the people to be protected must do, the more successful the countermeasure. Automatic ("passive") measures do not require the person to do something, and manual ("active") measures require that they do.

6. There is nothing sacred about any specific model for determining countermeasures. Whichever model is used should serve as a sorting device, a checklist that assists the user.

7. Consideration of the cultural, social, and political forces will sometimes determine success or failure.

8. Choice must be based on effectiveness in helping to reduce the end results (death and injury)—not always on preventing an accident.

The following poem shows the importance of stressing one countermeasure over another:

### The Parable of the Dangerous Cliff

Twas a dangerous cliff, as they freely confessed,
   Though to walk near its crest was so pleasant;
But over its terrible edge there had slipped
   A duke, and full many a peasant.
The people said something would have to be done,
   But their projects did not at all tally.
Some said, "Put a fence 'round the edge of the cliff,"
   Some, "An ambulance down in the valley."

The lament of the crowd was profound and was loud,
   As their hearts overflowed with their pity;
But the cry for the ambulance carried the day
   As it spread through the neighboring city.
A collection was made, to accumulate aid,
   And the dwellers in highway and alley
Gave dollars or cents—not to furnish a fence—
   But an ambulance down in the valley.

"For the cliff is all right if you're careful," they said;
   "And if folks ever slip and are dropping,
It isn't the slipping that hurts them so much
   As the shock down below—when they're stopping."

So for years (we have heard), as these mishaps occurred
   Quick forth would the rescuers sally,
To pick up the victims who fell from the cliff
   With the ambulance down in the valley.

Said one, to his plea, "It's a marvel to me
   That you'd give so much greater attention
To repairing results than to curing the cause;
   You had much better aim at prevention.
For the mischief, of course, should be stopped at its source,
   Come, neighbors and friends, let us rally.
It is far better sense to rely on a fence
   Than an ambulance down in the valley."

"He is wrong in his head," the majority said;
   "He would end all our earnest endeavor.
He's a man who would shirk this responsible work,
   But we will support it forever.
Aren't we picking up all, just as fast as they fall,
   And giving them care liberally?
A superfluous fence is of no consequence,
   If the ambulance works in the valley."

The story looks queer as we've written it here,
   But things oft occur that are stranger.
More humane, we assert, than to succor the hurt,
   Is the plan of removing the danger.
The best possible course is to safeguard the source;
   Attend to things rationally.
Yes, build up the fence and let us disperse
   With the ambulance down in the valley.[1]

## CHANGING HUMAN BEHAVIOR

It is generally agreed that a majority of accidents are caused or at least greatly influenced by human behavior. Therefore, attempts to prevent accidents focus upon changing human behavior by one or more of the following ways. It should be noted that such attempts usually begin with education and continue down through the others if the preceding one is not effective. For example, if education fails, then coercion is tried; when that fails, legal sanctions are endorsed. This whole process may take years or decades before an effective countermeasure is found or developed.

   *Education.*   Organized safety education is of recent origin and it is impossible to pinpoint the origin of the first safety instruction taking place. It is known that *McGuffey's Readers* included a number of references to safe practices. Since then many forms of safety education have appeared for all accident types.

An evaluation of any safety instruction should answer at least the following questions concerning a safety lesson, topic, or course: (1) To what extent have the stated objectives of instruction been met? and (2) Is the safety instruction better than the one it will supplant? Safety instruction attempts have had mixed reviews. Some studies report success in thwarting accidental injuries while others indicate failure and recommend that the instruction should be either revised or abandoned.

*Advising.* The effectiveness of this approach may be dependent upon the prestige of the person giving the advice. The prestige is related to the person's presumed experience, knowledge, and judgment. Examples of advising include: tornado and hurricane alerts, a state governor advising holiday travelers to obey speed limits, and traffic alerts during busy times alerting drivers to heavy traffic and traffic accidents.

*Commanding.* The adherence to a command also depends upon whether the commander has authority. Examples include: a policeman directing you to drive through a red light, a lifeguard whistling a person to stop running on the swimming pool deck, and a speed limit sign showing 55 mph.

*Appealing to values.* This appeal focuses upon the saving of a life or avoiding an injury. Examples of such appeals include: posters or signs showing and saying something about accident prevention and slogans such as "the life you save may be your own."

*Inducements.* This is an offering of something valued in return for safe behavior. Examples in industry are gifts (e.g., pens, trophies, camping equipment, etc.) given at the end of an accident-free period of time. Sometimes pictures and names appearing in a newspaper for safe behavior serve as an inducement.

*Coercion.* This is the opposite of inducement and means the threat of harm to the person. Examples of coercion include any threat by a parent to a child, whether it be a spanking or detainment in the child's room for the weekend if the child is misbehaving so as to risk the chance of an injury. Warning tickets given by a policeman serve as a threat to violators.

*Legal sanctions.* This is using force to make a person safe. This means changing behavior by requiring or prohibiting a certain type of behavior, by law or regulation. These include traffic laws such as running red lights, speeding, or driving while intoxicated. These are more politically acceptable than laws directed at protective behavior, such as required safety belt use or mandatory motorcycle helmet use. Having a law or regulation is not an assurance that accidents will decrease. Experience with the drinking driver problem and violations of the 55 mph speed limit law show that problems exist. Legal sanctions are usually the last effort for changing behavior to reduce accidents and injuries.

### Changing or Establishing an Attitude

Acquiring or modifying an attitude is *not* done, according to a great deal of evidence, by the sole use of persuasive communication (e.g., repetition of "drive cautiously" or "please be careful").

An effective method of influencing an attitude is called "human modeling." A person can observe and learn attitudes from many sorts of human models. In one's younger years, one or both parents serve as models and later other members of the family may play this role. Teachers may become models for behavior, but the varieties of human modeling do not stop at the home or school. Public figures, prominent sports people, famous scientists or artists may become models. It is not essential that people who function as human models be seen or known personally— they can be seen on television or in movies. In fact, they can even be read about in books. This latter fact serves to emphasize the enormous potential that literature has for the determination of attitudes and values.

The human model must, of course, be someone whom the person respects, or as some writers would put it, someone with whom he or she can identify. The model must be observed (or read about) performing the desired kind of behavior. Having seen the action, whatever it may be, the person also must see that such action leads to satisfaction or pleasure on the part of the model (e.g., a movie star smiling while fastening his or her safety belt).

The modification of attitudes undoubtedly takes place all the time in every portion of an individual's life.

## HADDON MATRIX

William Haddon, Jr.[2] developed a strategy system to aid in the identification of countermeasures. Though originally developed to cope with the traffic accident problem, the concept and matrix can be applied to any type of accident. The strategy is to reduce losses due to injuries rather than merely to prevent injuries. Haddon states that even when an accident cannot be prevented, there are many ways to prevent or reduce the frequency and severity of injuries which result from an accident.

Haddon suggests approaching the problem of reducing injuries by considering the three major phases that determine the final outcomes. These three phases are shown in Table 8-1 with examples of countermeasures related to crashes, burns, electrocutions, poisonings, and drownings.

The *first phase*, or pre-event phase, consists of many factors which determine whether an accident will take place. Elements that cause people and physical and/or chemical forces to move into undesirable interaction are included here. For example, probably the most important human factor in the pre-event phase is alcohol intoxication in almost all accident types.

In the past, the emphasis in accident prevention has been on human behavior

**TABLE 8-1 Examples of Tactics for Reducing Injury Losses**

| TYPE OF EVENT | PRE-EVENT PHASE | EVENT PHASE | POST-EVENT PHASE |
|---|---|---|---|
| Impacts (e.g., from falls) | Alcoholism programs<br>Handrails on stairs | Fire nets<br>Padding on floors<br>Football helmets | Trained ambulance crews<br>Well-equipped ambulances<br>Pneumatic splints |
| Exposure to heat | Child-proof matches<br>Eliminating floor heaters<br>Venting explosive gases | Flame-retardant clothing<br>Reducing surface temperature of heaters and stoves<br>Sprinkler systems in buildings | Burn centers<br>Skin grafting<br>Rehabilitation |
| Exposure to electricity | Covered electric outlets<br>Insulation on electric handtools and wiring | Circuit breakers<br>Fuses | Cardiopulmonary resuscitation<br>Equipment and training |
| Ingestion of poison | Child-proof medicine containers<br>Separation of CO from passenger compartments of autos | Making cleaning agents inert or less caustic<br>Packing poisons in small, nonlethal amounts | Poison information centers<br>Detoxification centers |
| Immersion in water | Fences around swimming pools<br>Draining ponds | Life jackets<br>Training to tread water or swim | Lifesaving training<br>Teaching mouth-to-mouth resuscitation techniques to general population |

Source: Susan P. Baker and William Haddon, Jr., "Reducing Injuries and Their Results: The Scientific Approach," *The Milbank Memorial Fund Quarterly/ Health and Society*, Fall 1974.

and attempts to change it. Accidents are usually regarded as someone's fault, rather than as a failure that could have been prevented by some change in the system. For example, if a boy, while cutting the grass with a power rotary lawn mower, ejects from the mower a stone which cuts a bystander, the resulting injury (the cut from the stone) is likely to be blamed on the boy operating the mower, rather than being attributed to the fact that a rotary mower many times will have no protective device to avert the ejection of stones and debris. Such devices are now required, but are often taken off.

Thus, the mower can contribute to the initiation of the accident, either by placing excessive demands or restrictions on the operator, or through mechanical inadequacies or failure. For example, in automobile crashes, steering, tire, and brake failures sometimes initiate crashes but seldom are searched for after the crash.

Other pre-event countermeasures relate to the environment, and there the principle of separation plays an important role. For example, children can be separated from cleaning agents containing caustic ingredients through the use of child-resistant containers and by storing containers in locked compartments out of reach of children.

The *second phase*, or event phase, begins when physical and/or chemical forces exert themselves unfavorably upon people and/or property. Countermeasures preventing harmful effects even when excessive energy (mechanical, chemical, thermal, etc.) is contacted are part of this second phase. Examples of event phase countermeasures for motor vehicle accidents include "packaging people" for crashes through the use of safety belts, padded dashes, and collapsible steering wheel columns. Nontraffic examples are boxing gloves, safety shoes, hard hats, helmets, lead x-ray shields, nets for acrobats, and gloves for laborers.

This second phase is to soften contact regardless of the cause. Stressing this phase follows the idea that because accidents will happen, let's protect humans and property the best we can. Tradition, on the other hand, has stressed the pre-event phase rather than the event phase.

The *third phase*, or post-event phase, involves salvaging people and/or property after contact with excessive energy (mechanical, chemical, thermal, etc.) has taken place. Early detection of aircraft crashes through transducers that start broadcasting a special signal at the time of a crash is an example of the third phase, as are fire detection systems (heat or smoke), SOS and MAYDAY signals, and the use of forest fire lookout towers.

In case of serious injury it is important to provide expert medical care as quickly as possible. Transportation for the injured, trained ambulance personnel, and emergency room staffs are appropriate countermeasures which are a part of this phase.

Haddon's other matrix consists of putting the three phases (pre-event, event, post-event) and the three epidemiological factors (human (host), agent, environment) together in a matrix which provides a greater practical and theoretical utility in categorizing countermeasure options. See Tables 8-2, 8-3, and 8-4.

It should be clear, however, that both of these matrices still encompass accident prevention efforts. The tables give examples of countermeasures for motor vehicle accidents, drowning, and suffocation in abandoned refrigerators. Not all of the possible countermeasures are given in the tables. Those given are for examples.

**TABLE 8-2  Countermeasures. Accident Type: Motor Vehicle.**

| Phases / Factors | Pre-event | Event | Post Event |
|---|---|---|---|
| Host | Driver education | Driver "packaging" | Proper first aid and emergency care of bleeding |
| Agent | Automobile safety inspection of brakes, tires, etc. | Collapsible steering wheel to avoid impaling or crushing driver's chest | Accessible and low cost of vehicle-damage repair |
| Environment | Adequate signs and signals | Breakaway posts and sign poles | Emergency telephones and adequate emergency systems |

Adapted from William Haddon, Jr., "A Logical Framework for Categorizing Highway Safety Phenomena and Activity," *Journal of Trauma*, March 1972, by permission of the author.

**TABLE 8-3   Countermeasures. Accident Type: Drownings.**

| Phases \ Factors | Pre-event | Event | Post Event |
|---|---|---|---|
| Host | Swimming instruction | Life jackets | Visible swimwear |
| Agent | No swimming pool | Shallow pool | Underwater lights |
| Environment | Barriers and fences | Lifelines | Rescue systems |

Adapted from Park E. Dietz and Susan P. Baker, "Drowning Epidemiology and Prevention," *American Journal of Public Health*, April 1974.

## THE TEN STRATEGIES

There are various additional ways to sort out options and tactics for reducing human and other damage. Haddon identified ten logically based strategies that are available and a guideline in formulating countermeasures.[3] All the strategies may be used for reducing the damage from all types of accidents.

These ten basic strategies, each with illustrative tactics, are:

1. To prevent the creation of the hazard in the first place. *Examples:* prevent production of boats, guns, snowmobiles.
2. To reduce the amount of the hazard brought into being. *Examples:* reduce speed of vehicles, lead content of paint, make less beverage alcohol (a hazard itself and in its results, such as drunken driving).
3. To prevent the release of the hazard that already exists. *Examples:* bolting or timbering mine roofs, impounding dangerous toys.
4. To modify the rate of spatial distribution of release of the hazard from its source. *Examples:* brakes, shutoff valves.

TABLE 8-4   Countermeasures. Accident Type:
Discarded or Abandoned Refrigerator Suffocation

| Phases / Factors | Pre-event | Event | Post Event |
|---|---|---|---|
| Host (human) | Tell children to stay away from discarded refrigerators because they are not "playthings" and they can kill | If a child is missing, a first place to look is in refrigerators | Resuscitation training for parents and older children |
| Agent | Manufacturers install permanent trays in refrigerators which don't allow room for children to crawl into them | Manufacturers install an interior wall section which a child's force can puncture to allow ventilation | Escape worthiness, (i.e., door can be opened from within by a force of 5 pounds) |
| Environment | Imposed penalties for discarding refrigerators without removing hinges and door | Manufacturers install an alerting device which would indicate occupancy and use (light or buzzer) | A first place to look for missing children is in refrigerators |

5. To separate, in time or space, the hazard and that which is to be protected. *Examples:* walkways over or around hazards; evacuation; the phasing of pedestrian and vehicular traffic, whether in a work area or on a city street; the banning of vehicles carrying explosives from areas where they and their cargoes are not needed.

6. To separate the hazard and that which is to be protected by interposition of a material barrier. *Examples:* gloves, containment structures, child-proof poison-container closures, vehicle air bags.

7. To modify relevant basic qualities of the hazard. *Examples:* using breakaway roadside poles, making crib slat spacing too narrow to strangle a child.

8. To make what is to be protected more resistant to damage from the hazard. *Examples:* making structures more fire- and earthquake-resistant, giving salt to workers under thermal stress, making motor vehicles more crash resistant.

9. To begin to counter the damage already done by the environmental hazard. *Examples:* rescuing the shipwrecked, reattaching severed limbs, extricating trapped miners.

10. To stabilize, repair, and rehabilitate the object of the damage. *Examples:* posttraumatic cosmetic surgery, physical rehabilitation for amputees and others with disabling injuries (including many thousands paralyzed annually by spinal cord damage sustained in motor-vehicle crashes), rebuilding after fires and earthquakes.

Two points should be kept in mind in using these strategies: (1) they provide guidelines for possible control programs; they do not provide a formula or guide for specific cases. These should be dealt with on an individual basis; and (2) the strategies do not center on causation but instead on the entire realm of how to reduce damages.

### Ten Strategies Example

Because of their importance, sports injuries will be used to illustrate approaches based on *Haddon's ten basic strategies for preventing injury.*[4]

The *first strategy is to prevent the creation of the hazard in the first place*, for example, by not manufacturing sports equipment that is apt to cause injury. This strategy might be applied to trampolines, an important source of spinal cord injuries. After the American Academy of Pediatrics recommended in 1977 that school use of trampolines be banned, there was a drop of more than 60 percent in the number of trampoline head and neck injuries treated in hospitals participating in the Consumer Product Safety Commission's National Electronic Injury Surveillance System (NEISS).

The *second strategy is to reduce the amount of hazard that is created*, for example, reducing the height from which people can fall or jump, limiting the speed capability of snowmobiles, or limiting the speed of beginning skiers by providing slopes with only small vertical drops in relation to the lengths of the trails. Exposure can be curtailed through shorter periods of play or by permitting hunting only on certain days. Reducing the number of players who participate in a particular sport is another example, illustrated by limiting participants to members of a specified age group.

The *third strategy involves either preventing or reducing the likelihood of the release of a hazard.* Examples include not allowing boxers to fight and designing hunting weapons that will not discharge inadvertently. In ancient times, the cessation of gladiatorial contests provides an additional example, as would the ending of bull fighting in Latin countries. Reducing the likelihood of the release of the hazard is often a more practical approach; an example is packing and grooming ski slopes to reduce hidden obstacles that might cause skiers to fall.

The *fourth strategy is to modify the rate or spatial distribution of release of the hazard from its source.* Examples include release bindings on skis, controlled release of dammed-up water to protect boaters downstream, and the use of shorter cleats on football shoes so that the foot can rotate easily without transmitting a sudden force to the knee. Changes in football rules have outlawed spearing and face-tackling; these techniques use the head as a primary contact point, and the forces on the head and neck are likely to exceed injury thresholds. Yet, more than one-third of high school football players in Minnesota continued to use these maneuvers a year after they were banned, and one player in five reported concussion symptoms during the playing season.

The *fifth strategy is to separate, in time or space, the hazard and its release from that which is to be protected.* Starting avalanches during times when ski slopes are closed, an example of temporal separation, decreases the likelihood that avalanches will occur when skiers are on the slopes. Placing benches and other equipment farther from playing areas reduces the frequency of "out of bounds" injuries that commonly occur when players run into them. Spatial separation is also illustrated by storing pistols used for target shooting at the shooting range rather than at home, and by providing paths for bicyclists, joggers, and people walking that are separate from roads for motor vehicles.

The *sixth strategy is to separate the hazard from whatever is to be protected by interposing a material barrier.* In many sports, the head, face, eyes, chest, or other body parts need to be protected from balls, bats, or other players. A review of sports-related injuries and deaths among people ages five to fourteen revealed that 38 percent of the deaths involved baseball. Being struck on the chest by the baseball with subsequent cardiac arrest appeared to be the predominant cause. This suggests a need for chest protection for young baseball players. Eye protection devices for racquetball and squash can prevent many eye injuries, the most common serious injury associated with such racquet sports. Facial and dental injuries among hockey and football players have been substantially reduced by face masks. Protective helmets are appropriate to many sports, such as football and horseback riding, where head injuries are a serious problem.

The *seventh strategy is to modify the relevant basic qualities of the hazard.* Illustrations include recent adoption of a softer ball in squash rather than the previously used hardball, padding the outer edge of racquets and using balls large enough so that the bony socket of the eye affords some protection. The pointed ends of hockey sticks, once a major source of facial injuries, are now rounded to make them less injurious. Gymnasium walls should be designed without protrusions and either made of energy-attenuating materials or padded in areas where players can strike them. Breakaway goalposts and slalom poles that yield on impact are further examples.

The *eighth strategy is to make that which is to be protected more resistant to damage from the hazard.* Conditioning of the musculo-skeletal system is an important means of reducing the likelihood of injury. Grouping school athletes by skills, physical fitness, and physical maturity rather than age has reportedly reduced injury rates. Exercise and therapy to reduce osteoporosis are promising approaches of special relevance to older people participating in athletic and recreational activities.

The *ninth strategy is to begin to counter damage already done.* Athletes who may have sustained spinal cord injuries, for example, need to be carefully supported when they are moved in order to reduce the likelihood of paralysis. Football players with concussion symptoms should not be returned to play on the same day because of the potential for progressive neurological debilitation. One study found that most high school players who experienced loss of consciousness returned to play the same day. (Communication systems and readily available emergency and definitive care are clearly important but often inadequate, except in some major urban centers and in states with good emergency systems.

The *tenth strategy is to stabilize, repair, and rehabilitate the injured person.* Reconstructive surgery, physical and mental rehabilitation, and modification of the environment to accommodate the handicapped help to minimize adverse outcomes of serious injury.

*These ten strategies and examples of illustrative tactics suggest the wide variety of measures that can reduce the likelihood and severity of injuries, as well as the severity of the consequences of injury once it has occurred. In choosing among potentially useful preventive measures, priority should be given to the ones most likely to effectively reduce injuries. In general, these will be measures that provide built-in automatic protection, minimizing the amount and frequency of effort required of the individuals involved.*

## NOTES

1.  Author unknown.
2.  William Haddon, Jr., "A Logical Framework for Categorizing Highway Safety Phenomena and Activity," *The Journal of Trauma*, 12 (1972), 193–207.
3.  William Haddon, Jr., "Advances in the Epidemiology of Injuries As a Basis for Public Policy," *Public Health Reports*, 95 (1980), 411–21, and William Haddon, Jr., "The Basic Strategies for Reducing Damage from Hazards of All Kinds," *Hazard Prevention*, 16 (1980), 1.
4.  Susan P. Baker et al., *The Injury Fact Book* (Lexington, MA: Lexington Books, 1984), pp. 94–97.

# 9

# Motor Vehicle Accidents

## AUTOMOBILE ACCIDENTS

The magnitude and severity of the motor vehicle safety problem is not readily perceived by individual motorists in their day-to-day driving. The reasons for this lack of perception are not hard to find: most accidents are not catastrophic and usually "happen to someone else." In addition, the chance of being killed on an average ten-mile trip is extremely small—about one in three million—and cannot be considered a high risk by most drivers and passengers.

It is these short-term risks that influence the individual motorist's reaction to traffic safety, but it is the long-term statistics which produce a problem of major importance. Based on recent fatality rates, about one out of every sixty infants born today will die in a motor vehicle accident and on the average two out of three persons may expect to suffer a motor-vehicle injury during their lifetime.

BOX 9-1 *FIRST TRAFFIC ACCIDENT*

New York City, May 30, 1896 . . . Henry Wells of Springfield, Massachusetts, driving a Duryea Motor Wagon, collided with a bicycle, ridden by Evylyn Thomas. It was the first accident involving a motor vehicle to occur in America. Miss Thomas went to the hospital with a broken leg. Wells spent the night in a jail cell.

BOX 9-2  *FIRST TRAFFIC FATALITY*

> Central Park West and 74th St., New York City, September 13, 1899 . . .
> As Henry H. Bliss, a real estate broker, stepped off a streetcar he was run over
> by an automobile driven by Arthur Smith. Bliss died later in Roosevelt Hospi-
> tal. It was the first documented traffic fatality. Arthur Smith was arrested and
> held on one thousand dollars bail, but there is no record of what happened to
> him.

Motor vehicle crash injuries, along with some fifty thousand fatalities annually, represent a staggering drain on the nation's health and economy, one which could get even worse. The increasing presence on the roads of smaller, less protective cars, along with the repeal of motorcycle helmet-use laws in many states, are contributing to the current and expected increases in the death and injury toll.

An example of the loss in terms of economics is:

- The costs of crash injuries are, among health problems, second only to cancer. The cost of injuries outranks that of coronary heart disease, and greatly out-ranks the cost of stroke, the other leading killers of Americans.[1]

BOX 9-3

> Each person in the United States, on average, can expect to be in a crash at
> least once every ten years. For the individual, the question then becomes, how
> serious will one's crashes be?
>
>    —*Fatalities.* The odds of death are that one out of every sixty people born
>    will die in a crash.
>
>    —*Injuries.* The odds of injury are that one out of every twenty people born
>    will suffer a severe injury in a crash.
>
>                                     — *National Highway Traffic Safety Administration*

### Human Factors

*Age.*  Teenagers kill and injure themselves and other people on the highways at rates far higher than those of other drivers. More deaths per licensed driver are associated with the crashes of 18-year-olds than with any other age group. Next to the 18-year-olds, the 16-, 17-, and 19-year-olds had the highest rates of deaths per licensed driver; the figures then decline rapidly as drivers grow older.

Teenage drivers are more often involved in fatal crashes at night, especially weekend nights. Alcohol use is higher among drivers in these hours because of the increased number of parties and bar hours on Friday and Saturday nights. This age group is often characterized as risk-takers.

Another explanation is that young drivers are new and inexperienced drivers.

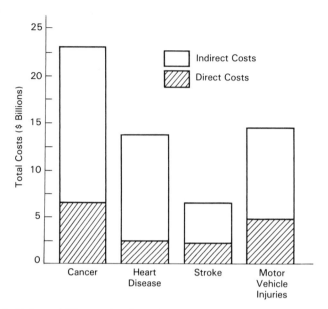

**FIGURE 9-1** Estimated Direct and Indirect Costs Associated With Incidence of Cancer, Coronary Heart Disease, Motor Vehicle Injuries, and Stroke (in Millions of 1980 Dollars). From *The Incidence and Economic Costs of Major Health Impairments: A Comparative Analysis of Cancer, Motor-Vehicle Injuries, Coronary Heart Disease, and Stroke* by Nelson S. Hartunian and Charles N. Smart (Lexington, Mass.: Lexington Books, D.C. Heath and Company, Copyright 1981, D.C. Heath and Company).

Also, young drivers are more frequently exposed to hazardous times and locations. Not all youthful drivers are involved, but many accidents involving youths are closely related to feelings of hostility and rebellion and to the acting out of these feelings, especially among male drivers.

*Sex.* Teenaged males have much higher rates of driver involvement in fatal crashes than females. For males the rate peaks at eighteen, whereas for females it is highest at age sixteen.

*Alcohol.* In the United States alcohol use is the single most frequently noted human factor in fatal crashes. It has been known for years that more than half of all fatal crashes in the United States involve a driver who has been not just drinking, but drinking in sufficient quantity to have a blood alcohol concentration (BAC) at or above 0.10 percent. The use of alcohol combined with driving is the largest single contributor to motor vehicle crashes resulting in fatalities not only to the drunken drivers themselves but to adults and children in or struck by their vehicles.

### Alcohol and the Human Body

An understanding of the nature of alcohol and its interaction with the human body is helpful in understanding its role in motor vehicle accidents. The active ingredient in distilled spirts, wine, and beer is ethanol, one of several types of alcohols. Ethanol is also called ethyl alcohol, grain alcohol, and more commonly, just "alcohol."

A "typical" drink, about three-fourths of an ounce of alcohol, is provided by a "shot" of distilled spirits (one and one-half ounces of 100 proof alcohol), a glass of fortified wine (three and one-half ounces of 20 percent alcohol), a larger glass of table wine (five ounces of 12 percent alcohol), or a pint of beer (sixteen ounces of 4.5 percent alcohol).

Absorption of alcohol into the body occurs through the simple process of diffusion: alcohol does not have to be digested before entering the blood. The rate of absorption of alcohol depends on the quantity taken, its concentration, and especially on the other contents of the gastrointestinal tract. Food in the tract delays absorption. When alcohol is taken with a heavy meal, up to six hours may be required for complete absorption.

Alcohol is eliminated from the body almost entirely through the process of oxidation. Typically, the rate of elimination is about 0.015 percent per hour. Roughly speaking, the average person eliminates, each hour, one of the "typical" drinks described above. No practical means of significantly speeding up the elimination of alcohol has been discovered yet.

There are many methods of measuring the amount of alcohol in the blood. The most accurate and reliable of these test the blood directly, rather than some other fluid (e.g., urine). Modern breath tests can be quite precise in the measurement of breath alcohol.

Alcohol intoxication is most commonly apparent through observation of the behavioral and emotional effects of alcohol consumption. Although these effects vary among individuals and among cultures, there is a universal pattern of reaction to drinking, beginning with feelings of relaxation and pleasure and progressing to heightened emotionalism and disturbances in psychomotor functioning.

The behavioral and emotional effects of alcohol consumption are caused by the effects of alcohol on the brain. The measurement of BACs is really an attempt to determine, indirectly, the amount of alcohol in the brain.

Just how much alcohol must be ingested for acute alcohol intoxication to occur varies from person to person. Important factors are body weight, contents of the stomach, physical health, and the tolerance the individual has developed to the effects of alcohol.

*Age.*  Both the youngest and oldest persons have been found less frequently than others among drinking drivers. The youngest drivers, however, appear to have a much greater alcohol-crash risk after drinking (especially in the low BACs) than persons of other age groups. Inexperience with both drinking and driving has been suggested as a reason for the higher involvement of young drivers in alcohol-related crashes. Youths are more sensitive to even small amounts of alcohol than are older, more experienced drinkers. Despite this, heavy alcohol use is more frequent among persons under age twenty-five.

*Sex.* One of the best differentiators of drinking drivers is sex. Males are involved far more frequently than females in alcohol-related crashes. This is thought to be a consequence of social customs which call for males to do most of the driving, especially at night when most drinking–driving occurs.

*Risks.* Statistics indicate that one out of every two persons will be involved in an alcohol-related crash during their lifetimes. This is most likely to happen on a weekend when one out of every ten drivers is drunk. Sadly, only one in 2,000 drunk drivers will be arrested.

A disproportionate number of teens will be involved in alcohol-related accidents. Drivers under age twenty make up only nine percent of the population, but they are involved in 18 percent of accidents in which alcohol is a factor. This is one of the main reasons many states have raised the minimum legal drinking age.

Most states have set .10 percent alcohol in the blood as the level at which a person is considered drunk. Utah and Idaho have set a level of .08 percent. However, studies indicate that younger drivers with much lower blood alcohol levels often are involved in crashes.

At a .10 percent alcohol level a person would have difficulty walking or coordinating the movements needed to operate a vehicle; even at just .08 percent senses, memory, reaction time, and mood are all adversely affected. A 100 pound adult would reach this level with three drinks over a two hour period. It doesn't make much difference whether he or she drinks three beers, three mixed drinks, or three glasses of wine—they all contain the same amount of alcohol. When the blood alcohol concentration reaches .10 percent, an adult driver is six to seven times more likely to have an auto accident.

Once the alcohol is consumed it takes about one hour for the body to metabolize the alcohol; that is, to oxidize and remove the alcohol content of each drink. Therefore a person who consumed three beers between 7 and 8 PM would not be sober until 11 PM.

As few as two drinks in one hour can impair driving ability unless the drinker waits two hours before driving. If alcohol is taken into the body faster than it can be removed, the blood alcohol level climbs and so does the potential for an accident. The faster drinks are consumed, the greater the decrease in driving ability.

### Environmental Factors

*International.* Death totals of different nations must be compared cautiously because of differences in the volume and kinds of traffic, numbers of vehicles, population density, definitions of death, and other factors.

The United States mileage death rate is generally the lowest among other comparable countries of the world.

*Region.* The states within the south, southwest, and Rocky Mountain regions generally tend to have higher mileage death rates than other regions within the United States.

BOX 9-4    *NINE MOST DANGEROUS STATES IN WHICH TO DRIVE*
*(based on mileage death rates)*

| 1. West Virginia | 5. Alaska |
|---|---|
| 2. New Mexico | 6. Montana |
| 3. Louisiana | 7. Nevada |
| 4. Mississippi | 8. South Carolina |
| | 9. Florida |

— National Safety Council, *Accident Facts*, 1984

*Urban-rural.* Motor vehicle deaths occur more frequently in rural places, but injuries occur more frequently in urban places. The Interstate System has been shown to be safer than other road types.

*Day and Month.* Motor vehicle death totals vary sharply for different days of the week and different months of the year. Deaths are highest on Fridays, Saturdays, and Sundays. Deaths are at their lowest levels in January and February and increase to their highest levels in July and August.

*Time of Day.* Time of day is an important factor. More than one-third of the fatalities occur between 10:00 PM and 4:00 AM. Alcohol-impaired driving, which is more common at night, contributes significantly to the greater severity of nighttime crashes.

*Major Holidays.* Generally, both deaths and death rates are higher during the holidays than they are during comparable nonholiday periods. The National Safety Council annually predicts and records holiday death tolls for these major holidays: Memorial Day, Fourth of July, Labor Day, Thanksgiving, Christmas, and New Year's. Newspapers usually announce reports from the National Safety Council concerning numbers of motor vehicle fatalities.

BOX 9-5    *UNUSUAL BUT TRUE*

PRESTON, England (UPI)—Allan Wilkinson took his mother-in-law shopping. She fell out of the car while it was still moving.

Wilkinson, 40, quickly backed up the car—and ran over her left leg. Then he went forward and ran over her right leg.

BOX 9-6

There's a line on the ocean where by crossing you can lose a day. There's one on the highway where you can do even better.

— *Anonymous*

*Road Conditions.* Even though most motor vehicle accidents occur on dry road surfaces, skidding on wet or icy roads results in vehicle control loss and resultant injuries.

If there is an object near a roadway, sooner or later it will be struck. The streets and highways are dotted with them—bridge abutments, guardrails designed for strength rather than safety, and sign and light poles embedded in concrete—are only a few examples.

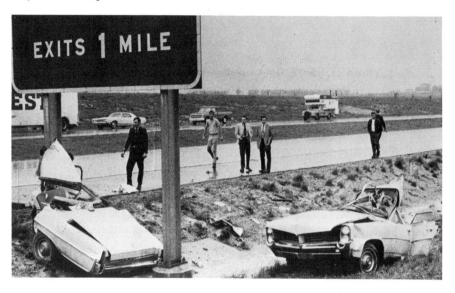

**FIGURE 9-2** This car was sliced into two halves by a rigid, unyielding signpost on a so-called "modern" highway—with fatal consequences for the occupants. Photo courtesy of the Insurance Institute for Highway Safety.

*Small Cars.* In every type of crash situation, the occupants of small cars fare worse than the occupants of large cars. For example, ejections from cars during crashes happen substantially more often in small cars than in larger cars due to the small cars' structural inadequacies to keep occupants contained. Small cars involved in fatal crashes are far more likely to roll over than large cars. Even if all vehicles were the same size, the death rate would be greater if all vehicles were small because smaller cars simply have less room for energy to be absorbed and occupants to decelerate in a crash. Small cars are not less dangerous because of their maneuverability —subcompacts have more insurance claims than larger cars.

### Effects

There are two collisions in a motor vehicle crash. In the first collision, the car strikes another car, a tree, or similar object. This first collision only involves the car; the occupants are not injured. However, because a body in motion tends to remain in motion (Newton's Law), the occupants continue traveling forward at about the

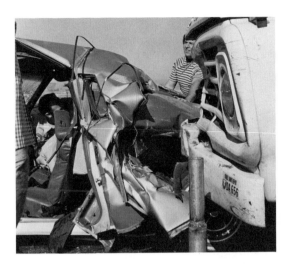

**FIGURE 9-3** In every type of crash situation, occupants of small cars fare worse than occupants of larger vehicles. Photo courtesy of the Utah Highway Patrol.

same velocity as the car was traveling. The second collision occurs when the occupants strike the car's interior or are ejected from the car and strike the road or other outside objects; the injuries to the occupants occur during the second collision.

The vehicle does not actually stop all at once, but slows down as the front end collapses under the force of the collision, so that at about 30 mph it takes a car about one-tenth of a second to come to a complete stop. At that speed, the front end is often crushed, but the passenger compartment usually remains intact. Because the crushing of the front end absorbs energy, the longer this impact takes and the more controlled the collapse of the vehicle, the greater the potential is for survival.

So, if the passenger compartment remains intact at 30 mph, why is it that there are as many deaths and injuries at this speed as any other? This is where the "second collision" comes in. While the front end of the car is collapsing and the vehicle is slowing down, the person inside the car is still moving forward at 30 mph. One-fiftieth of a second after the car has stopped, the person slams into the dashboard and windshield. While the car takes one-tenth of a second to stop, the human takes only one-hundredth of a second. So, in a 30 mph crash into a wall, a subject weighing 150 pounds will continue forward with a force of about thirty times his weight, or about 4500 pounds.

The injuries to children are especially severe. If a child were being held by an adult, then the forward force would be thirty times the child's weight; if the child weighed twenty pounds, then he would be moving with a force of six hundred pounds—a weight few adults can hold, especially when applied suddenly. The adult's weight, moving forward with the force of several thousand pounds, would press against the child's body. This is known as the "child crusher syndrome."

The degree of injury is related to such variables as the type of vehicle driven

# What Happens in a Collision

## 1st, The Car Collision

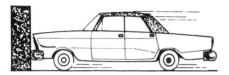

When a car hits a solid barrier, it doesn't stop all at once. The bumper stops immediately, but the rest of the car continues to move forward.

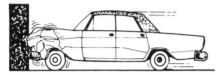

The car slows down as the crushing of the front end absorbs some of the force of the collision.

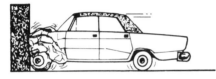

At 30 mph, the car takes about 1/10 of a second to come to a complete stop. The front end is crushed, but the passenger compartment usually remains undamaged.

## 2nd, The Human Collision

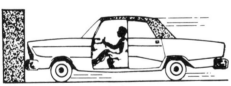

On impact, the car begins to crush and to slow down. The person inside the car has nothing to slow him down, so he continues to move forward inside the car at 30 mph.

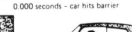

0.000 seconds - car hits barrier

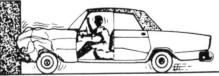

Within 1/10 of a second, the car has come to a complete stop, but the person is still moving forward at 30 mph.

0.100 seconds - car stops

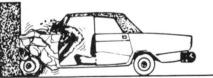

One-fiftieth of a second after the car has stopped, the person slams into the dashboard and windshield. This is the human collision. The car takes 1/10 of a second to stop; the human takes only 1/100 of a second.

Courtesy: US Department of Transportation, National Highway Traffic Safety Administration.

0.120 seconds - person hits car interior

**FIGURE 9-4** What happens in a collision. Source: National Highway Traffic Safety Administration.

and the number of vehicles involved. Let's assume a match between a Ford LTD and a Honda Civic in a head-on collision. Since the Ford, with a weight of about four thousand pounds, would have the weight advantage when traveling at 30 mph, it would be slowed to about 10 mph by the collision; a 150 pound passenger would crash into the interior surface of the car with a force of about three thousand pounds. However, experts say that if he had the advantage of a seat belt or an air bag, he should survive.

On the other hand, the Honda, weighing about two thousand pounds, would experience a nearly instantaneous change in velocity from 30 mph moving forward to 10 mph moving backwards. A subject weighing 150 pounds would hit the interior of the car with a force of about six thousand pounds. Survival would be questionable.

It is not just the force of the impact which causes injury, but what the passenger hit inside the vehicle. Hard surfaces create injuries similar to hammer blows, while sharp surfaces function like knives. The windshield can induce especially nasty wounds; it is not unusual to see victims who have been scalped, or have had portions of their faces avulsed.

Studies indicate the areas of the body most commonly injured are the head, neck, chest, and abdomen. More than half of the fatal and life-threatening injuries come from the victims' bodies hitting the steering wheel and column, instrument panel, the windshield, and areas of the dashboard such as protruding knobs and heating/air conditioning vents.

So there are actually two collisions in an automobile accident. The first collision damages the vehicle, which is costly, while the second damages the human, which can be deadly.

In studying the second collision, it was found that people died from four main causes: (1) ejection, (2) striking the car interior, (3) invasion of the occupant's space, and (4) person-to-person collisions.

*Ejection.*    This is the most common cause of motor vehicle deaths. Occupants are killed as they are thrown onto the road, against a pole or tree, or into the path of their own or another car.

*Striking the Interior.*    Examples of injuries include: protruding radio knobs and cigarette lighters penetrating the skull, or rear-view mirrors breaking off and leaving a spike to embed.

*Invasion of Space.*    This may come from several sources. For example, the steering column may thrust into the driver's sternum, crushing it and possibly perforating the heart or aorta. The hood may be shoved into the vehicle or guardrails may act like a spear by being driven into the vehicle's interior.

*Person-to-Person.*    Serious injuries can occur by being thrown into other people in the car.

### Types of Motor Vehicle Accidents

The National Safety Council uses a classification scheme which proves useful in the identification of motor vehicle accidents:

*Collision between Motor Vehicles.* This involves collisions of two or more motor vehicles. Motorized bicycles and scooters, trolley buses, and farm tractors or road machinery traveling on highways are motor vehicles.

*Noncollision Accidents.* Includes all types of noncollision accidents.

*Pedestrian Accidents.* Includes persons struck by motor vehicles, either on or off a street or highway, regardless of the circumstances of the accident.

*Collision With Fixed Object.* Includes collisions in which the first harmful event is the striking of a fixed object such as a guardrail, abutment, impact attenuator, etc.

*Collision With Pedalcycle.* Includes collisions between pedalcycles and motor vehicles on streets, highways, private driveways, parking lots, etc. The National Safety Council defines a pedalcycle as a vehicle propelled by human power and operated solely by pedal.

*Collision With Railroad Train.* Includes collisions of motor vehicles (moving or stalled) and railroad vehicles at public or private grade crossings. In other types of accidents, classification requires motor vehicle to be in motion.

*Other Collisions.* Examples include collisions with animals, animal-drawn vehicles, street cars.

### Injuries

Motor vehicle crashes are among the leading causes of severe injuries.

Hospital-treated brain injuries to victims alone are estimated at more than 180 thousand annually or almost half of the total in the United States. A brain-injured person who survives may suffer permanent neurological impairment, even to the extent of never regaining consciousness.

The spinal cord is the principal pathway by means of which the brain and the rest of the body maintain communication. When the cord is injured, the results are catastrophic, and commonly include paraplegia, quadriplegia, or death. Crashes are one of the main causes of paralyzing spinal cord injuries every year in the United States. Also a large number of cases of severe and permanent brain damage are sustained in crashes.

The leading cause of noncosmetic facial surgery in America is injury sustained in motor vehicle crashes. In fact about 114 thousand severe facial lacerations and twenty-five thousand severe facial fractures are sustained each year.

A very commonplace yet inadequately understood neck injury sustained in crashes is often called "whiplash." The term covers a range of damage to the complex structures of the neck.

### Motor Vehicle Crash Prevention

Not all the answers to the motor vehicle crash problem are yet known. The following approaches are not all-inclusive.

*Teenage Drivers.*[1]    Considering the magnitude of the crash problem associated with teen drivers, several approaches might reduce the number of motor vehicle crashes:

- Raise the minimum age of licensure to eighteen. Looking at the lifestyle of teenagers and their parents, it is obvious that withholding licenses until age eighteen may make gains in safety, but may result in loss of mobility, convenience, and employment. This area requires considerably more study and discussion to determine if the gains outweigh the losses. A modification could be to allow only "essential" driving by 16- and 17-year-olds (e.g., to and from work). This could be one way of offsetting the inconvenience or hardship for many teenagers and their parents in raising the age of licensing.

- Prohibit teenagers from driving during late evening and early morning hours. Almost half the fatalities of drivers less than eighteen years old take place from 8:00 PM to 4:00 AM. One study found that curfew laws restricting the nighttime driving of young drivers substantially reduced motor vehicle crashes.

- Evaluate high school driver education. A vast majority of the high schools in the United States offer driver education. Over 50 percent of the states use successful completion of driver education as a condition for licensing minor age drivers.

    Some raise the question as to whether driver education is part of the motor vehicle solution or whether it is contributing to the problem of crashes. By increasing the number of teenage drivers through driver education, it has the ironic effect of actually creating more teenage crash victims.

    On the other hand, teenagers who have taken driver education have fewer traffic violations than those who have not. Some experts feel that the blame for the high fatality rates among youth is not on the driver education course itself, but its timing. They feel delaying driver education a year or two may very well be a possible solution to the issue of high school driver education's effectiveness in reducing motor vehicle crashes.

- Raise the drinking age. States that have raised their legal minimum drinking age in recent years have had a substantial reduction in nighttime fatal crashes. Raising the legal minimum drinking age to twenty-one in all states would have an important impact in reducing motor vehicle deaths.

*Drunk Driving.*    A report completed by the National Highway Traffic Safety Administration reveals that programs to reduce motor vehicle crashes by "cracking down" on drunk drivers in order to remove them from the roads at best have achieved short-term reductions in crashes. Even then, as the experience of the most successful programs legislated in Great Britain, France, and elsewhere have shown, the effects "began to diminish" shortly after such programs were initiated. Crashes approached prior trends within a few months or, at most, a few years of the start of the program.

The report credits the initial, positive effect of these deterrence programs to publicity and news coverage.

According to the report, it is the public's perception of severe consequences if caught, not the severity of the punishment if caught and convicted, that results in whatever limited success legal crackdowns have. This is an important conclusion because it has been popularly assumed that all that is necessary to "solve" the drunk driving problem is the threat of very tough penalties.

The report raises serious questions about the efficacy and cost-effectiveness of past attempts to reduce the drunk driver crash problem.

It has long been believed that to effectively combat the drinking driver problem, more severe penalties and stricter enforcement are the answer. H. Laurence Ross, author of *Deterring the Drinking Driver*[2] says that laws and policies should focus on three elements to be effective:

1. Likelihood of apprehension must be perceived to be high. Roadblocks and breath testing may be one means of establishing such a threat if the roadblocks are set up frequently enough.
2. Swiftness of administering penalty must be assured. Some states have moved to make penalties automatic by setting mandatory sentences.
3. Severity of penalty need not be extreme. The mere retraction of the driver's license for a few weeks might be a noticeable and more effective threat for drinking drivers in the automobile dependent American society. According to Ross' research, increasing the severity of punishment has had no effect.[2]

*Avoiding the Drunk Driver.* Persons under the influence of alcohol often drive in a way that can indicate their drunkenness before getting close enough for a collision. Be alert for drivers who are driving too fast or too slow. Frequently when drivers realize they have had too much to drink and should not be driving, they become overcautious and drive so slowly that they cause accidents. Be alert to drivers who cross the center line—even momentarily. Get as far away from them as you can. Drunk drivers may also be observed changing lanes without warning and making turns without signaling. Wide turns, driving over curbs, and ignoring traffic signs or signals may also indicate a drunk driver. Let these drivers pass if they are behind you, and allow enough distance for a cushion of safety between yourself and these drivers so that you have time to adjust to their erratic moves.

Here are a few facts about assessing someone's ability to drive after drinking:

1. A person can be drunk and not stagger or slur his or her speech.
2. Many people can hide the fact that they are drunk simply by being quiet and sitting still.
3. Most people will not take any action in attempting to stop another person from driving while under the influence of alcohol.

4. The only way to sober up is to allow time to do it. Neither coffee nor cold showers will speed up the oxidation of alcohol in the body and make the person sober more quickly.

Even with the effort to crack down on drunk drivers, it will be impossible to remove all of them from the roads. They will continue to drive. Nevertheless, several steps to protect yourself and your family can be taken:

1. Use safety belts. This may be the most effective protection against the drunk driving menace.
2. Never get into a car with a person who has been drinking.
3. When going to a party, bar, or a restaurant, use the concept of the "designated driver." A nondrinker should do the driving.
4. Avoid the most dangerous driving times—between 8:00 PM and 4:00 AM on Friday and Saturday nights.
5. Practice defensive driving. This means keep a lookout for erratic driving behavior and be ready to take evasive action.

*55 mph Speed Limit.*  During the two years before the 55 mph speed limit went into effect (1972 and 1973), traffic fatalities averaged over fifty-four thousand a year. For the years after the enactment of the 55 mph speed limit law, the average dropped well below that figure. Although other safety and fuel conservation measures contributed to this reduction, safety experts estimate that over one half the fatality reduction can be directly attributed to the slower, more uniform flow of traffic produced by the national speed limit. The American Epilepsy Foundation has indicated that the 55 mph speed limit has been the single most effective preventative for new cases of epilepsy because it has reduced (by ninety thousand each year) the number of head trauma injuries resulting from automobile accidents.

The traffic safety literature is replete with statistical analyses of the effect of speed and speed changes on accidents and injuries. A widely cited study indicates that:

- Accident severity increases as speed increases, especially at speeds exceeding 60 mph.
- The fatality rate is highest at very high speeds and lowest at about the average speed.
- The greater the variation in speed of any vehicle from the average speed of all traffic, the greater its chance of being involved in an accident.

### Injury Control

Millions of traffic crashes occur each year which do not result in death or serious injury. The safety features that permit motorists to ride out a crash without serious injury consist of: (1) safeguarding occupants in the vehicle, known as "occupant packaging"; (2) improving vehicle design so that the passenger compartment will not be dangerously penetrated or crushed; and (3) removing roadside obstacles or replacing them with "cushioning" devices.

### Occupant Restraints

Safety belts are now available to almost all passenger car occupants. According to National Highway Traffic Safety Administration studies, safety belts are 50 to 65 percent effective in preventing fatalities and injuries. This means that about fifteen thousand lives could be saved annually if all passenger car occupants used safety belts at all times.

Fastened safety belts, during a crash, distribute the forces of a rapidly decelerating body over a larger area of the body while stretching to absorb some of the forces. In addition, belts hold you in place while the car crashes and slows down. When the car stops moving, the person is still moving but at a greatly reduced speed. The remaining forces of deceleration are then absorbed safely by the body and the belts. In short, the person slows down with the car rather than continuing to travel at the same speed the car was traveling on impact. And because the person is being held in place by the belts, he or she will not be involved in a serious second collision, a person-to-person collision, or ejection from the automobile.

*Accidents Involving Fire or Submersion.*    You may have heard that if you are involved in an accident resulting in fire or submersion in water, you may be trapped inside the car if wearing safety belts. In reality, the fears behind this myth have little basis in fact. The chances of being involved in an accident of this type are extremely low since less than one-half of one percent of all accidents result in fire or submersion of the vehicle. Even if fire or submersion does occur, it usually occurs after the initial crash. If you were protected from serious injury by safety belts during this initial crash, the chances of remaining conscious and capable of escaping from the car quickly would be very good.

*Protection for Short Trips.*    Some people believe that it is important to fasten safety belts only for long trips at high speeds on freeways or turnpikes. This is another myth. Short trips of less than twenty-five miles to the local shopping center,

BOX 9-7  *UNUSUAL BUT TRUE*

Charles Barbor and Robert Bolden were trying to find their way along the foggy country roads around Charlottesville, Virginia. One more left turn, they reckoned, would put them on the right track. So, they turned on a bumpy but straight road.

Then they saw a headlight—only one. Unfortunately, the road belonged to the Southern Railway. The left turn had put them on the track, all right, but not the right one. Both men suffered minor injuries.

– National Safety Council, *Family Safety*

BOX 9–8  *UNUSUAL BUT TRUE*

> In Brescia, Italy, two motorists driving in a dense fog crashed head-on—literally—with a crack of skulls.
>
> Trying to peer through the fog, both men were driving with their heads sticking out of the car windows. They met head-on as they passed each other. Neither was seriously hurt.
>
> — National Safety Council, *Family Safety*

around town, or to work comprise about 95 percent of all trips made. The facts are that three out of four accidents occur within twenty-five miles of home, 80 percent of all accidents occur at speeds of less than 40 mph, and the accident rate is much greater on city streets than on highways.

Fatalities have been recorded at speeds as low as 12 mph. Since the more driving exposure you have the more likely you are to be involved in an accident, it is just as important to fasten safety belts for short trips as it is for long trips.

*During Pregnancy.*  Studies have shown that pregnant women are much safer if protected by safety belts in an accident. The American Medical Association's Committee on Medical Aspects of Automotive Safety has stated that both the pregnant woman and the fetus are safer, provided the belt is worn as low on the pelvis as possible. The use of a shoulder strap in addition provides an extra safety factor.

*Safety Belt Laws.*  Recognizing the lifesaving potential of safety belts, about thirty countries or provinces have established mandatory safety belt use laws. The American Seat Belt Council has reviewed the experience of each country and found that where safety belt usage was required and properly enforced, it has increased dramatically and remained high and crash injuries have declined (although not as steeply as expected).

*Child Restraint Use.*  Although adult safety belt laws are in effect in only a few states, all states do have child passenger restraint laws. Child restraint usage is estimated to be 80 to 90 percent effective in preventing fatalities and injuries. Over twenty brands of child safety seats that pass federal standards are now on the market.

*Why Are Safety Belts Used?*  Studies have shown that between 7 and 30 percent of drivers actually use safety belts. There is no adequate explanation as to why some people use safety belts and others do not. Some research indicates that non-users view safety belts as being inconvenient, uncomfortable, and ineffective in reducing the risk of injury or death. These studies fail to report information about basic motivations, or the origin of attitudes and beliefs in the wearing of safety belts.

Other studies associate usage with having taken a driver education course or

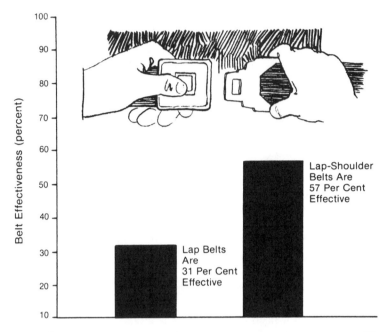

**FIGURE 9-5**  If you are involved in a crash and wearing a lap-shoulder belt, you are 57 percent less likely to be injured or killed than if you are not wearing a safety belt.

with having had a relative or friend injured in an automobile accident while not wearing a safety belt.

Still another study reported that family members tend to have similar patterns of safety belt use. In other words, the use or nonuse of safety belts runs in families. Children are more likely to use them if one parent and especially if both parents use safety belts.

This study also found that those using safety belts tended to use other preventive health behaviors (e.g., dental checkups, abstaining from smoking, exercising, and limiting caloric food intake). People who use safety belts thus tend to have good health habits in general.

Those who feel that they can have some degree of control over their lives wear safety belts as a way to increase their chances of survival; whereas those who view their life as dictated by fate, luck, or other factors beyond their control tend not to use safety belts.

### Vehicle Design

The second lifesaving aspect of crash survivability lies in designing the vehicle to absorb and deflect collision forces so that the passenger compartment remains a safe haven for occupants. Examples include: front-end, energy-absorbing devices; structural reinforcement; padding; effective head-rests; hood-penetrating windshield deflection.

### Roadside Hazards

The third element of crash survivability is devoted to the removal of road-side hazards. It has been said that if there is a dangerous obstacle near the roadway, sooner or later it will be struck. The streets and highways are dotted with them—bridge abutments, guardrails designed for strength rather than safety (see Figure 9-6), and sign and light poles embedded in concrete. Efforts have been made, primarily on high-speed roadways, to remove dangerous objects to provide clear recovery space, install breakaway signs and light supports, flatten slopes, and improve guardrails and median barriers. These improvements have contributed substantially to reductions in traffic accidents, injuries, and fatalities. It has been found that with the breakaway supports and crash cushions, occupants survive collisions with little or no injury and frequently only minor damage to the vehicle.

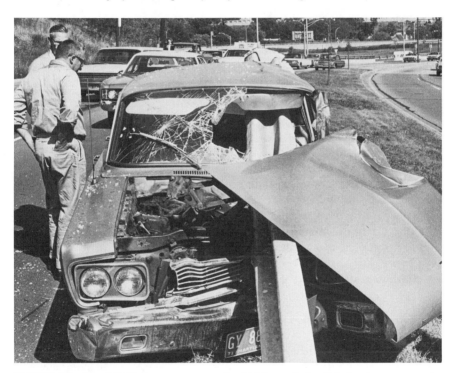

**FIGURE 9-6** Guard Rail? A common example of highway "safety" design that creates rather than reduces danger. This blunt-end guardrail speared a car through the passenger compartment. Photo courtesy of the Insurance Institute of Highway Safety.

## MOTORCYCLE ACCIDENTS

The rapid increase in the number of motorcycles registered in the United States over the last decade, coupled with a high fatality rate for motorcyclists compared with drivers of other vehicles, has generated considerable concern among those in highway safety. Much of the hazard associated with motorcycles can be attributed to the nature of the vehicle itself; compared with automobiles, motorcycles are less stable, are less visible to other road users, and offer less protection to the driver in the event of a crash.

Motorcycles are a real part of the traffic. They are here to stay and with the light-weight motorcycles, their mobility, economy of use, and ease of operation, they are becoming even more popular.

The automobile driver is the motorcyclist's worst enemy. In these collisions, the motorcyclist is not always to blame. Many people have observed that drivers of larger vehicles do not always realize that motorcycles, and especially motor scooters and motor bicycles, are also motor vehicles and should be treated as such. In many cases, automobile drivers claim they simply did not see a motorcyclist in time to avoid an accident. Excessive speed for given conditions is a main contributor to motorcycle accidents.

In terms of miles driven, the motorcycle is the most dangerous type of motor vehicle. In fact, no major cause of death has experienced an increase as great as death due to a motorcycle crash.

### Human Factors

Considering that motorcyclists are afforded little or no protection at the time of the impact, it is amazing that they survive as well as they do. Certainly the youth-fulness of the motorcycle accident driver must contribute to his survival. All studies show that most victims are young—under twenty-five years of age.

Female drivers have one-half the risk of serious injury of male drivers, and male cyclists are involved in more accidents than females. Females appear to be susceptible to injury as passengers.

The majority of motorcycle crashes involve inexperience, failure of another driver to perceive the two-wheeled vehicle, or use of alcohol.

### Environmental Factors

Most of the research studies on motorcycle accidents have been done on populations and accidents in the "cycle" states; that is, those states where motorcycles are dominant because of favorable weather conditions conducive to year-round riding (e.g., California, Arizona, Florida). In "cold" states the motorcycle is mostly used during warmer months, with fatal crashes occurring most often in the summer. The most dangerous hours of the day have been identified as those between 4:00 PM and 6:00 PM. The most dangerous day is Saturday. It has been reported that the rate of serious injury is lowest in January, and highest in June, July, and August. Statistical differences among states are determined primarily by two factors: (1) amount of motorcycle travel, and (2) helmet use.

Most victims are within five miles of their residence when involved in an accident, and this is explained by the fact that most riding occurs within five miles of their residence. Most of the accidents occur on dry roads. This is to be expected since motorcycles are not driven much on wet or icy roads.

### Motorcycle Crash Prevention

Some people feel that nothing can be done to make motorcycles safe, and it has even been suggested that they be abolished or severely restricted. At the other extreme, motorcyclists commonly feel that their constitutional freedoms are being infringed upon, especially regarding helmet use.

There exists among traffic safety specialists a controversy as to whether motorcycle safety education programs belong in the high school driver education curriculum.

The Motorcycle Safety Foundation was established to promote, foster, and encourage motorcycle safety and education. This agency has developed educational materials.

Among other pre-crash countermeasures are:

1. Special motorcycle license recognizing those with skills and knowledge necessary for safe motorcycling.
2. Bright-colored fluorescent vest mandatorily worn to aid motorists in spotting the cyclist.
3. Establish a minimum age of drivers.
4. Control the speed of cycles.

### Injury Control.

Studies suggest that the risk of fatal injury to a motorcyclist in a collision is significantly reduced by the wearing of a helmet. The risk of serious head injury is 30 percent less for those who wear helmets.

The well-designed helmet provides two protective features: it distributes concentrated forces over larger areas of the head, and it reduces force levels transmitted to the head. Individuals and organizations committed to the reduction of motorcycle injury losses must work more actively toward the acceptance and use of this effective and inexpensive method of injury protection for the operator and passenger.

Motorcycle helmets are a form of "crash packaging"; they are manufactured to reduce the injurious forces that commonly reach a cyclist's head in a collision. The trend toward repeal of motorcycle helmet use laws by the states has brought with it huge increases in deaths associated with motorcycle crashes. Besides a helmet, leather clothing, gloves, long trousers, and boots all offer protection and are strongly suggested for motorcyclists.

The injury burden of crashes is falling on young males. The economic burden,

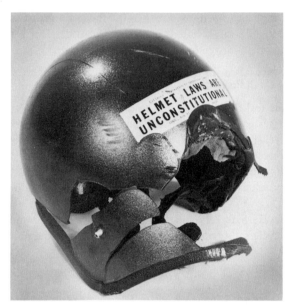

**FIGURE 9-7**   When motorcycle helmet laws are repealed, a huge increase in deaths associated with motorcycles occurs. Photo courtesy of the National Safety Council, *Family Safety*.

however, is falling not on the dead and injured but mainly on taxpayers and insurance policyholders who are supporting the extensive emergency, hospital, and rehabilitation resources required to care for the brain-damaged, paraplegic, and quadriplegic cyclists.

## PEDESTRIAN ACCIDENTS

People inside automobiles are relatively protected in a collision. But almost every pedestrian who is struck is hurt. The pedestrian is vulnerable and without protection. He does not stand a chance against a vehicle weighing about two tons.

Alcohol is heavily involved in adult pedestrian fatalities. One study showed that more than 50 percent of the fatally injured pedestrians tested had blood alcohol concentrations over 0.10 percent.

Crossing between intersections causes most pedestrian deaths in residential areas. The young and middle-aged pedestrians are most often negligent, while the elderly are the most law-abiding age group, yet the elderly are involved in the highest percentage of fatal accidents. It has also been noted that drivers of motor vehicles with less than fifteen years of driving experience are most often involved in pedestrian accidents.

### Effects

Pedestrians account for a sizable portion of highway fatalities and injuries. National Safety Council figures indicate that in recent years over ten thousand pedestrians have been killed annually and 120 thousand have received disabling injuries. Pedestrian fatalities have increased over the past decade. It has been estimated that 4 percent of all automobiles will strike a pedestrian at some time, and of all those struck, about 6 percent will die.

Because the motor vehicle is the main agent of injury, attention has been directed to its modification to reduce the seriousness of pedestrian accidents. The consequences of a pedestrian accident are dependent upon such factors as vehicle design, vehicle speed, pedestrian height and age, and pedestrian posture at impact.

The injuries to the body are primarily in the form of broken lower limbs and pelvis. Damage to the abdomen and thorax is common, and concussions are frequent. Pedestrians are not often "run over" by cars, but rather "run under" or "lifted up and over." A "second crash" effect takes place when the victim rebounds off the vehicle and impacts with the roadway (pavement) or side of the road.

### Human Factors

Pedestrians involved in accidents can be categorized into three age groups: the young, who are involved in about half of the pedestrian accidents, with those between four and eight years old being the most vulnerable; the elderly (sixty-five years or older), who are involved in under one-fourth of the cases; and the fifteen to sixty-four year group accounting for the remainder of accidents, with those between twenty-one and fifty years old involved in only 20 percent of the accidents. The involvement of males in pedestrian accidents is higher at every age than that of females.

Nine-tenths of the pedestrians fatally injured in a recent year were nondrivers. Their not being familiar with the automobile could explain the large number of accidents involving persons in the young and the elderly age groups. A child's vulnerability to being involved in a pedestrian accident seems to be more acute when the problems of family illness, mother's preoccupation, overcrowding, and absence of playground facilities are present. Knowledge of the area does not seem to be an influencing factor in pedestrian accidents. More residents of areas are injured than nonresidents; however, their exposure rate is higher in the area of their residence. For young children under five years of age, most accidents occur within one hundred yards of home; those aged eleven to fifteen years are involved in accidents within one-quarter of a mile from home.

### Environmental Factors

Pedestrian fatalities and injuries are primarily an urban problem. While about 70 percent of motor vehicle fatalities occur in rural areas, the majority of pedestrian deaths (roughly two-thirds) occur in urban areas. Severe injury or death is more likely in rural areas because of the higher impact speed in these areas. Likelihood of fatality is greater on roadways of four or more lanes.

Far more pedestrians are injured during the months with more hours of darkness (November through February). Fatalities occur most often on Saturdays. The peak hour for pedestrian fatalities occurs about an hour after sunset.

### Pedestrian Accident Prevention

Researchers have concluded that pedestrian injuries will not be effectively reduced by traditional safety campaigns that concentrate on changing pedestrian behavior because such programs fail to recognize that the pedestrians most likely to be killed or injured are those whose behavior is hardest to influence. They warn that the prominence of driver negligence indicates that even the prudent pedestrian risks being struck as long as he shares his route with motor vehicles.

Banning parking of cars near intersections and crosswalks allows a broader visual field for both drivers and pedestrians. Reflectorized clothing and crosswalk illumination increases visibility for pedestrians. Having all vehicles fitted with audible warning devices to alert pedestrians when the vehicle is backing up is also suggested as a preventive measure.

## BICYCLE ACCIDENTS

There has been a resurgence of interest in bicycling. Multispeed gearing, improved lightweight construction, stress on physical fitness, and saving gasoline have made the bicycle more appealing to adults.

Unfortunately, the dramatic increase in the number of cyclists has brought an equally dramatic increase in the number of bicycle injuries and fatalities. The Consumer Product Safety Commission estimates that more than 371 thousand persons received bicycle-related injuries serious enough to require hospital emergency room treatment (note that most of these do not involve an automobile), and as many as one million injuries required professional medical treatment.

Loss of control is a major problem in bicycle accidents. This may result from some human action such as riding double, stunting, or making an unsafe maneuver. Other important causal factors are mechanical and structural problems and entanglement of body parts in the bicycle.

Bikers are notoriously unresponsive to traffic control measures. This may be explained by the fact that the largest segment of the riding public is composed of children who have not been taught the rules of the road and the hazards inherent in traffic violations. It should be noted, however, that the fifteen to twenty-four year old group is heavily involved in accidents and that this group usually knows the rules of the road and the inherent hazards.

About 90 percent of all bicyclist deaths involve collisions with motor vehicles. Nonfatal injuries, however, generally result from falls, which are rarely reported.

### Human Factors

A thousand bicyclists—most of them teenagers and children—are killed every year in this country. Despite the recent increases in adult bicycle riding, the accident problem predominantly involves children. However, accidents with motor vehicles are prevalent among young adults. It is reported that male riders are nearly four times as likely to be involved in bicycle accidents as females. This probably reflects differences in exposure. One concern is the large number of children who ride their bikes at night, despite the rarity of lights; it is interesting to note, however, that this has resulted in few injuries. Another problem noted is that some children have bikes too large for them to handle properly.

### Environmental Factors

Injuries and death occur more frequently in urban than in rural areas. As most of the riding is during daylight hours, most of the injuries occur during daylight hours and during clear weather.

The peak time for bicycle accidents begins during "after school" hours (3:00 PM to 8:00 PM).

Two-thirds occur during the five-month period from May through September.

### Bicycle Accident Prevention

Since many bicycling injuries among children appear to be related to immature skills and judgment, two potential countermeasures would be to delay the learning process until age six, seven, or even later, when these abilities are more developed, and to provide specific formal training.

Many believe that major emphasis should be placed on biker education programs. Such programs are designed to teach cyclists of all ages the rules of safe riding and to induce them to observe these rules. Cyclists are shown that they are required to observe the same rules as those that prevail for motorists. It is therefore important to familiarize every cyclist with local traffic regulations.

The basic safety rules:

1. Do not carry passengers.
2. Observe traffic regulations and stop signs.
3. Use hand signals to indicate turning and stopping.
4. Ride single file.
5. Do not ride from between parked cars.
6. Keep to the right side of the road.
7. Keep both hands on the handlebars.
8. Do not speed in busy intersections.
9. Avoid crowds.
10. Give right of way to pedestrians and automobiles.
11. Do not ride when tired or ill.

12.   Avoid stunt riding, racing, and zig-zagging in traffic.
13.   Do not "hitch" rides.
14.   Use caution at all intersections and driveways.
15.   Make bicycle repairs off the road.
16.   Dismount and walk across heavy traffic.

High priority must be given to use reflective materials on wheels and pedals. Handbrakes appear to be more effective than pedal-operated brakes, except for children who usually lack the strength to depress a handbrake.

Unfortunately, educational programs alone are not enough to reduce substantially the frequency of bicycle accidents. Many areas have designed special provisions for bicycles to try to reduce the number of potential conflicts between different kinds of vehicles. For example, construction of bike paths on separate rights of way, and the channeling of bicycle, pedestrian, and automobile traffic on shared facilities.

Grade separations at intersections have been provided in some cities. Channelization will decrease the risk involved in bike riding. This is done through special bicycle lane lines and offset median crossings.

### Injury Control

Measures suggested to reduce the death and injury rate might include the use of helmets, especially helmets designed primarily to withstand blunt impacts. Over 90 percent of fatalities are from contact with motor vehicles; therefore another considertion is to have motor vehicle modifications to make front-end impacts with bicyclists less violent. Another aspect is the problem of extended rear-view mirrors on the right sides of small trucks which serve a lethal injury to some bicyclists. These mirrors might be replaced or improved to make them less dangerous.

## COLLISIONS WITH ANIMALS

Many believe more deer are killed by collisions with vehicles than by deer hunters. This belief is founded upon the number of dead deer alongside the highway being more visible than those at a deer camp during hunting season.

However, not seen nor reported are those deer deaths when no human is injured and vehicle damage is minor. Reports by drivers account for fewer than half the carcasses found along the road. Also, many deer are hit by a car, then hobble away to die unnoticed some distance from the highway.

Deer are especially unpredictable, but if a driver is alert for the potential hazard of a deer dashing into his path without warning, and adjusts his or her speed accordingly, collisions can be avoided. Heeding deer crossing signs by reducing speed is highly encouraged.

Nationally, it is estimated that well over a hundred thousand deer are killed annually by motor vehicles.

Deer are attracted to roadways for feeding, an activity undertaken chiefly during the hours of darkness in the spring of the year. The road shoulder offers highly palatable grasses partially because of the extra runoff water from the pavement.

If one deer is seen, it often means more deer are present. It is believed that the shadow behind the deer created by the headlights startles the deer when it moves, so that it bolts out into the path of the vehicle. Some experts recommend steering toward the deer. Deer will change direction and bounce back across the road when confused. They usually retreat in the direction from which they came. At night the reflective eyes of deer and any other animal are a cue to the driver to be alert.

The main concern are collisions resulting in human death and injury. People are killed by deer going through the windshield or while swerving to miss a deer only to collide with another vehicle or an off-road object. When a deer appears in front of you, the best driving technique is to steer straight ahead—the deer may move. Plus, blinking your car's headlights on and off dim may help prompt the deer to move.

Other animals hit by motor vehicles include horses, cattle, sheep, pigs, and a host of others. These are capable of doing a great deal of damage to an automobile and its occupants. Smaller animals and birds do little damage but may cause the driver to swerve causing a collision.

## NOTES

1. This section is based upon Insurance Institute for Highway Safety, *Policy Options for Reducing the Motor Vehicle Crash Injury Cost Burden* (Washington, D.C.: Insurance Institute for Highway Safety, 1981).
2. H. Laurence Ross, *Deterring the Drinking Driver*, pp. 102–4.

# 10

# Falls

It is not the falling but the landing that hurts. To most people, falls seems to be in-significant occurrences because they do not realize that falls represent the most serious threat to life around the home and are exceeded as a cause of accidental death only by motor vehicle accidents. Surveys indicate that about twelve thousand people in the United States die annually from injuries sustained in accidental falls. Each year one person in twenty receives emergency room treatment because of a fall.

## HUMAN FACTORS

### Age

The death rate from falls increases markedly with age. Over half of all deaths from falls are of persons seventy-five and older who comprise only 4 percent of the population. By age the incidence of injuries resulting from falls contrasts sharply with their deadliness: more than two-fifths of those injured in nonfatal falls are under fifteen years of age and only one-tenth are sixty five and older. In other words, injuries from falls are a problem of youth while death from falls is a problem of the elderly. It is clear that while children are more predisposed to falls than the

BOX 10-1 *UNUSUAL BUT TRUE*

> Keith Batchelder, who is fifteen months old, crawled out of his crib and out a window of his family's fifth-floor apartment in Bensenville, Ill.
> Keith fell about forty-five feet and landed in a flower bed. He suffered only a slight bruise on his left leg.
>
> — National Safety Council, *Family Safety*

elderly, the fall of an elderly person is far more serious than that of a younger person.

The large number of injuries resulting from falls among children is attributable to their mobility and adventurous activities. Children under five have a much higher death rate than do older children. This may be the result of a predisposition to severe injury-producing incidents and a greater inability to withstand trauma. Falls can be particularly serious when a child is less than one year of age. At this time the brain is growing rapidly and the skull has a thinner wall than at any other time of life. Most injuries are sustained in the head region, perhaps because there is a greater weight in the upper half of the infant's body. The young child is exposed to hazards with which he has had no prior experience. For example, during the crawling stage the child frequently climbs upon and then falls from furniture. Then, while learning to walk, he often trips.

### Sex

Death rates due to falls are much higher among males than among females in all age groups. The "shuffling tendency" in old men often results in tripping falls and has been attributed to muscle weakness and the inability to lift the feet. Injuries are greater among females, but this sex difference may be reflecting differences in exposure and activity.

### Physical Conditions

*Elderly.* As people begin to age, chronic problems set in. Chronic problems that may affect the elderly can be broken down into three areas:

1. Muscular-skeletal. These can be arthritis-related changes, which result in decreased strength both in hand-grip strength and also more generalized in lower back, legs, and arms. It is estimated that 80 percent of the population by age sixty-five has some degree of arthritis. Spinal changes occur from a variety of causes (e.g., osteoporosis-decalcification of bones), as well as a slowing down of the protective reflexes that protect the trunk and head from damage.
2. Cardio-vascular. There are two common conditions that can result in a reduction in the cerebral flow of blood: orthostatic hypotension, which results in a decrease in blood pressure—an individual who changes position too fast (e.g., standing up rapidly) may stumble, lose orientation to space, or in extreme

cases faint; hypertension, which results in an increase in blood pressure—an individual may have a series of small strokes, some of which may result in the person falling.

Falls occur due to a cutoff of blood to the brain when a person has his or her head back and looking upward.

3. Sensory changes. These changes may include: decrease in visual acuity; decrease in hearing; calcification of bones in the middle ear (resulting in vertigo).

Falls are a severe problem for the elderly population, since falls often result in the fracture of a bone. Often this fracture may involve the head of the femur (hip), which heals slowly. Osteoporosis, a bone disease which affects women more than men, is a condition in which the bones become increasingly porous and brittle.

Falls that cause only slight injury to younger persons may result in serious injury or even death for the elderly. In part this is because of the loss of bone density that occurs with aging. Compared with a 30-year-old, a 70-year-old woman has lost 25 to 30 percent of her bone density; a 70-year-old man loses 15 to 20 percent.

*Children.* Toddlers and slightly older children have poorly developed locomotive skills, a lot of curiosity, and limited strength and coordination. They often climb into dangerous positions, lose their balance, and fall.

*Alcohol.* There has been a misrepresentation that "drunks never get hurt when they fall because they are so relaxed." This does not mean that people can avoid injury if they are relaxed. In fact "drunks" will fall more often due to their drunkenness.

## ENVIRONMENTAL FACTORS

### Region

Death rates due to falls are higher in the northern states than southern states. This is true in summer as well as winter, thus eliminating the longer and icier northern winters as an explanation. Falls occur more frequently in urban than rural areas, with farm dwellers having the lowest rates. It has been suggested that poor housing conditions in the city account for the higher metropolitan rates. Examples of conditions include rickety stair construction, no stairway treads, dim lighting, and clutter.

### Location

The National Health Survey reports that about 60 percent of fall injuries occur at home with 60 percent of these inside the house. This high proportion of falls in the home reflects the great amount of time spent there by young children and by the elderly.

About one-fourth of the fatalities occur in falls on the same level (e.g., the floor, ground, sidewalks, or street). Falls on stairs, from ladders, and from one level to another are the other leading locations. Most studies show a predominance of falls taking place in the afternoon hours—this parallels the hours of greatest activity in the home, where falls are most prevalent.

*Falls in the Home.*   Areas within the home where falls are prone to happen:

1. Bathrooms. Many accidents occur when someone slips in a wet tub or shower. Accidents also occur when a bathroom floor is wet and the individual is barefoot. Accidents occur on dry floors when a throw rug slips out from under an individual's feet, because it may not contain or may have a worn slip-resistant backing.
2. Kitchens. Floor-related accidents may occur when the floor is wet from water or floor polish. They also may occur when the floor is dry and covered with foreign matter.
3. Laundry Rooms. Falls in this room are generally related to slipping on a wet surface.
4. Furniture. There are an astounding number of falls related to furniture which result from slips and trips where the victim impacts against a table or bed (especially bunk beds) or other piece of furniture.
5. Floors. Many falls appear related to changing surfaces, such as going from a carpeted surface to a resilient surface, or from a dry to a wet surface.
    The victims are usually walking on wet floors, and occasionally the wetness involves a cleaning or polishing agent. The most common areas of accidents are those with sources of water. On dry floors, the floors are usually polished; victims either are running, moving quickly, changing direction, or stepping from one floor surface to another.
6. Stairs. These falls occur on both interior and exterior stairs and are often related to lapses in the victim's attention, distractions, carrying objects, and unstable or cluttered stair surfaces.
7. Other. Cats tangle themselves around people's legs, especially in the dark. As a result, tripping over the family cat can produce injuries. Clothing such as flared or "bell bottom" trousers, clog and platform shoes have also caused falls.

## EFFECTS

Deaths from falls often evolve from injuries to the head. With a head injury, the crucial question is the state of the brain rather than the state of the skull. Skull fractures are in themselves of little importance, unless they press on the brain or unless they are accompanied by leakage of cerebrospinal fluid. Cerebrospinal fluid serves as a shock absorber for the brain and spinal cord.

The two primary types of brain injury are: (1) bruising when the head forcibly strikes a blunt object (e.g., ground, floor). This contusion causes swelling, which in turn causes pressure on the brain. The pressure disrupts the brain's normal functions. (2) Laceration of the brain tissue from fragments being depressed inward into the skull and brain.

Fractures (a break in a bone) also result from falling. Extensive bleeding can accompany a major fracture, especially those of the pelvis and femur. This blood loss may be slow. The following list demonstrates the amount of blood that can be lost within six hours after a fracture:

1. Pelvis—2 to 4 pints
2. Femur—1 to 2 pints
3. Tibia-Fibula—½ to 1¼ pint
4. Radius-Ulna—½ to 1 pint
5. Humerus—⅓ to ¾ pint
6. Ribs—¼ pint

A startling concept is that 50 percent of all persons impacting against a hard surface with a velocity of 18 mph will be killed. This is equivalent to a fall of eleven feet.

Ordinarily anyone who falls from higher than the sixth floor of a building will be killed, but not always. Several factors may influence the outcome of a free fall: (1) the vertical distance fallen; (2) the position of the body on landing; (3) the kind of landing material; (4) the duration of impact; and (5) the general condition of the fall victim.

Of all those, the position of the body on landing may be the most important factor that determines survival in addition to the distance of the fall.

The most common position on impact after a free fall is feet first. Severe in-injuries occur to feet, ankles and legs. In a seated position injuries to the pelvis and spine are common. When the head strikes first there is a high association with neck,

BOX 10-2 *UNUSUAL BUT TRUE*

> While working in her garden in Hyde, England, Mrs. Hilda Taylor broke a bone in her foot. Hobbling around the house two days later she fell and broke the other foot. Then while her husband, Eric, was making her breakfast, he fell over the family dog and broke a bone in his foot. The next night he fell again. You guessed it! He matched his wife by breaking the other foot.
>
> — National Safety Council, *Family Safety*

BOX 10-3 *UNUSUAL BUT TRUE*

> While on vacation, Bill Taylor of Scarborough, England, took his family to a path by the North Sea where he had fallen and broken his leg three years before.
>
> His wife and three daughters were amused as he turned actor to demonstrate just how it happened. It was a realistic performance—too realistic. Taylor fell in the same way in the same place. This time he broke his other leg in two places.
>
> — National Safety Council, *Family Safety*

shoulder, and chest injuries, in addition to those of the head; this form of landing has the highest fatality rate.

But landing in a flat, spread out position reduces the force of impact on all body parts. This sparing factor may be sufficient to permit survival.


## FALL PREVENTION

There is no single universal safety device on which to base a fall prevention campaign. As in all accidents, many factors can cause a fall.

Here are preventive measures that can reduce the risk of injury:

*Floors.* All foors should be kept as dry as possible, since water and other liquids can greatly increase the risk of slipping. It is important to check the backing surfaces of throw or area rugs to make sure that they are rubberized and not worn from frequent laundering.

*Tubs and Showers.* Securely mounted grab-bars would be a real safety addition to any home and should be installed in public places (e.g., motels). Tub and shower surfaces, if not slip-resistant, should be fitted with slip-resistant applications. Safety mats are available, but pose problems in cleaning and wearing out.

*Stairs.* Any carpeting applied to stairs should be tight fitting. In selecting carpet, avoid those that have a pattern that may cause perceptual confusion. It can be very helpful to have the ends of stairs marked in such a manner as to distinguish one step from another. On exterior steps that are exposed to the elements of weather, it is useful to use slip-resistant treads. These treads should not protrude in such a way as to pose a tripping hazard.

Individual steps should have a consistent height and length and should not have too steep an angle. Risers should not be greater than eight inches and treads not less than ten inches. Beware of protruding nosings (front edge) on steps which can trip people.

If possible, handrails should be continuous and on both sides of a staircase. It is useful if the rail is slightly textured for those who have weak grip strength in their hands. Public buildings with wide staircases should always have a stair rail available. It may be necessary to provide a continuous rail in the middle of the staircase that is anchored to the steps. It is advisable to consider a lower second rail with a smaller dimension for small children.

Lighting should be adequate with switches at the top and the bottom of stairs, and reflections should be minimal. Stairs should be kept clean of obstructions (e.g., toys, pets) and dirt.

*Furniture.* In both public and home environments one needs to be aware of hazards associated with furniture (sharp edges, projecting legs, etc.). Bunk beds with side rails, furniture with a more stable base for children, and chairs that are easy for the elderly to get out of are suggested.

## INJURY CONTROL

A positive relationship exists between physical fitness and resistance to fall injuries. Recommended practices during an actual fall include: relaxing muscles since injury is more likely with contracted muscles; rolling onto a softer part of the body (e.g., the thighs); and landing on the balls of the feet and letting the bent knees absorb the blow before rolling (this is the secret that allows a parachutist to come down onto hard ground without damage to himself).

BOX 10-4   *UNUSUAL BUT TRUE*

> Pvt. Terry Bennett, of the Army's elite Golden Knights parachute team, fell some 8,000 feet when her chute failed near Ft. Bragg, N.C.
> She landed in a muddy field and miraculously suffered only a dislocated elbow and two broken bones in her wrist.
>
> — National Safety Council, *Family Safety*

BOX 10-5

> The greatest altitude from which anyone has bailed out without a parachute and survived is 21,980 feet. This occurred in January 1942 when Lt (now Lt-Col) I. M. Chisov (USSR) fell from an Ilyushin 4 which had been severely damaged. He struck the ground a glancing blow on the edge of a snow-covered ravine and slid to the bottom. He suffered a fractured pelvis and severe spinal damage.
>
> Vesna Vulovic, a 23-year-old airline hostess, survived when her DC-9 blew up at 33,330 feet over the Czechoslovak village of Ceska Kamenice on January 26, 1972. She was hospitalized for 16 months after emerging from a 27-day coma, having broken many bones.
>
> — *Guinness Book of World Records*

Studies have suggested that in some cases fluoride and calcium or estrogen therapy may strengthen bone and therefore reduce the severity of injuries in falls. However, such regimens carry risks of side effects that must be considered. Exercise for the elderly can increase muscle strength and balance.

In case a person does take a severe fall—or fears one—a backup system can take away worry. Some communities have alarm systems so that people can call a central number to check in daily. If there is no call, someone investigates. Another type of alarm summons help if the toilet does not flush for eight hours. Many people simply keep in daily touch with neighbors or friends.

# 11

# Drownings

Approximately seven thousand Americans die each year from drowning, making it the third leading cause of accidental death. Drowning statistics do not reflect the whole problem. An estimated seventy thousand people are near-drowning victims each year. Even this figure does not give the whole picture, because in many instances the victim recovers and the incident is not reported.

The term "drowning" usually refers to those victims who die by submersion in the water or other liquid.

## HUMAN FACTORS

Several factors bear heavily on the incidence of drowning as they relate to human factors:

*Alcohol.* Reports of drownings range from 10 to 47 percent where victims were under the influence of alcohol. Because intoxication by alcohol does affect one's judgment, it makes boating, water skiing, swimming, and other aquatic activities more dangerous. Incidences of intoxicated individuals going swimming at night in deep water, or jumping off a bridge indicate that alcohol is a significant factor in some drowning cases. Little attention has been given to this factor in most public education programs aimed at reducing the toll of drowning.

*Age.* The "teenager" is the age group that is chiefly involved in drownings. More than 60 percent of the victims are under twenty-five years of age. This may reflect a greater degree of exposure to the danger and for longer periods of time than in other age groups. A sizable percentage of the victims are children under the age of four.

*Sex.* Eighty-five percent of the victims are male. This may reflect the greater exposure of males to aquatic sports and recreational activities, as well as the fact that they are usually more venturesome and risk-taking than females.

*Ability.* About two-thirds of the drowning victims do not know how to swim. Good swimmers do drown and this might be partially explained by the victims' overconfidence or poor judgment.

*Hyperventilation.* This is a technique used by swimmers trying to prolong their stay under water. They think that by hyperventilating, they get more oxygen into their blood; but this is not the case. Carbon dioxide in the blood provides the major stimulus to breathing, and while those three or four deep breaths do not significantly increase the amount of oxygen normally present, they do reduce the carbon dioxide, which may block the built-in warning signals that tell a swimmer to surface for air. The result can be a blackout or drowning.

Hundreds, and possibly thousands, of good swimmers have drowned because they have not understood the effects of deep breathing before underwater swimming for distance. Drowning prevention rests in counseling swimmers not to hyperventilate before an underwater swim.

BOX 11-1

> The world record for voluntarily staying underwater is 13 minutes 42.5 seconds by Robert Foster of Richmond, California, who stayed under 10 feet of water in San Rafael, California, in 1959. He hyperventilated with oxygen for 30 minutes before his descent. The longest breath-hold without oxygen was 6 minutes 29.8 seconds by Georges Pouliquin in Paris in 1912. It must be stressed that record-breaking of this kind is extremely dangerous.
>
> — *Guinness Book of World Records*

*Hypothermia.* Quite often, drowning will result directly from hypothermia. It should not be assumed that hypothermia is found only in frigid climates for it can occur even in relatively warm waters. The thermal conductivity of cold water is twenty times greater than that of air, and heat loss can be substantial in victims submerged in water.

*Exhaustion.* This is among the most frequently reported factors involving those drowned. Exhaustion most often occurs in swimmers, skin- and scuba divers, as well as among those attempting to rescue another person.

*Food in stomach.* Water safety experts have long advised a swimmer to wait at least one hour after eating before swimming. Most people assume the reason for this traditional advice is to avoid "stomach cramps" that may disable a swimmer and cause drowning. Scientific evidence is contradictory. On one hand, reports from those who have experienced cramps while in the water and studies of eating prior to swimming in competition indicate that there are no adverse effects. However, other evidence indicates that if a person has eaten a lot, is in poor health, or has a cardiovascular problem, eating just prior to swimming presents a potential problem. After food is eaten the stomach muscles need an adequate supply of oxygen-carrying blood. If strenuous exercise is begun shortly after eating, the heart may not be able to supply both stomach and skeletal muscles.

*Activity of victim.* As can be seen in Table 11-1, many drowning victims never intended to get wet, much less become submerged. Water attracts people of all ages and all degrees of familiarity with its dangers.

**TABLE 11-1 Drownings by Activity**

| ACTIVITY | PERCENTAGE |
| --- | --- |
| Swimming | 24.9 |
| Playing in or near water | 18.4 |
| Wading | 11.5 |
| Standing, walking near water | 11.0 |
| Motor vehicle occupant | 7.2 |
| Boating | 7.0 |
| Fishing from boat | 6.9 |
| Attempting rescue | 2.9 |
| Taking bath | 2.0 |
| Skin and scuba diving | 1.8 |
| Other | 6.4 |

Source: National Safety Council, *Accident Facts.*

## ENVIRONMENTAL FACTORS

In the United States the death rate from drownings has remained fairly constant during the past several decades. The hazard of drowning varies greatly in different parts of the country, depending on factors such as proximity and utilization of bodies of water and on the climate. Japan, where much of the population is associated with fishing and aquatic sports, has the highest drowning rate in the world. Alaska has the highest rate in the U.S. because of the low water temperature and occupational (e.g., fishing) exposure common in Alaska.

*Region.* Death rates due to drowning not involving boats have generally been highest in the Rocky Mountain and Southern states and lowest in the Northeast.

*Location.* The places where the largest numbers of drownings occur are rivers, lakes, ponds, and oceans. This may reflect simply where the largest number of unsupervised exposures occur. Ocean drownings are not as frequent as those in rivers and lakes, perhaps because of the more frequent supervision by lifeguards on ocean beaches.

For infants and children the most frequent place is in the bathtub or in swimming pools. A similar preponderance of drownings in bathtubs is found among the elderly. This may reflect the fact that the very young and the very old are less likely to be engaged in aquatic sports or recreational activities, or it may indicate that infants and children need more supervision in the bathtub and that the elderly are more prone to heart attacks, strokes, or falls (should this occur in a bathtub, drowning could be reported as the cause of death).

*Month.* More than half of all drownings take place during June, July, and August. Less than 10 percent occur from December through February. This reflects the fact that a much larger number of persons are on or in the water during the summer months. In other words, the chance of drowning increases in warm weather because of the increase in aquatic activity.

*Day and Hour.* About 40 percent of drownings occur on Saturdays and Sundays and about two-thirds in the afternoon or early evening hours. This pattern reflects the increase in recreational water activity and use of alcohol on weekends.

*Water Conditions.* In about half the cases the water is calm, water temperature is at least $65°F$, and the weather is clear.

Cold water is more dangerous than cold air because water drains heat away from the body twenty times as fast as air (air at $70°F$ feels warm while water at the same temperature feels cold). In cold water the skin temperature will drop to within three degrees of the water temperature in two minutes. A heart attack results in some people. Blood supplies to the arms and legs are reduced, making it more difficult to swim.

The average person immersed in water at $32°F$ will be unconscious in fifteen minutes or less. In $40°F$ water he will last thirty minutes; in $50°F$ water he may last sixty minutes; in $60°F$ water he could remain conscious for about two hours.

## EFFECTS

The process of drowning is as follows: It begins as a person struggling to keep afloat. When a person is submerged, they may try to hold their breath; but eventually the victim inhales water. When the larynx feels water intruding, it immediately closes through an automatic muscular contraction known as a laryngospasm, which effectively seals off the airway and protects it from further aspiration so effectively that no more than a small amount of water reaches the lungs. The larynogospasm will continue for an unspecified period of time (assuming the person is not removed from the water), during which the victim dies from suffocation. Eventually the larynogospasm usually relaxes, allowing water to enter the lungs.

Drownings can be classified into four basic types:

1. *Dry drowning.* An estimated 10 percent of all victims drown without aspiration of water because of prolonged larynogospasm. Because no water enters the airway, dry drowning responds readily to mouth-to-mouth resuscitation, and victims of this type of near-drowning account for 90 percent of those successfully resuscitated.

2. *Wet drowning.* About 80 percent of drownings are of this type. After the larynx relaxes, the lungs become partially flooded with water.

    Fresh water in the lungs enters the bloodstream and has a profound effect on blood cells, resulting in destruction of the blood cells, which swell and burst; also the heart may develop ventricular fibrillation.

    In salt water drownings, water is taken from the bloodstream and into the lungs. As much as one-quarter of the total blood volume is lost as fluids move into the lungs. The victim drowns in his own fluids as much as in the salt water itself.

3. *Immersion syndrome.* This refers to sudden death from cardiac arrest as a result of contact with very cold water.

4. *Secondary drowning.* This drowning type describes the case of a victim who is rescued or saves himself yet dies a few minutes or up to ninety-six hours or more after the incident of secondary complications. Aspiration pneumonia is a late complication of near-drowning episodes, occurring after forty-eight to seventy-two hours have elapsed. It is recommended that near-drowning victims be hospitalized or at least closely monitored.

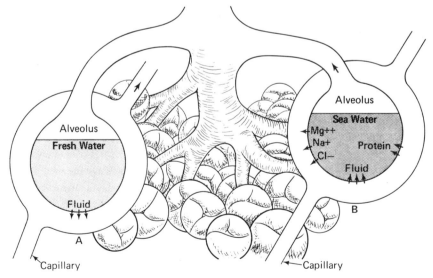

**FIGURE 11-1** In fresh-water drowning, water passes into the circulatory system; in salt-water drowning, fluid passes from the circulation into the lungs. Adapted from *Patient Care*, June 15, 1972, p. 79.

## DROWNING PREVENTION

### Swimming

Learning to swim is essential for survival in the water. Almost 90 percent of drownings occur only ten yards from safety. Parents often are unsure of how old a child must be before he or she can learn to swim. The Council for National Cooperation in Aquatics (CNCA) has issued a statement that the minimum age for organized swimming instruction be set at age three, and that it is imperative that parents be made to realize that even though preschoolers may learn to swim, no young child, particularly the preschooler, can ever be considered "water safe" and must be carefully supervised when in or around water. The CNCA is a group that includes the American National Red Cross, the National Safety Council, the National Recreation and Parks Association, and others.

Parents can encourage younger children to feel comfortable around water, beginning with carefully supervised bathtub play. Most realize that learning to swim is a long, continuing process.

Good swimming ability, although obviously helpful and desirable, by no means completely protects one from the risk of drowning. Indeed, in some instances overestimating one's swimming ability or one's lifesaving ability (many die trying to save others) can result in a drowning.

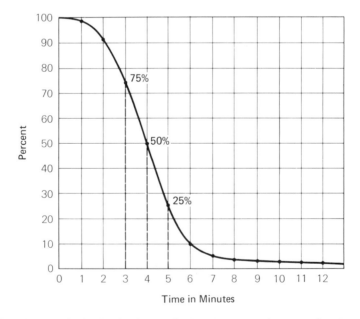

**FIGURE 11-2** A graph plotting the chance of a victim's recovery (by percent) against the time elapsed after breathing has stopped. This assumes that competent artificial respiration is administered.

### Supervision

No single action will prevent all drownings. One measure, however, could prevent a large number—competent adult supervision. Leaving children temporarily unattended is a major cause of drowning. Professional lifeguards should be required at all swimming areas other than those at private residences.

### Barriers Against Trespass

Fences and walls should not be expected to halt all trespassers. Such barriers can, however, keep out small children and make trespassing by older children more difficult.

### Pre-existing Illness

Those who suffer from seizure disorders are especially vulnerable to drowning. Physician counseling for every person who experiences periodic lapses of consciousness due to seizures and acute circulatory ailments should be advised about the special hazards posed by aquatic environments. Such people should be advised to bathe in the smallest possible amount of water, for it is in the bathtub that exposure is most frequent and the danger least evident.

### Swimming Aids

Swim rings, inner tubes, sea horses, and air mattresses are referred to by some as "drowning equipment." Flotation equipment is usually no threat to the capable swimmer who slides off a wet mattress or loses his hold on an inner tube. For the poor swimmer, such equipment allows the individual to have fun but, by giving him or her a false sense of security, may cause them to go beyond a safe depth.

## INJURY CONTROL

These countermeasures deal with a person who is in the water and in distress.

*"Drownproofing" vs. Treading.* "Drownproofing" is a floating method devised to keep a person afloat in several different situations (e.g., long hours in water, while suffering a cramp, severely injured, etc.). The method is based on the principle that with a full breath of air in the lungs almost all persons are lighter than water. An average head weighs close to fifteen pounds, so if a man floats vertically about five pounds is in the air, and with women, about eight pounds. A man then is expending energy to hold five pounds of weight out of the water. "Drownproofing" method is to drop down into the water for a rest of eight to ten seconds between breaths and float like a jellyfish, then come up for air as needed with little effort.

However, studies performed on people subject to low water temperatures demonstrate specific locations of heat loss from the body. Most heat is lost from

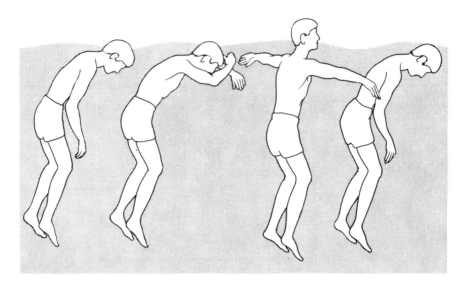

**FIGURE 11-3** Drownproofing technique increases heat loss from the body if used in cold water (70° or less).

the head and neck, the sides of the chest, and the groin area. It was noted that swimming substantially increases heat loss and thus the risk of hypothermia. It has been concluded that the "drownproofing" technique in cold water is not recommended and is dangerous because of heat loss from the head and other body areas.

Therefore, a preferred method of conserving body heat for victims immersed in cold water does require some type of flotation device. This method relies on the heat escape lessening posture (HELP position) in which the victim draws knees up under the chin, presses arms to the sides, and remains as quiet as possible. For three or more persons, it is suggested that life jackets be tied behind the back and that the groin and lower body areas be pressed together. This method keeps the head out of the water.

*Diving Reflex.* The diving reflex is a reaction of the body and has been found to exist in mammals other than man (e.g., seals). Basically it is a reaction of the body to immersion of the facial area in cold water which results in an oxygen conserving action by the body. The body reacts by shunting blood from the extremities to the brain, heart and lungs, permitting a person to be without an external oxygen source for longer periods of time. There have been many cases of survival from cold water drowning where the time in the cold water exceeded the concept of four to six minutes normally indicating clinical death. These victims have been resuscitated after forty-five minutes in cardiac arrest. Once the water temperature falls below 70°F, death may be delayed. The colder the water, the better the victim's chances are for survival if properly resuscitated.

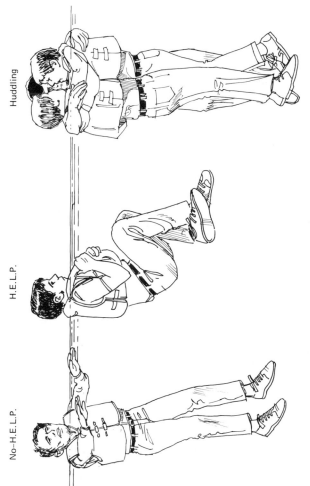

No-H.E.L.P.          H.E.L.P.          Huddling

**FIGURE 11-4** Flotation Survival Techniques. Source: U.S. Coast Guard

135

*Personal Flotation Devices (PFD).* In official U.S. Coast Guard language, there is no such thing as a "life jacket"; instead there are Personal Flotation Devices or PFDs.

Four types of PFDs are approved by the Coast Guard for use on recreational boats, and each type offers its own advantages. All wearable PFDs are designed to keep you afloat and your head and mouth out of the water. Most modern PFDs are comfortable and durable, and some types can be worn under regular clothing.

Type I PFDs are designed to turn an unconscious person from a face-down to a vertical or slightly backward position. They provide at least twenty pounds of bouyancy (a typical adult weighs less than fifteen pounds in water, depending on factors such as body fat and clothing worn). Type I PFDs are best for use in rough water.

Type II PFDs are also designed to keep an unconscious person's face out of water, but they provide less buoyancy (about 15.5 pounds). They are most frequently used in recreational settings where the chances of rescue are better. They come in a variety of models and are among the least expensive PFDs.

Type III PFDs will keep a conscious person afloat with his face out of water. They provide the same range of buoyancy as Type IIs, but are designed so that a conscious person must place himself in a vertical position. The Type III PFD will then hold him that way with no tendency to turn face down. Type IIIs are lightweight, designed for ease of movement, and come in many colors and styles, including vests and jackets.

Type IVs are approved devices designed to be thrown to a person in the water, but not worn. These include flotation cushions and ring buoys. Type IVs provide at least 16.5 pounds of buoyancy and are acceptable for use in canoes, kayaks, and boats less than sixteen feet long. Type IVs are *not* intended for use by nonswimmers or children.

PFDs not only help keep people afloat, they also can help in protecting them from hypothermia while in the water. By rolling into the HELP position (Heat Excape Lessening Posture) while wearing a PFD, heat loss in water can be reduced by about 60 percent.

*Clothing in the water.* Many people have been taught that they should immediately strip off their clothing if immersed in water—that "heavy" clothes will drag a person down. This is not true. Clothing can help save a person in a drowning situation. It traps air, which provides insulation against the cold water and helps prevent hypothermia. The trapped air will also help keep the victim afloat. Fabrics made of leather, natural fibers, and most rubber or plastic compounds are less dense than water and will aid flotation. Even materials denser than water will help as long as they contain trapped air.

*Rescue.* The adage of "reach, throw, row, then go" offers the best sequence for attempting to rescue a person from water. Frequently a single drowning accident is turned into a double or triple one by the unskilled or inadequate efforts of incom-

Type I: Life Preservers *Must be labeled: "Designed to turn unconscious wearer face up in water." Must be colored orange or red.*

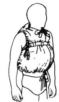 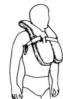

160.002[1]
Kapok (Jacket Type)
Minimum buoyancy:[2]
Adult—25 lb.
Child—16½ lb.

160.055
Plastic Foam
(Bib Type)
Minimum buoyancy:[2]
Adult—22 lb.
Child—11 lb.

Type II: Buoyant Vests *Must be labeled: "Designed to turn unconscious wearer face up in water."*

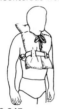 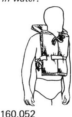 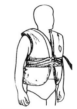

160.047
Kapok or Fibrous
Glass (Bib Type)
Minimum buoyancy:[3]
Adult—16 lb.
Medium child—11 lb.
Small child—7¼ lb.

160.052
Plastic Foam
(Bib Type)
Minimum buoyancy:[3]
Adult—15½ lb.
Medium child—11 lb.
Small child—7 lb.

160.064
Foam-filled
Vests
Minimum buoyancy:[3]
Adult—15½ lb.
Medium child—11 lb.
Small child—7 lb.

Type III: Special Purpose Water Safety Buoyant Devices *Must be labeled: "Designed to keep a conscious person in a vertical or slightly backward position in the water."*

 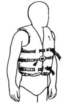 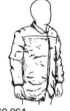

160.064
Foam-Filled Vests
Minimum buoyancy:[3]
Adult—15½ lb.
Medium child—11 lb.
Small child—7 lb.

160.064
Ski Vests
Minimum buoyancy:[3]
Adult—15½ lb.
Medium child—11 lb.
Small child—7 lb.

160.064
Sleeved Jackets
Minimum buoyancy:[3]
Adult—15½ lb.
Medium child—11 lb.
Small child—7 lb.

[1] *Coast Guard approval number: 160 indicates life-saving equipment, second three numbers specify the kind of equipment. Manufacturer's numerals follow.*
[2] *Child: under 90 lb.*
[3] *Medium child: 50-90 lb.; small child: under 50 lb.*

**FIGURE 11-5** Personal flotation devices–summary of U.S. Coast Guard designations. Adapted from *Consumer Reports*, August 1974, p. 613.

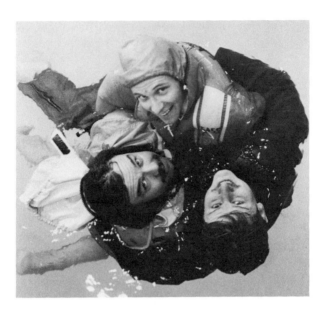

**FIGURE 11-6**   Clothing can help save a person in a drowning situation. This drawing shows the Huddle position in cold water. Photo courtesy of the National Safety Council, *Family Safety.*

pletely trained individuals to save drowning persons. When anyone is floundering in the water, it is prudent not to grapple with him because in his desperation he will have epinephrine (adrenalin) to augment his strength. It is always best to give him a pole or rope.

Whether or not the rescuer is a good swimmer, there is a concept of improvising flotation aids which can be applied to most rescue attempts. When no standard rescue equipment is available, the rescuer can usually find something that floats to hold up an exhausted swimmer or floundering victim of a water mishap until he is rescued or has recovered enough strength to kick or paddle his way to safety. There are lots of things that float—gallon vacuum jug, ice chest with clamp-on lid, canoe paddle, fallen tree branch, spare tire in a car's trunk are examples. An interesting disclosure is that victims seldom cry out or thrash about in the water; this may be a factor in drownings when lifeguards are present.

*Swimwear.*   Persons in a drowning situation disappear, and the difficulty of locating a body underwater may be a contributing factor to drowning. Clothing manufacturers could construct clearly visible swimwear. Perhaps a luminescent material or coloring the swimwear yellow or orange would aid detection of the submerged.

*Submerged automobile.*   Each year people are rescued from cars that have plunged into water, but many passengers do not survive. The annual number of car submersions is not great. Probably only 200 to 300 of the thousands of traffic fatalities are drownings. Because of the drama involved with each case, each is attended by much publicity. Some uninformed drivers resist wearing safety belts because they feel that their exiting from their submerged vehicle may be hampered. Actually, being securely belted is likely to prevent the driver and other occupants from being seriously injured or knocked unconscious. The chances of getting out of a submerged car are better for the uninjured.

When a car is driven into deep water it will float like a boat for a short time. Then, of course, it will sink, and the heavy end will go first. If one or more windows are open at the time of the submersion, and the car is not collision damaged, the occupants merely have to open the door and swim to the surface. Rescue of the injured, nonswimmers, children, and any panic-stricken passengers may be necessary.

Cars with all the windows closed are different. In deep water, there will be great pressure on the doors and windows, making it almost impossible to push the doors open. A large air bubble will be maintained for many minutes within the car. Rolling down a window will relieve the pressure on the door, but exiting must be done quickly. Electric windows pose a problem and usually necessitate breaking the glass to get equal pressure before a door can be opened.

*Lighting.* Underwater lighting in a swimming pool aids location of an immersed body. Spotlights on boats could avert collisions and could also be of assistance in locating floating persons who would otherwise drown.

## BOATING

Here are the major types of accidents and what can be done about them.

*Capsizing and sinking.* About half of all small-boat fatalities are of this type. Improper loading and overloading are probably the chief factors in capsizing. The records are full of cases in which too many people set out in a boat built for fewer persons; one person moves, and the boat turns over. According to the Coast Guard, you can roughly estimate the number of people that can be safely taken aboard a small boat by multiplying its length by its width and dividing that figure by fifteen. Federal law now requires that each new boat carry a capacity plate stating its maximum safe weight load. The number of seats in a boat is not a reliable indicator of how many people it can safely carry. Additionally, the operator's view may be obstructed and the boat improperly handled.

*Collision.* The most frequent kind of boating injury results from one craft striking another, or a floating object, or a person. Some operators of boats do not look where they are going, while others do not know the "rules of the road"—on which side to pass another boat, who has the right of way, how to signal intentions.

*Falling Overboard.* Slipping while refueling or pulling up an anchor, while pulling in fish or firing guns, or while simply standing up are the main causes of falling overboard. Heavily implicated is the use of alcohol. Most accidents of this type could be prevented by adhering to this rule: Never stand up in a small boat. Also, do not ride the gunwales and do not jump in to rescue someone unless all other approaches have failed.

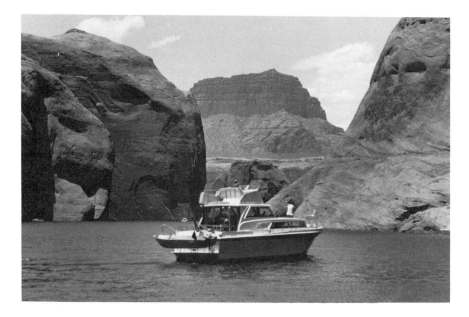

**FIGURE 11-7**  Boating is a pleasureable experience, but can be dangerous. Photo courtesy of Gerald Peterson, UDOT.

**TABLE 11-2  Types of Boating Accidents Related to Fatalities**

| RANK ORDER | TYPE OF ACCIDENT |
|------------|------------------|
| 1 | Capsizing |
| 2 | Falls Overboard |
| 3 | Collision with Fixed Object |
| 4 | Flooding |
| 5 | Collision with Another Vessel |
| 6 | Sinking |
| 7 | Striking Floating Object |
| 8 | Grounding |
| 9 | Struck by Boat or Propeller |
| 10 | Fire or Explosion of Fuel |
| 11 | Other Fire or Explosion |
| 12 | Falls within Boat |
| 13 | Other Casualty; Unknown |

Source: U.S. Coast Guard, *Boating Statistics.*

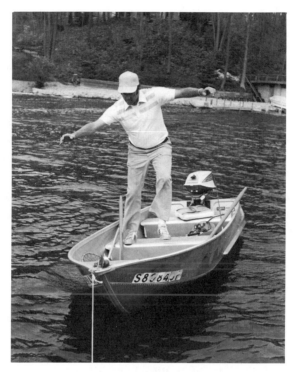

**FIGURE 11-8** Standing up in a boat and falling overboard is a main cause of boat-related drownings. Photo courtesy of the National Safety Council, *Family Safety*.

*Unsafe boats.* Boats wear out and break down just like automobiles, and many accidents can be attributed to such malfunctions as broken steering cables, fuel-line problems, and stalled engines.

*No lifesaving devices.* Requirements for lifesaving equipment on recreational boats have been established by the U.S. Coast Guard. Previous Coast Guard requirements for recreational boats applied only to motorboats, but now sailboats, canoes, and rowboats come under Coast Guard jurisdiction. The authority for boating requirements comes under the Federal Boat Safety Act. The most significant part of this act is the establishment and enforcement of minimum safety standards. For example, load capacity, safe powering, flotation in a swamped or damaged condition (see Figure 11-9), a "good Samaritan" clause (provides protection to someone giving assistance to a boat in trouble), safety education, and enforcement are provisions found in the Federal Boat Safety Act.

*Ignorance.* Novices frequently start their boats in gear, causing them to lurch forward; they anchor from the stern, instead of the bow, a maneuver which can drag the boat under. The Coast Guard has a home-study course available along with

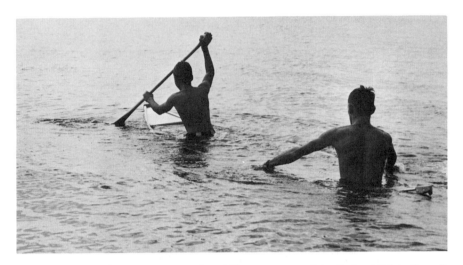

**FIGURE 11-9** Stay with the boat—it floats! Photo courtesy of the National Safety Council, *Family Safety.*

lecture slide shows for the beginning boater. Extensive courses are available from them and the Red Cross.

*Skin- and scuba diving.* Violations of accepted safety rules contribute to most skin- and scuba-diving fatalities. Most authorities agree that participants should be not less than sixteen or seventeen years of age. Stamina and swimming ability should rank high as drowning deterrents.

# 12

# Fires

The United States continues to have one of the worst fire death records of the industrialized world, vying with Canada during the last two decades for the unenviable distinction of reporting the highest human losses. Fire in the U.S. kills about six-thousand people annually and disfigures about 90,000 others and costs more than $6 billion in property damage.

The U.S. fire death rate is high because the number of fires is high. During one hour there is a statistical likelihood that more than three hundred destructive fires will rage somewhere in the U.S. At least one person will have died.

More than a million burn injuries each year require medical attention or restriction of activity.

Fire is a burning that destroys or changes what is burned and usually produces heat, flame, light, and sometimes smoke. All fires require the three basic ingredients and burn according to the same principle (see Figure 12-1). Fires behave in different ways, however, depending on the nature of the ingredients involved.

The three ingredients necessary for every fire are:

1. *Fuel.* Fuel can be organic, such as wood, or inorganic, such as metal. It can be in the vapor or solid state, although many times only the vapor state is involved in the combustion process. For example, gasoline, a liquid, is commonly thought of as a fuel; but it is only the vapors that are involved in the burning process. Combustion of finely divided metals is a process that does not in-

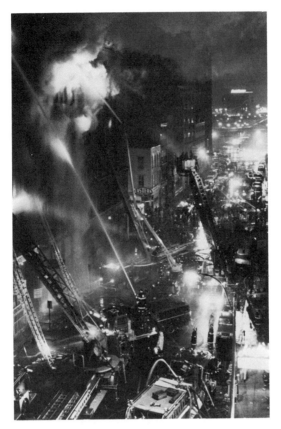

**FIGURE 12-1** The United States and Canada lead the world in fire losses. Photo from *The Boston Globe*, courtesy of the National Fire Protection Association.

volve the vapor state. Steel wool, for example, will burn or oxidize rapidly in the presence of heat and oxygen.

2. *Heat.* Heat is necessary to initiate oxidation. No matter where the heat originates, the combustion process cannot proceed without it.

3. *Oxygen.* Oxygen is almost always obtained from the surrounding atmosphere, which contains about 21 percent oxygen.

The process of burning can be described as follows: When a fuel becomes hot enough, its vapors mix with oxygen in the air, causing a chemical reaction that releases heat, flame, and smoke. The vapor, not the fuel itself, is what burns. A fire spreads because the heat feeds into new fuel and raises it to the ignition point. To extinguish a fire one removes one of the ingredients—by cooling the hot fuel or by separating the fuel and the oxygen.

Each fuel has its own "ignition temperature." The ignition temperature is the temperature to which a fuel must be heated in order for its vapors to combine with

### Chemistry of Fire

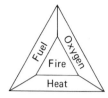 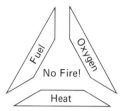

**Oxygen**    — The air we breathe. It is also self contained in some plastics and gun
  **+**        powder.

**Fuel**    — May exist in anyone of three forms, such as: a solid (wood, paper), a liquid
(gasoline, alcohol), or a gas (acetylene, hydrogen). Since oxygen is a gas
  **+**        the fuel must also be in a gaseous state for chemical combination; or
simply, for combustion to occur.

**Heat**    — Is made up of both temperature and quantity. There must be a sufficiently
high temperature, but there must also be a sufficient quantity of heat.
Heat converts the fuel into a gaseous state to combine with the oxygen.
One match will not ignite a log but a thousand matches burning together
  **=**        would probably provide enough heat (quantity) to ignite the log. The
temperature of a thousand matches is the same as for one but the quantity
is greater.

**Fire**    — The result of combining oxygen, fuel and heat, the three sides of the
triangle.

          Remove any one of the three sides of the triangle and the fire ceases to
exist.

**FIGURE 12-2** Chemistry of fire. Adapted from *Safety Journal*, American Telephone and Telegraph Company.

the oxygen and start to burn. The ignition temperature may also be called the "kindling point."

Solid fuels (ordinary combustibles) do not produce vapors until they are heated to their ignition temperature. At this temperature, the vapors given off combine immediately with oxygen and burning begins. The ignition points of some solids are: cotton sheets—464°F., paper—about 450°F., wood—about 500°F. As a comparison of temperatures, a match flame has a temperature of about 2000°F.

Flammable liquids are, by far, one of the most hazardous materials found. These include any number of solvents, ethers, alcohols, fuels, and cleaning solutions. It is important to minimize the use of, or preferably completely eliminate, flammable liquids wherever possible. For example, nonflammable liquids can be substituted in many cases for flammable cleaning solutions and solvents.

Flammable liquids give off vapors at temperatures lower than their ignition temperatures. For example, gasoline begins to give off vapors at about −45°F., but its ignition temperature is about 536°F. Kerosene gives off vapors at about 100°F., but its ignition temperature is 444°F. Although the vapors will not combine with oxygen and start burning on their own at these lower temperatures, they are capable of starting to burn when a flame or spark quickly heats them to their ignition temperature. Often the vapors, though invisible, are present and can easily be ignited. The vapors usually travel near the floor.

Most common heat sources usually produce temperatures higher than the ignition temperatures of most common fuels. Thus they can easily raise the fuel to its ignition temperature. For example, the heat produced by a match flame or an electric arc is about 2000°F., and the heat produced by a lighted cigarette ranges from about 550°F. to 1350°F. They are well above the ignition temperatures of paper, wood, cotton, gasoline—the common fuels.

Plastics exhibit a wide range of reactions when exposed to fire. Almost all plastics are somewhat flammable.

Burning starts in different ways, depending upon the ingredients involved. Ordinary burning begins when heat—usually from friction, a flame, a spark, or a heated surface—is high enough to ignite the vapors of a fuel. Electrical current is another way. Spontaneous heating occurs when a fuel increases its own temperature without drawing heat from its surroundings. In other words, it "heats by itself." This usually happens through fermentation or chemical action. Spontaneous heating of a material to its ignition temperature results in spontaneous ignition. The fire starts "by itself." Fuels that have a high spontaneous ignition are oily clothing or rags, silk and other fabrics, and damp hay. Explosion and fire occur when something is ignited in a confined space such as a container, room, or building, causing quick chemical changes that make the fuel gases expand rapidly with great force. Some examples are firecrackers, rockets, and blasting caps. Aerosol cans may also explode if heated.

Flammability (how easily and how fast something burns) depends on the ingredients involved. The kind of fuel affects flammability. Some fuels have lower ignition temperatures than other fuels and, therefore, burn more easily. For example, paper is easier to burn than metal. Some fuels burn very slowly (asbestos

**TABLE 12-1  Causes of Residential Fires and Fire Deaths**

| CAUSE | PERCENTAGE OF FIRE DEATHS |
|-------|---------------------------|
| Smoking | 37 |
| Cooking | 7 |
| Incendiary/suspicious | 7 |
| Heating | 6 |
| Electrical | 4 |
| Appliances | 3 |
| Open flame, spark | 3 |
| Other | 6 |
| Unknown | 27 |

Source: National Safety Council, *Accident Facts.*

and cement), sometimes only smoldering and never really flaming, while others burn very quickly (soft wood and paper). The shape and form of the fuel also affects flammability. Usually a light, airy form burns more easily than a heavier, more solid form. For example, a crumpled-up newspaper sheet burns more easily than the folded sheet of newspaper. The rate and period of heating is another influence. Long exposure time to heat increases the possibility of burning. For example, a log surrounded by heat from paper and kindling is much more likely to ignite than a log that has a match held against it for a few seconds.

In general, fires spread very quickly. As a fire burns, it gives off heat. This heat warms other fuels in the area to their ignition temperatures and they begin to burn. As a fire grows, it can produce so much heat that it even heats fuels that are a distance from the fire.

## HUMAN FACTORS

*Age.* The very old and the very young are high risk groups. The death rate from fire among children under five and the elderly over sixty-five is three times that of the rest of the population. Though together these young and old make up only 20 percent of the American population, they account for 45 percent of the fire deaths.

The decreased agility of older people makes them especially vulnerable to the hazard of having their clothing ignited by fire. In addition, because of their infirmities, the elderly often find it very difficult to escape from a burning building. The danger to very small children lies in their being left at home alone or with inadequate supervision, plus their difficulty in escaping from burning buildings.

*Sex.* Death rates are higher among males than females. Nationwide, males outnumber females almost two to one as fire death victims.

## ENVIRONMENTAL FACTORS

*Region.* Statewide fire death rates are highest in Alaska and states in the East, especially the Southeast, and lowest in the western half of the United States. The availability and use of wood for fuel and building materials may play a role in regional differences.

*Locale.* Overall, the fire death problem seems more severe both in large cities and in rural communities than in mid-sized communities (50,000 to 100,000 population). More than 80 percent of the fatalities occur in the home. On an annual basis, roughly one percent of homes are damaged or destroyed by fire. Nonmetropolitan areas' high rates might be attributed to a lack of fire departments, local rather than central heating, and a shortage of emergency medical services.

*Month.* The majority of household fires occur from December through March, when the weather is cold, the hours of darkness long, and heating and lighting systems most utilized.

BOX 12-1

> Henry Wadsworth Longfellow's wife was preparing to seal some locks of their children's hair with wax when her flimsy dress caught on fire. She died. The poet tried to save her; his face was badly burned in the process. It was probably to hide the scars that he grew his famed full beard.

## EFFECTS

Most of fire's victims die by inhaling smoke or toxic gases well before the flames have reached them. In fact, most fire victims never see the flames. A person caught in a burning building may have from a few seconds to an hour to escape, to reach an area of refuge, or to be rescued.

Sources vary in their estimates of what percentage (from 50 to 80 percent) of the six thousand fire deaths are related to smoke inhalation. Of the nearly fifty thousand fire victims admitted to hospitals each year, smoke or thermal damage to the respiratory system may occur in as many as 30 percent.

There are four dominant modes of inhalation injury in a fire: (1) asphyxia due to oxygen deficiency (2) asphyxia due to carbon monoxide excess; (3) thermal injury; and (4) smoke poisoning.

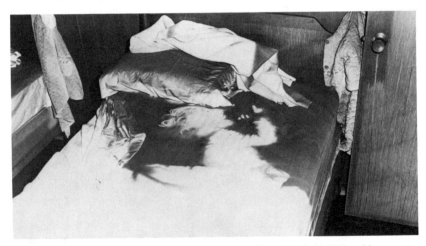

**FIGURE 12-3** Most fire victims never see the flames. Photo by O. H. Willoughby, courtesy of the National Fire Protection Association.

*Asphyxia due to oxygen deficiency.* The depletion of the oxygen supply can be extremely dangerous. Normally 21 percent by volume of the air we breathe is oxygen. If that figure drops to 15 percent breathing becomes labored, dizziness and headache set in, and muscular control is difficult. At 10 percent extreme nausea is experienced and paralysis may be established. At 6 to 7 percent collapse and unconsciousness are inevitable, and below that figure death will occur in a few minutes. Furthermore, at 12 to 15 percent irreversible brain damage may result.

*Asphyxia due to carbon monoxide.* Often called the silent killer, carbon monoxide is one of the most common and dangerous poisons. It is dangerous because it is a gas that is colorless, tasteless, odorless and nonirritating; and it can kill within minutes, depending upon the concentration in the air. It is found in all fires. Generally a hot, fast fire, with plenty of oxygen, will produce a minimum of CO; while a slow, relatively cool fire, with a limited amount of available oxygen, will produce more.

Carbon monoxide passes unchanged through the lungs and combines with hemoglobin (the oxygen-carrying pigment in red blood cells) producing carboxyhemoglobin. This deprives the cells of the body of necessary oxygen, since CO's affinity for hemoglobin is about 200 to 250 times greater than that of oxygen. Thus, the red blood cell is unable to carry as much oxygen as it normally could.

Effects of various concentrations of carbon monoxide range from mild headache to death, and are described briefly in Table 12-2.

Carboxyhemoglobin has a bright red color, and this has led people to say that you can diagnose CO poisoning by noting "cherry red" coloration of the victim's lips, nail beds, and skin. It has been shown, however, that the cherry red color

**TABLE 12-2  Symptoms of Carbon Monoxide Poisoning**

| PERCENT CARBOXY-HEMOGLOBIN | SYMPTOMS |
| --- | --- |
| 10% | Shortness of breath on mild exertion, headache with throbbing temples |
| 20% | Shortness of breath on mild exertion, headache with throbbing temples, nausea, vomiting |
| 30% | Severe headache, irritability, impaired judgment, dizziness, nausea, vomiting |
| 40–50% | Severe headache, confusion, collapse, nausea, vomiting |
| 60–70% | Loss of consciousness, convulsions, respiratory failure. Death if exposure continued |
| 80% or greater | Rapid death |

Source: Anthony S. Manoguerra, "Carbon Monoxide Poisoning," Emergency: The Journal of Emergency Services, January, 1980. Reprinted with permission.

occurs only with carboxyhemoglobin levels that are not compatible with life. It is essentially only seen on autopsy.

Carbon monoxide poisoning is not a minor accident that can be quickly passed over. The victim requires assessment and observation of respiratory and cardiac status, regardless of how unaffected he may initially appear. No minimum level of carbon monoxide has ever been determined to be safe. Even minor exposure can result in permanent central nervous system damage.

Children fare less well than adults with CO poisoning; it is not unusual for a youngster, especially an infant, to have severe symptoms including unconsciousness, while adults subjected to exactly the same exposure may show little effect. Women, because they have a greater tendency to be anemic, tend to fare less well than men. A person at complete rest is likely to be less affected than someone who is fairly active at the time of exposure.

Every CO exposure should be treated as an emergency. Because carbon monoxide is an odorless, colorless gas, it is easy to forget that when a victim is discovered, he or she must be removed from the CO setting lest the first responder also become a victim of carbon monoxide poisoning.

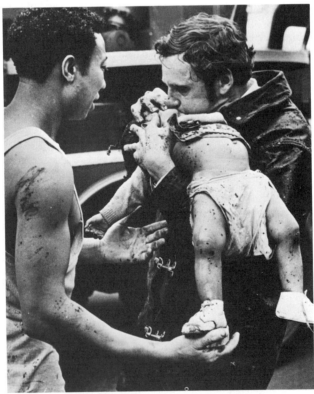

**FIGURE 12-4** Artificial respiration for fire victim. ©1970 *Buffalo Courier-Express*; photo by Ron Moscati.

*Thermal injury.* Extremely high temperatures as a result of exposure to fire conditions can cause an immediate reaction in humans. Temperatures above 300°F can cause death in minutes. The air temperature near the ceiling of a burning room may reach 1,000°F. or more, but most of the heat inhaled is dissipated in the nasopharynx and upper airway.

Thermal (heat) injury is almost always limited to the upper airway (nose, mouth, pharynx, larynx). Only those victims who inhale live steam sustain actual lung damage from inhalation of heat. The upper airway damage is due to second and third degree burns which result in blisters, charring, and swelling due to capillary leakage and edema.

Death can occur when the mucous membranes lining the respiratory system secrete fluids and thereby fill the lungs with liquid. A victim of heat inhalation can drown in his own liquid. Damage in the upper respiratory tract may cause swelling with gradual stoppage of the air passages, suffocation, and death.

Like burns of the skin, swelling does not occur immediately after injury, and the risk of airway obstruction is greatest twelve to twenty-four hours after the burn.

*Smoke poisoning.* Nearly three hundred separate toxic products have been identified in wood smoke. The ever-present plastic products in today's homes produce these same types of toxins. The gases produced include: sulphur dioxide, nitrogen dioxide, hydrogen chloride, hydrogen cyanide, phosgene, and aldehydes. There is evidence that the combined hazard of two or more toxic gases is greater than the sum of the hazards of each.

The immediate effect of toxic gases is the loss of bronchial epithelial cilia (hairlike projections) and decreased alveolar surfactant resulting in decreased lung volume. Surfactant is a chemical in the alveoli of the lung that is responsible for the stability of the alveoli (tiny air sacs in the lungs).

*Panic.* Though not a physical product of fire, panic often occurs when fire breaks out and has been the cause of injuries and deaths due to trampling or jumping from windows too high off the ground.

*Burns.* The most familiar aspect of fire damage to a human is burn damage. Burn damage to human skin is described by its depth which is spoken of in terms first, second, and third degree.

First-degree burns are characterized by redness of the skin. Pain and swelling can occur, but only the outer layer of the skin (epidermis) is affected.

Second-degree burns result when the epidermis has been destroyed by heat,

BOX 12-2

In 1832, Dupuytren, the French surgeon, classified burns as to degrees, such as first degree, second degree, third degree.

and when there is partial destruction of the underlayer of skin (dermis). These burns are characterized by painful blisters and a red, moist appearance.

Third-degree burns are marked by excessive destruction of both layers of the skin and sometimes destruction of muscle, fat, and even bone tissue. Infection is the main problem and is the cause of death in most cases of extensive third-degree burns. Third-degree burns are usually characterized by charring of the skin, which may be black or dark brown, cherry-red, or milk-white, hard, dry, and leathery. Soot may make a burn appear to be third degree.

Most burns are a combination of the three degrees. Often the degree of burn is very difficult to detect even by the experienced experts because the skin varies in thickness (depending upon its location on the body) and because of the victim's age, and because burns are frequently of mixed exposure to the source of heat.

**TABLE 12-3   Effects on Skin in Contact with Surfaces at Different Temperatures**

| TEMPERATURE (°F) | SENSATION OR EFFECT |
|---|---|
| 212 | Second-degree burn on 15-second contact |
| 180 | Second-degree burn on 30-second contact |
| 160 | Second-degree burn on 60-second contact |
| 140 | Pain; tissue damage (burns) |
| 120 | Pain; "burning heat" |
| 91 ± 4 | Warm; "neutral" (physiological zero) |
| 54 | Cool |
| 37 | "Cool heat" |
| 32 | Pain |
| Below  32 | Pain; tissue damage (freezing) |

Source: R. F. Chaillet et al., *Human Factors Engineering Standard for Missile Systems and Related Equipment,* U.S. Army Human Engineering Laboratories, AD 623-731, Sept. 1965.

## FIRE PREVENTION

### Education

Among the many measures that can be taken to reduce fire losses, perhaps none is more important than educating people about fire. Americans must be made aware of the magnitude of fire's toll and its threat to them personally. They must know how to minimize the risk of fire in their daily surroundings. They must know how to cope with fire, quickly and effectively, once it has started.

Most fire service professionals agree that public education about fire has the greatest potential for reducing losses, and that there is a need for education of the public in fire safety. Most of these professionals believe that most fires occur because of public apathy toward good fire prevention practices.

The special target of educational efforts designed to prevent fire loss should be those fires caused by human action. It is estimated that over 70 percent of the building fires can be attributed to the careless acts of people.

The prevention of fires due to human carelessness is not all 'hat fire safety education can hope to accomplish. Many fires caused by faulty equipment rather than carelessness could be prevented if people were trained to recognize hazards; and many injuries and deaths could be prevented if people knew how to react to a fire, whatever its cause. As one writer has summed up the problem:

> A significant factor contributing to the cause and spread of fire is human failure—failure to recognize hazards and take adequate preventive measures, failure to act intelligently at the outbreak of the fire, failure to take action which would limit damage.[1]

BOX 12-3 *UNUSUAL BUT TRUE*

> Firemen raced to a fire in Columbus, Ohio, and found firemen already there. In fact, the on-the-scene firemen had been there before the fire even started! The burning structure was Fire Engine House No. 10.
>
> — National Safety Council, *Family Safety*

Day in and day out, firefighters see the evidence of human failure. They see pennies in fuse boxes and 30-ampere fuses where 15-ampere fuses ought to be. They see the tragic consequences of trash or flammable liquids stored near furnaces, overloaded electrical circuits, gas heaters improperly vented. They find the victims of fire who have died in their sleep because they failed to take the routine precaution of always sleeping with bedroom doors closed. They find the charred bodies of those who took a fatal gamble with fire: who opened a hot door, who dashed through smoke instead of crawling along the floor, who might have survived the gauntlet if they had held a wet cloth over nose and mouth. Organizations like the National Fire Protection Association and the National Safety Council have based their fire safety messages on these common failings. Firefighters and others have brought these messages into the homes and classrooms of America. And still, thousands of Americans die needlessly every year.

A cynic might remark that this widespread ignorance shows that Fire Prevention Week, school programs in fire safety, and all the posters and pamphlets on fire prevention are wasted efforts. Yet, we do not know how much worse the annual fire record would be if there were no educational efforts. Moreover, we do know that public education programs can dramatically reduce fire losses. Studies provide evidence of this.

### Inspection

Many have found a checklist to be effective in inspecting a home for fire hazards. The list below is just an example of what can be done; it is by no means comprehensive.

1. Is smoking in bed strictly forbidden?
2. Are matches and lighters kept out of reach of children?

3. Do you make sure all electrical appliances purchased have the Underwriters' Laboratories tag attached?
4. Do you use the correct size fuse (15 amp for lighting) in each circuit of the fuse box?
5. Are all the extension cords exposed and not run under rugs and furniture?
6. Do you have heating equipment checked by a competent service man regularly?
7. Do you keep rubbish cleaned out of the attic, basement, closets, garage, and yard?
8. Is paint kept in tightly closed metal containers?
9. Are gasoline and other flammable liquids stored in safety cans and kept out of reach of children?
10. Do you prohibit the use of gasoline, kerosene, or similar materials for cleaning purposes?
11. Do all family members know how to report a fire?
12. Is there a prearranged escape route from the home in case of fire?
13. Are there sufficient outlets for all appliances to prevent overloading the electrical wires?
14. Are curtains that are located near a stove made of nonflammable material? If not, are they securely fastened to prevent them from blowing over the flame?
15. Is the gas stove equipped with a gas pilot in good working order?
16. Is there a recently inspected fire extinguisher in the home?
17. Are flammable materials, such as oily rags, kept in a closed metal container?
18. Are furnace, chimney, and flues cleaned regularly?
19. Are solid doors on bedroom doors and at tops of stairways?
20. Are fires rekindled with gasoline or kerosene forbidden?
21. Are flammable liquids labeled as such?
22. Are curtains, drapes, upholstery, and carpets selected with flammability in mind?
23. Is portable heating equipment used with special caution?
24. Are extension cords used in lieu of permanent wiring?
25. Are home furnishings and bedding selected on the basis of ignition possibilities?

### Building Design and Codes

The two most important codes from the standpoint of fire safety are the building code and the fire prevention code. Typically, two-thirds to three-fourths of the provisions of a building code apply to fire safety, as do all the provisions of a fire prevention code. There are ample examples of tragic fires in buildings that met all local building code requirements. Another problem with the codes is the diversity among cities. What works in one town will not in another—and many times for no good reason at all.

A law is effective only to the extent that it is enforced, and so it is with a fire prevention or building code. Many serious building fires have been the result not of code deficiencies, but of lax enforcement. A fire-resistant floor, for example, is an insufficient barrier to smoke and fire if the architect allows gaps in the floor or a workman punches a big hole in the floor to allow a pipe to pass through.

Vigilance is needed in the review of plans and in inspection during construction. Once construction is finished, compromises in fire safety may be hidden from view. The training of inspectors is, in many places, inadequate.

### Product Design

It is not just the large structures of the built environment that need improved design if fire losses are to be reduced. Many products need design improvement. Heating and cooking equipment, faulty wiring, and electrical appliances are major fire causes.

The National Commission on Product Safety has identified color television sets, floor furnaces, hot-water vaporizers, and unvented gas heaters as specific fire or burn hazards. Others include electric blankets, dryers, hotplates, extension cords, space heaters, and many others.

## INJURY CONTROL

### Smoke Detectors

Home fires are especially dangerous at night when the occupants are asleep. Most casualties are victims of smoke and toxic gases—they are not burned and they never saw the fire's flames.

The National Fire Prevention and Control Administration has encouraged the installation of smoke detectors in all homes. Smoke detectors have the potential of reducing home fire deaths by over 40 percent.

BOX 12-4  *UNUSUAL BUT TRUE*

> A smoke detector in Fairfield, Conn., was lying under the Christmas tree as a gift. A fire broke out, the device sounded an alarm, which woke up the sleeping Bulakites family, all of whom escaped from the house unharmed.
>
> — National Safety Council, *Family Safety*

Smoke detectors help the home occupants by giving early warning so they can escape. Also, the earlier the fire is discovered, the less property the fire can destroy before it is extinguished.

Many communities have adopted legislation requiring smoke detectors in all new and existing homes.

Ranging in price from ten to fifty dollars, smoke detectors are reaching all-time high sales.

People are interested in smoke detectors, and the two most often asked questions are:

1. Which type of detector is best?
2. Where should the detectors be located in the home?

*Types of detectors.* When selecting a smoke detector, the first consideration is listing by a nationally recognized testing laboratory, such as Underwriters' Laboratories, Inc.

There are two types of household smoke detectors: photoelectric and ionization.

*Photoelectric smoke detectors* use a light source and light sensitive cell in a darkened chamber. The light source produces a light beam. The photoelectric detector goes into alarm when smoke enters the darkened chamber and reflects the light beam into the light sensitive cell.

*Ionization smoke detectors* use a radioactive material to make the air within the sensing chamber conduct electricity. The alarm sounds when smoke interferes with the flow of electrical current in the ionization chamber. The radiation source presents no health hazard to the home's occupants.

Ionization detectors best sense the fires that produce very small or invisible smoke particles. Photoelectric detectors sense smokey, smoldering fires best—those that produce larger smoke particles. The National Bureau of Standards has concluded that properly installed photoelectric or ionization detectors are both adequate in home fire lifesaving potential.

Only the smoke detector gives early warning of both smoldering and flaming fires. Heat detectors do not give early warning of the smoldering fire nor do they respond to the flaming fire as quickly as the smoke detector.

Battery-operated units give round-the-clock protection, if a responsible person has maintained the battery. All UL-listed battery units are designed so the batteries last at least one year, if operated according to manufacturer's instructions. As the battery weakens and needs replacement, warning chirps or beeping sounds occur for at least a minute for a minimum of seven days. Some units have a red flag to signal a weak battery.

Some electric-powered units can be plugged into an electric outlet. Be sure the outlet used cannot be turned off by a wall switch and is not the same circuit as heavy electrical appliances that may blow a fuse if they catch fire. Some electric units may be directly wired into the home electrical system. This will usually require the services of an electrician.

Either a battery- or electric-powered unit is effective if it is properly installed and maintained.

*Placement of detectors.* The most important location to install the smoke detector is the hallway outside the sleeping area. Homes with more than one group of bedrooms should have detectors installed in each sleeping area.

Homes with more than one floor level should have a smoke detector on every

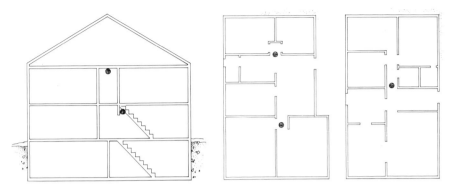

**FIGURE 12-5** Smoke detectors: recommended locations. Source: FEMA

level. Installing a smoke detector in each bedroom increases protection, particularly when there are smokers in the home.

Data from tests conducted for the National Bureau of Standards have been used to develop a "life safety index." A single smoke detector in the sleeping area provided over three minutes to escape through the normal exit in over 35 percent of the test fires. The three-minute escape was increased to 89 percent of the test fires when smoke detectors were on every floor level.

Because smoke rises, the best place to install a detector is on the ceiling or high on an inside wall just below the ceiling.

*Sleeping areas.* Detectors should be installed close enough to the bedrooms so that the alarm can be heard if the doors are closed. Do not install a smoke detector within three feet of an air supply register that might blow the smoke away from the detector. A detector should not be installed between the air return to the furnace and the sleeping area as the smoke will be recirculated and diluted resulting in a delayed alarm.

*Basement.* The detector should be located in the basement ceiling at the bottom of the stairway for the best protection.

In order to minimize false alarms, avoid installing the smoke detector where it will be exposed to cooking or furnace fumes, fireplace smoke, or dust.

### Evacuation

Most parents would be upset if their child's school did not hold regular fire drills, but few parents have ever had a fire drill at home, where fires are most likely to occur and where 90 percent of fire deaths occur.

Fire experts recommend that a family discuss fire escape plans and then have periodic fire drills for all family members. First, impress upon everyone the danger of home fires and the importance of repeated drills. Most local fire departments have pamphlets and other information about the seriousness of fires. Explain that the major danger from a fire is not the flames but the deadly gases and smoke that accompany it. Point out the necessity of getting to fresh air and getting out quickly, as every second can mean the difference between life and death. The family fire escape plan should include the following procedures:

1. Everyone should sleep with his bedroom door closed at night. A closed door can delay the spread of fire and keep out deadly gases and smoke for the few extra minutes needed for escape. Sleep with a window partially open so that a fire cannot pull all the oxygen from the room.

2. Draw a floor plan of your home and mark an escape route and alternate route from each room in the house. Explain how to exit through windows, breaking the glass with a heavy object: Exits from second-story windows may require a rope or folding ladder. Never go out a window head first; back out of the window and hang from the sill with your hands before dropping to the ground. Dropping from a window should be a last resort.

3. Give special consideration to very young children and elderly persons when mapping escape routes.

4. Agree on a way in which any family member can sound an alarm—pounding on walls, yelling, whistling, etc.

5. Instruct family members not to waste time getting dressed or collecting prized possessions.

6. Make sure that every family member knows how to test a door. If panels or knobs are warm, keep door closed and use alternate escape route. If not, brace foot and hip against door and open cautiously to prevent superheated air from blowing it open.

7. If you are forced to remain in a room, stay near a slightly opened window. Place towels (wet, if possible) or cloths in the door cracks. To reach the other side of a smoke-filled room, crawl with your head about 18 inches above the floor. Cover the nose and mouth with a pillow or wet cloth, or hold your breath. (There is mounting evidence that the danger of respiratory damage can be diminished by use of a wet cloth.)

8. Decide on a meeting place outside the house where everyone will assemble as soon as they are outside.

9. Call the fire department as soon as everyone is out of the house. Use a neighbor's phone or a call alarm box. Speak clearly and plainly, making sure you give your full name and address.

10. Hold a practice drill once you have set up escape routes; then repeat drills periodically (every six months).

The National Fire Protection Association and the Fire Marshals Association of North America have devised a program called Operation EDITH (Exit Drills In The Home). In a community that adopts Operation EDITH, well publicized efforts are made to encourage families to devise—and rehearse—plans for getting the family out of the house in the event of a fire.

### High-Rise Building Fire Escape

Several safety steps are well worth taking if spending any length of time in a high-rise building. These guidelines on what to do defensively if disaster strikes are appropriate for most high-rise buildings.

It is wise to survey the corridors with the object of learning the locations of emergency stairways. Two should be located and the number of doorways that separate them from your room should be noted. (If it should be necessary to locate these exits during an emergency, in all likelihood one would be on hands and knees, unable to see or read door numbers and signs.)

If the building has a fire alarm system, find the nearest fire alarm. Try the windows to see if they will open, and look out the window to see what is outside. Escape may be possible, but remember that dropping from more than two floor levels usually results in injury.

If a fire is found in the building, you will probably be alerted by an alarm, yelling, a phone call, sound of fire engines, or even the smell of smoke.

If the door to the hall is hot, it should not be opened. Remain in the room with the door firmly shut. If there is a bathtub it should be immediately filled with cold water (might be needed for fire fighting), and all heating and air-conditioning units should be turned off, as they might vent smoke into the room.

Stuff wet towels around cracks in the doorway and ventilation ducts.

Windows should not be broken, but slightly opened. If the windows do not open, you may have to break one out with a chair or drawer. If fresh air enters and the room is smoky, the room vent should be turned on to help rid the room of smoke and toxic vapors.

Signal to others that you are in the room by hanging a sheet out the window.

If the main room becomes smoke filled, retreat to the bathroom (if there is one) and close the door.

If the door to the hall is cool, open the door and proceed on hands and knees if necessary to an exit stairway, *not* to an elevator. Be sure to take your room key with you in case you have to return to your room. Upon reaching a stairwell, again feel the door before opening it. If the stairwell is not smoke filled, proceed down unless previously instructed to go to the roof. If heavy smoke is encountered during stairway descent, return to the room.

You may want to keep a small flashlight in case you need to exit through smoke or darkness.

### Home Fire Extinguishers

If you walked into your living room tonight and saw the drapes on fire, what would you do?

You should:

- get all the people out of the house *fast*
- call the fire department *fast*

Then—and only then—if the fire is small and if your own escape route is clear should you fight the fire yourself with a fire extinguisher. You may be able to put out the fire or at least hold damage to a minimum. Do not take chances. Get the people out and call the fire department first.

If you can attack a fire fast enough, your success with a fire extinguisher may depend upon one or more of the following:

- your ability to quickly identify the type of fire,
- the availability of the right kind of extinguisher for that particular type of fire.
- your knowledge of how to use the extinguisher, and
- how well the extinguisher has been maintained.

### Selecting an Extinguisher

There are three classes of fires. Your ability to identify the type of fire quickly may save your home—or your life. The reason is that most extinguishers are designed to fight particular classes of fires. Some fight only one class, some fight two classes; only one home-type extinguisher fights all three classes of fires.

- Class A is fire in ordinary combustible materials (paper, wood, cloth, and many plastics).
- Class B is fire in flammable liquids, gases, and greases.
- Class C is fire in electrical appliances and equipment (faulty wiring, as in a TV).

Fire extinguishers are labeled to indicate the class or classes of fires they are designed to fight. However, there are drawbacks to purchasing several kinds (A, B, or C) of extinguishers. They might get mixed up and out of place, or there might be the sort of fire that is inappropriate for the type of extinguisher available.

To avoid this problem, experts generally recommend the all-purpose Class ABC extinguishers for use all around the home. They will work on any kind of fire likely to be encountered.

The unit's weight is a basic indicator of capacity. A recommended model should contain at least five pounds of extinguishing material. A model containing six pounds is better and one of ten pounds is better still.

The numerical rating that is on the extinguisher is another indicator of its ability: The higher the rating, the more fire the extinguisher will put out. On a five-pound ABC extinguisher there might be a rating of 2A-20BC. A six-pound model might carry a 4A-40BC rating. This tells you that the six-pound model is capable of extinguishing twice as much fire as the smaller one.

Select a model that has a pressure dial on the top so it can be checked every couple of months to make sure that the cylinder has not developed a slow leak.

The number of extinguishers needed depends on the nature and size of the area you need to protect. The kitchen, where many home fires occur, is a logical site for one. Another should be placed in the bedroom area or where there is a fireplace. The garage, basement, and car are other ideal locations for an extinguisher.

**TABLE 12-4  Fire Extinguishers for the Home**

| TYPES OF EXTINGUISHER | CLASSES OF FIRE |
|---|---|
| *Water* <br> Freezes in low temperature unless treated with antifreeze solution. <br> Usually weighs over 20 pounds and is heavier than any other extinguisher mentioned. | Fights class A fires only |
| *Standard Dry Chemical Also called Ordinary or Regular Dry Chemical (Sodium Bicarbonate)* <br> Clean residue immediately after using the extinguisher so that sprayed material will not be affected. | Fights class B and C fires |
| *Purple K Dry Chemical (Potassium Bicarbonate)* <br> Has greatest initial fire-stopping power of the extinguishers mentioned for class B fires. <br> Clean residue immediately after using the extinguisher so sprayed material will not be affected. | Fights class B and C fires |
| *Multipurpose Dry Chemical (Ammonium Phosphates)* <br> Only extinguisher which fights all three classes of fires. <br> Clean residue immediately after using the extinguisher so sprayed material will not be affected. | Fights class A, B and C fires |

Class A is fire in ordinarily combustible materials (paper, wood, cloth, and many plastics).
Class B is fire in flammable liquids, gases, and greases.
Class C is fire in electrical appliances and equipment (faulty wiring, as in a TV).

Source: General Services Administration.

### Using an Extinguisher

Do not keep the extinguisher too close to where a fire might occur. Mount it by the door to that room so you have the option of attempting to put out the blaze or fleeing. If used on a cooking pan fire, stand several feet away, otherwise the pan could be blown off the stove and the fire could spread. With other fires, get as close

**TABLE 12-5  Common Household Fires and How to Fight Them**

| TYPE OF FIRE | WHAT TO DO |
|---|---|
| Food in the oven | Close the oven door. Turn off the heat. |
| Smoke from an electric motor or appliance | Pull the plug or otherwise turn off the electricity. If flaming, use water after the electricity is off. |
| Smoke from a television | Keep clear; the picture tube may burst. Call the fire department. Shut off power to the circuit. |
| Small pan fire on the stove | Cover with a lid or plate. Turn off the heat. |
| Deep fat fryer | Turn off the heat and cover with a metal lid if you can approach it. Don't attempt to move the appliance. Don't fight the fire. Evacuate, then call the fire department. |

Source: National Fire Prevention and Control Administration.

as possible without jeopardizing yourself before pulling the trigger. Extinguishers expel their material quickly—in eight to twenty-five seconds for most home models containing dry chemicals. Direct the nozzle at the base of the fire and sweep across it. Always keep a door behind you so that you can exit if the fire gets too big.

## OTHER SPECIAL FIRE AND BURN PROBLEMS

### Fireworks

About sixty-five hundred persons annually seek emergency room treatment for injuries associated with fireworks. About one in ten of these injuries is severe enough to require hospital inpatient treatment. In recent years fireworks have been responsible for about four deaths annually.

Most injuries occur to children. About four out of five victims are male. Obviously, the most frequently injured part of the body is the hand and fingers and the most common injury is burns.

Bystanders are the ones most likely to be hurt from fireworks. The implications are that the firework user is negligent because of "horseplay" or ignorance about the potential damage which a firework can do.

The federal government does prohibit the sale of the most dangerous types of fireworks. These include cherry bombs, aerial bombs, M-80 salutes and larger firecrackers containing more than 0.77 grains (less than one-eighth teaspoon) of powder. Also banned are mail-order kits designed to build these fireworks. Despite this banning, the majority of accidents are linked to legal fireworks.

An example of a legal, but very dangerous firework is the well-known "sparkler." A child either burns himself and/or others or jabs others while playing with the "sparkler."

Another complaint against fireworks is that they cause thousands of fires and millions of dollars in property losses.

Most states forbid the sale of fireworks except to licensed pyrotechnists. Every Fourth of July a few deaths, some severe burns, and sometimes loss of sight result from the unauthorized use of explosives which unscrupulous merchants still sell to children and thoughtless parents.

Such accidents cannot be entirely eliminated until adults fully understand the dangers of explosives and the absolute necessity of preventing children from playing with them. Many people now celebrate the Fourth by attending controlled firework displays managed by specialists and sponsored by the community. Certainly this practice is more in keeping with the spirit of the occasion and the requirements of safety than are the dangerous practices associated with the holiday.

The Consumer Product Safety Commission offers the following recommendation:

> Fireworks are not toys for children. *Do not allow children to play with fireworks under any circumstances.* Even the "sparkler" burns at very high temperatures and can easily ignite clothing.

### Gasoline

Experts say that one gallon of exploding gasoline can equal the force of fourteen sticks of dynamite. Five gallons, says the American Automobile Association, can generate as much heat as 250 pounds of detonating dynamite, enough to completely demolish an auto or raze most homes.

It is the expanding vapors of gasoline that are extremely dangerous; even cold temperatures will not stop the process. An automobile's gas tank is sturdy and has a vent into the fuel system so vapors are returned to be safely converted into energy used in running the car. A can filled with gasoline, on the other hand, will release vapors to fill whatever space it happens to be in, such as the trunk or passenger compartment.

Gasoline should be immediately cleaned up from the floors of garages and wherever else it may have spilled.

Flammable liquids give off vapors at temperatures lower than their ignition temperatures. For example, gasoline begins to give off vapors at about $-45°F$, but its ignition temperature is about $536°F$. Although the vapors will not combine with oxygen and start burning on their own at these lower temperatures, they are capable of starting to burn when a flame or spark quickly heats them to their ignition temperature. Often the vapors, though invisible, are present and can easily be ignited. The vapors usually travel near the floor.

Containers for gasoline, if left open for an extended period of time in a confined area, can become as dangerous as bombs. Containers should be covered and kept in a cool place away from all sources of heat, such as a water heater or electrical or automotive motors.

High temperatures can make the liquid contents of a closed can expand, build up pressure inside the can, and create stresses, especially at seams and joints.

It is recommended that safety cans of one gallon or more capacity should have a flash-arresting screen at the outlet. Such screens prevent external fire or a spark from igniting vapors within the can while the gasoline is being poured.

Only the quantity of gasoline absolutely needed should be stored around the house or garage. Storage should be in a metal can of no larger capacity than $2\frac{1}{2}$ gallons, well away from the house.

A checklist of "do nots" includes:

1. Do not fail to leave an inch or two of headspace to allow for the expansion of gasoline at high temperature.
2. Do not store gas cans in the house; keep them in the garage, if it's well-ventilated, or in a tool shed or outbuilding away from the house.
3. Do not forget to secure a container against upsets when transporting it.
4. Do not allow children access to gasoline containers.
5. Do not drain a can "dry" or leave it uncapped to dry when you empty it.
6. Do not store any detachable extension within a container. And do not store a can with a metal extension capped and in delivery position.
7. Do not leave openings for filling, pouring, or venting uncapped except when filling the container or dispensing gas.

### Electrical Fires

Electricity is dangerous. It kills directly by shock—it kills indirectly by starting fires. Electricity starts fires in four ways:

1. *Overcurrent.* Too much electricity passing through wiring heats it to the extent that insulation and surrounding material begin to burn.
2. *High resistance fault.* Produced by an imperfect electrical path. Examples are poor contact points or frayed wiring, where localized heating occurs and fire starts.
3. *Arcing.* An arc—where a spark leaps across a gap—is a normal occurrence in electrical devices. Usually the tiny, glowing particles are confined within the device, but a short circuit in an extension cord can start a fire. Even a tiny spark in an ordinary switch can cause gasoline vapors to explode.
4. *Hot surfaces.* Many normally operating electrical devices and appliances have outside surfaces hot enough to ignite paper, wood, and cloth. Examples are light bulbs, heaters, irons, and toasters.

*The usual protective devices will not prevent electrical fires.* Fuses and circuit breakers are intended primarily to protect the house wiring. They may not detect an overload in an extension cord or a fault in an appliance. A short circuit will usually blow the fuse or trip the circuit breaker to shut off the power after the fault has already occurred. There is generally no built-in protection either for a high resistance fault or for hot surfaces. Only vigilance and constant attention to properly maintained electrical equipment will prevent electrical fires.

Here is how to prevent electrical fires.

*Do not overload the circuits.* If the fuse keeps blowing or if the circuit breaker frequently trips, the circuit is probably being overloaded.

*Never replace a fuse with one having a higher ampere rating.* Circuits in most older homes should use 15-amp fuses; in new homes, 20-amp fuses. Special heavy-duty circuits for electric stoves and other appliances may utilize 20- or 30-amp or heavier fuses.

*Keep appliance cords and extension cords in good condition.* Replace rather than repair if the insulation is frayed or brittle. Don't tack extension cords to walls as substitutes for permanent wiring, and don't lay them under rugs and carpets.

*Do not use an ordinary extension cord for any appliance which uses a great deal of electricity (toaster, iron, heater, etc.).* An appliance which uses more than 600 watts (5 amps) should be equipped with special, heavy-duty cords with 14 or 16 gauge wires.

*Do not use an appliance which is not working properly.*

*Keep appliances with hot surfaces away from things that can be ignited.*

*Keep paper and cloth away from light bulbs.*

*Provide a ground connection for the outside TV antenna.* Special fixtures and instructions are readily available from TV or hardware stores.

*Do not overload circuits.* To determine if the circuits in your home are being overloaded, add up the wattages of all the lights and appliances on each circuit. If the wattage of the appliances used at the same time exceeds 1,800 watts for a 15-amp circuit or 2,400 watts for a 20-amp circuit, the circuit is overloaded. Wattages are shown on the nameplate of all appliances.

## Woodburning Stoves

Injuries associated with coal- and woodburning stoves have risen over the past few years as more households use them for supplemental or alternative heating. The U.S. Consumer Product Safety Commission (CPSC) estimates that nearly ten thousand persons are treated annually in hospital emergency rooms for injuries associated with these stoves.

Fires associated with woodburning stoves are primarily a problem in one- and two-family dwellings. More than 90 percent of the fires occur in such places. The most common cause of fire is improper maintenance, including using wornout equipment. Installation of the stove too close to combustibles or placing combustibles near the stove is another leading cause. Sparks igniting the exterior of the building account for the third leading cause.

## Hot Water Faucet Scalds

Hot water burns a thousand people annually severely enough for hospital emergency room treatment in the U.S. Readily available hot water can be a serious burn hazard in the tub and shower, particularly for the young, aged, and handicapped who are less able to respond quickly and effectively to an emergency.

Hot water is responsible for more than one-fourth of the hospitalized burn cases in a New York state survey. These immersion scalds involve the lower portion of the body as a child steps into and then sits in a bathtub.

High water temperature is quite dangerous. For example, at 160°F it only takes one second to get a full-thickness (third degree) burn.

It is suggested that 130°F is the upper safe temperature. In one study of fifty scald patients, one-third died. A convenient home temperature is 110°F but 130° is a safe compromise for homeowners, especially for washing dishes and laundry.

BOX 12–5

---

Human flesh begins to burn at 113°F (45°C). Three seconds in 146°F (63°C) water, or one second of exposure at 160°F (71°C), or water at 133°F (56°C) for about thirty seconds can result in third-degree burn injury. At 180°F (82°C) third-degree burns result. Third-degree burns can happen after five minutes in 120°F water.

Even after direct contact with a heat source has ceased, human flesh will continue to simmer and burn for minutes afterwards.

Water heated to 140°F at the hot water heater may be only 130°F by the time it reaches the home's shower or bathtub. An ordinary kitchen meat or candy thermometer can be used for temperature measurements at a faucet.

Parents can test bathtub water temperature by sprinkling several drops on their inner forearm (similar to the technique of testing a baby's bottle of milk) before placing a child in a bathtub.

Never leave a baby or small child in a bathtub—or even the bathroom—for any reason at all without an adult in attendance. They can easily be burned if they turn on the hot water faucet or fall into a tub of hot water.

Your bathtub and shower should have a faucet that mixes hot and cold water. Another way to prevent hot water burns is to control the temperature at the hot water heater (maximum of 130°F.) or install thermostatic or pressure regulating control valves in showers.

## NOTES

1. Deuel Richardson, "The Public and Fire Protection," *NFPA Quarterly* (July 1962), p. 4.

# 13

# Suffocation

The National Safety Council recognizes two basic types of suffocation: (1) suffocation-ingested object and (2) suffocation-mechanical.

## SUFFOCATION-INGESTED OBJECT

Suffocation from ingested objects includes ingestion or inhalation of objects or food resulting in the obstruction of respiratory passages. Over three thousand people die each year from the ingestion of foreign bodies into the respiratory tract.

Death rates are higher for males than females. In children younger than one year, ingested objects are the leading cause of death and rank fourth for children aged one through four years.

Such accidents pose a major problem for children, but the incidence does increase with age beginning at about the fourth decade of life and reaching its peak at the sixth and seventh decades of life.

The sterotype of the ingested object victim is a person having a steak dinner combined with alcoholic beverages and often wearing dentures. The term "cafe coronary" was used to describe cases of sudden death in restaurants. At first the deaths all had been attributed to heart attacks, but later, at autopsy, they were shown to be the result of obstruction of the airway by food. One autopsy revealed apparent gluttonous eating since the portion of obstructing food was a piece of filet mignon measuring 3¾ by 3 by 1 inch.

The type of food most often associated with choking deaths in children is meat. Beef and hot dogs are the main offenders, but others include fish, candy, popcorn, beans, nuts, bread, peanut butter, and french fries.

BOX 13-1  *UNUSUAL BUT TRUE*

> When Dick Winslow appeared at Good Samaritan Hospital in Los Angeles, he complained that his throat was the problem—it had hurt for days. An X-ray provided the explanation: A Mickey Mouse watch—no strap, just the watch —was struck there.
>
> The doctors managed to get it out with forceps. Winslow said he figured the watchworks must have been in a glass of vitamin pills he swallowed days earlier.
>
> National Safety Council, *Family Safety*

Nonfood items responsible for choking in children include pacifiers, rattles, balloons, screws, and bolts. Objects that are flexible and round are especially dangerous.

Suffocation from ingested objects has been recognized for centuries as a cause of sudden accidental death. In recent years, attention has focused on the "cafe

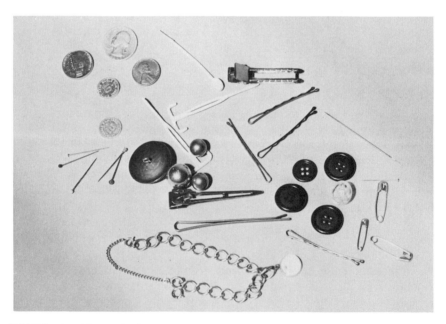

**FIGURE 13-1** Things children swallow and choke on. Photo courtesy of *Health News*, New York State Department of Health.

coronary" problems along with techniques and instruments for emergency care in the event of a choking.

Despite these advances, the incidence of fatal suffocation from ingested objects has remained relatively unchanged in the past twenty years. In one-third of the chokings the object is lodged above the glottis, and other people are present 85 percent of the time. This suggests a lack of awareness of the problem by the public.

The victim chokes suddenly and cannot breathe, turns blue or black, cannot speak, and dies in four or five minutes.

Four kinds of choking have been identified:

- Type 0: Choking all of us have experienced—the sensation of something in the airway relieved by coughing; it is not life-threatening.
- Type 1: Obstruction on the mouth side of the epiglottis (also known as the "lid" type because it may hold the epiglottis down over the larynx like a lid); it is life-threatening.
- Type 2: Life-threatening choking with airway obstruction on the lung side of the epiglottis (also known as the "plug" type because the obstruction closes up the trachea like a plug; a reflex laryngospasm may complicate the situation).
- Type 3: Subacute choking—a foreign body resides in the bronchi, but is not acutely life-threatening. For many cases the foreign body must be removed surgically.

The epiglottis is a thin, leaf-like valve guarding the opening of the trachea. It closes when food or liquids are present in the pharynx, except in an unconscious person when it may fail to work.

The work of Dr. Henry J. Heimlich and his development of the Heimlich Maneuver on the emergency care of the choking victim have been successful. His contributions include:

1. identifying the signs for early recognition of choking;
2. emphasizing a universal sign for food choking;
3. demonstrating specific manual maneuvers which can be life saving; and
4. providing wide dissemination of instructions for performing the simple maneuver known as the Heimlich Maneuver.

BOX 13-2 *UNUSUAL BUT TRUE*

A Seattle, Wash., man used a table knife in an attempt to dislodge a pill stuck in his throat and somehow ended up with the knife lodged in his chest cavity.

The man tried to rinse the pill down and to dislodge it with his finger before trying the knife. Doctors said he persisted in working the knife deeper into his throat because the pill caused a burning sensation that made it seem like it was still there. Miraculously, the knife did little damage and was removed successfully.

– National Safety Council, *Family Safety*

In fact, the stimulus for Heimlich to investigate his work in the field happened after reading the statistics from the National Safety Council that over three thousand Americans choke to death each year.

## SUFFOCATION-MECHANICAL

Suffocation-mechanical includes smothering by bed clothes, thin plastic materials, etc.; by cave-ins or confinement in closed spaces; and mechanical strangulation. About one thousand people are killed this way each year.

Mechanical suffocation is the third leading cause of death in children up to four years of age. Rates for males are generally higher than for females.

The advent of plastics has meant another hazard for children. Plastic bags (used by dry-cleaning and other industries) constitute the largest single way in which children die from mechanical suffocation. This occurs when the plastic bags are used as mattress protectors and come in contact with the child's face.

About the only measures taken to combat the plastic bag suffocation problem are printed warnings on some bags and public education, in the hope that parents will not use the plastic near young children.

Child cribs have for many years been a concern. The Consumer Product Safety Commission has crib regulations and standards to avert this suffocation problem. The problem arises when an infant's head slips through the slats, causing strangulation. Although safe models are now available; cribs have a long lifespan and attention should be drawn to the hazards of using older cribs.

Strangulation in children also has occurred when their throats are either trapped between crib slats and mattresses or hanged on ropes and cords, including cords holding pacifiers around their necks. Somewhat less common are entanglements between pieces of furniture, including parts of high chairs, in clothing, in closing windows, in old refrigerators, and under toybox lids.

# 14

# Poisoning

Poisoning is defined as a reaction to any chemical substance that may result in impaired health, permanent injury, or death. Poisonings occur by ingestion (e.g., aspirin, medications), contact (e.g., poison ivy), inhalation (e.g., carbon monoxide), or injection (e.g., snakebite, insect sting).

## INGESTED POISONING

Poisoning by ingestion occurs when any solid or liquid that tends to impair health or cause death is introduced into the body. Most of the poisons are commonly found in every household.

It would be almost impossible to list all poisons, because a great many substances are harmless if used in the proper way but are poisonous if used in the wrong way or in the wrong amount. Five million persons are poisoned annually. Of the victims, 90 percent are children.

### Effects

The ways in which poisons act are extremely varied and complicated.

*Primary effects.* The first primary effect, which is often cited, is the caustic effect: certain poisons (e.g., strong acids and alkalis) bring about a chemical destruction of the tissues by mere contact. The expression "burning" is appropriate here, since these substances actually cause lesions in the upper digestive tract. If the victim survives, he will have permanent scars.

A second primary effect of poisons is cytotoxicity: disturbance of the normal function of the cells of certain body tissues. This disturbance may result in the death of the cell. Although a disturbance of cellular metabolism of this kind can bring about a necrosis of the tissues similar to that produced by caustic substances, it can also be a temporary disturbance that may be reversible and may cure itself when the poison is eliminated.

A third primary effect concerns certain products to which some individuals are exceptionally sensitive. This sensitivity may be acquired or inherited.

### Human Factors

In the preschool ages poisoning has decreased markedly in recent years, but the danger is still greater among those under five years of age than at any other period of life. Death from accidental poisonings remains higher among males than among females at all ages.

A profile of poisoned children shows that they are more likely to be impulsive and overactive, and may be discipline problems for their parents. Children are most susceptible to accidental poisoning when family patterns are interrupted (e.g., moving, pregnancy, illness, death, or marital problems).

In order to understand how accidental poisoning occurs, it is essential to explore how poisoning is related to normal childhood development and behavior. Children under one year of age are relatively immobile and exist in a controlled environment. Once they begin to walk, however, their environment dramatically expands and becomes far less controlled. Young children become hungry and thirsty much more frequently than do older children and adults. They are attracted to objects that have a pleasant odor, are brightly colored, or are in familiar shapes. These same characteristics are used by manufacturers to make their products more marketable. Thus, many attractive objects that are potential toxins are available in the home. Since the young child's primary method of sampling is tasting, he or she is prone to ingest some of these potential toxins.

Pica (an abnormal craving for nonfood or unnatural food substances) is not fully understood. There are various theories as to why a child will eat a nonfood item (e.g., dirt, plaster, paint chips). Nutritional deficiencies were formerly thought to be responsible for the habit, but this theory has been challenged. A high level of anxiety in a child seems to be related to pica. At any rate, children will eat nonfood items—some more than others.

By age three, the child is adventurous. Studies have shown that a dangerous time is prior to meals while children are hungry and are waiting to be fed. Thirst is another problem; in the warm months, the ingestion of poisonous liquids increases as children drink such substances as petroleum products, paint solvents, and pesticides.

Children over three tend to be more selective in what they eat or drink, preferring things that taste good (e.g., flavored children's aspirin, vitamins).

Another factor in poisoning is parents calling medicines "candy" to induce children to take them during a sickness. To the child, this description is quite reasonable, since many drugs taste sweet and look like familiar candies. Furthermore, parents often take products out of the original containers and keep them in food containers (e.g., furniture polish in a soda bottle).

Still another factor which often leads to accidental poisoning of young children is the strong influence of imitation. They see parents taking a certain substance and want to be like mom or dad, so they too swallow whatever the parent did.

Nonreaders are the most likely victims. The written words "caution" or "warning" or "poison" mean nothing to the preschool child. It is thought that the traditional skull and crossbones may even attract children with its pirate connotation.

Adults often do not recognize the capabilities of small children. There are three basic stages of development in young children from six months to five years of age in which natural tendencies to explore and experiment create situations which lead to accidental poisonings. These three stages are:

- The Crawler, age six months to one year: Everything goes into her mouth. Her world is the floor and storage areas near the floor. Products she is most likely to find are household cleaners.
- The Toddler, age one to three years: They have the highest poisoning accident rate of any age group. Their world includes the closet, tops of tables, stoves, and counters. Many cleaning products, medications, and cosmetics are often found in these places.
- The Climber, age three to five years: It is at this stage of development that the child most often surprises his parents with his capabilities. Intrigued by high storage areas he has never been able to reach, he can be most ingenious in creating ways to reach them.

TABLE 14-1  Substances Most Frequently Ingested by Children Under Five Years of Age—Reported by Poison Control Centers

| RANK | SUBSTANCE | RANK | SUBSTANCE |
|------|-----------|------|-----------|
| 1. | Plants | 8. | Insecticides |
| 2. | Soaps, detergents, cleaners | 9. | Miscellaneous analgesics |
| 3. | Perfume, cologne, toilet water | 10. | Miscellaneous internal medicines |
| 4. | Antihistamines, cold medications | 11. | Fingernail preparations |
| 5. | Vitamins, minerals | 12. | Liniments |
| 6. | Aspirin | 13. | Household bleach |
| 7. | Household disinfectants, deodorizers | 14. | Miscellaneous external medicines |
|  |  | 15. | Cosmetic lotions, creams |

Source: National Clearinghouse for Poison Control Centers.

### Environmental Factors

It can generally be concluded in cases of accidental poisoning that the substances ingested were not only easily accessible but were also not in their proper locations (left on cabinet tops). The kitchen exceeds all other areas in the home as the place for accessible poisons, with the bedroom and bathroom following in prevalence.

It is also a fact that 95 percent of poisonings in children under five occur while they are under the supervision of parents or other adults.

### Poisonous Plants

A surprisingly small number of plant species account for the majority of plant poisonings. Furthermore, plants are the leading household poisoners, overtaking aspirin, which once was the leading child poisoner. Children who balk at spinach apparently have no hesitancy in sampling leaves from the family's potted plants. Small children do not have a highly developed sense of taste, so they are not able to recognize a bad-tasting plant and spit it out.

While most plants are not deadly, many can cause discomfort. The toxicity of some plants is conditional. Only certain parts of some plants, often the berries or bulbs, concentrate the toxin in dangerous amounts, and then perhaps only during certain times of the year.

Table 14-2 identifies some of the more prevalent poisonous plants. If the plant was ingested more than twelve hours before and no symptoms have appeared, there is no problem. Symptoms usually appear within four hours. Only with mushrooms are symptoms delayed for more than twelve hours.

Most people need help in plant identification. Some helpful sources might include: (1) a college or university botanist; (2) a local florist; (3) an older person who gardens and grows various types of plants; and (4) plant identification books. Popular plants' names can be misleading.

**TABLE 14–2  Common Poisonous Plants**

| PLANT | TOXIC PART | SYMPTOMS AND COMMENT |
|---|---|---|
| HOUSE PLANTS | | |
| Castor bean | Seeds | Burning sensation in mouth and throat. Two to four beans may cause death. Eight usually lethal. Death has occurred in U.S. |
| Dieffenbachia (dumbane), caladium, elephant's ear, some philodendrons | All parts | Intense burning and irritation of mouth, tongue, lips. Death from dieffenbachia has occurred when tissues at back of tongue swelled and blocked air passage to throat. Other plants have similar but less toxic characteristics. |
| Mistletoe | Berries | Can cause acute stomach and intestinal irritation. Cattle have been killed by eating wild mistletoe. People have died from "tea" of berries. |

**TABLE 14-2**  Continued

| PLANT | TOXIC PART | SYMPTOMS AND COMMENT |
|---|---|---|
| Poinsettia | Leaves, flower | Can be irritating to mouth and stomach, sometimes causing vomiting and nausea, but usually produces no other ill effects. |
| **VEGETABLE GARDEN PLANTS** | | |
| Potato | Vines, sprouts (green parts), spoiled tubers | Death has occurred from eating large amounts of green parts. To prevent poisoning from sunburned tubers, green spots should be removed before cooking. Discard spoiled potatoes. |
| Rhubarb | Leaf blade | Several deaths from eating raw or cooked leaves. Abdominal pains, vomiting and convulsions a few hours after ingestion. Without treatment, death or permanent kidney damage may occur. |
| **ORNAMENTAL PLANTS** | | |
| Atropa belladonna | All parts, especially black berries | Fever, rapid heartbeat, dilation of pupils, skin flushed, hot and dry. Three berries were fatal to one child. |
| Carolina jessamine, yellow jessamine | Flowers, leaves | Poisoned children who sucked nectar from flowers. May cause depression followed by death through respiratory failure. Honey from nectar also thought to have caused three deaths. |
| Daphne | Berries (commonly red, but other colors in various species), bark | A few berries can cause burning or ulceration in digestive tract causing vomiting and diarrhea. Death can result. This plant considered "really dangerous," particularly for children. |
| English ivy | Berries, leaves | Excitement, difficult breathing and eventually coma. Although no cases reported in United States, European children have been poisoned. |
| Golden chain (laburnum) | Seeds pods, flowers | Excitement, intestinal irrtation, severe nausea with convulsions and coma if large quantities are eaten. One or two pods have caused illness in children in Europe. |
| Health family (some laurels, rhododendron, azaleas) | All parts | Causes salivation, nausea, vomiting and depression. "Tea" made from two ounces of leaves produced human poisoning. More than a small amount can cause death. Delaware Indians used wild laurel for suicide. |
| Holly | Berries | No cases reported in North America, but thought that large quantities may cause digestive upset. |
| Jerusalem cherry | Unripe fruit, leaves, flowers | No cases reported, but thought to cause vomiting and diarrhea. However, when cooked some species used for jellies and preserves. |
| Lantana | Unripe greenish-blue or black berries | Can be lethal to children through muscular weakness and circulatory collapse. Less severe cases experience gastrointestinal irritation. |

TABLE 14-2 Continued

| PLANT | TOXIC PART | SYMPTOMS AND COMMENT |
|-------|-----------|----------------------|
| Oleander | Leaves, branches, nectar of flowers | Extremely poisonous. Affects heart and digestive system. Has caused death even from meat roasted on its branches. A few leaves can kill a human being. |
| Wisteria | Seeds, pods | Pods look like pea pods. One or two seeds may cause mild to severe gastrointestinal disturbances requiring hospitalization. No fatalities recorded. Flowers may be dipped in batter and fried. |
| Yew | Needles, bark, seeds | Ingestion of English or Japanese yew foliage may cause sudden death as alkaloid weakens and eventually stops heart. If less is eaten, may be trembling and difficulty in breathing. Red pulpy berry is little toxic, if at all, but same may not be true of small black seeds in it. |
| TREES AND SHRUBS | | |
| Black locust | Bark, foliage, young twigs, seeds | Digestive upset has occurred from ingestion of the soft bark. Seeds may also be toxic to children. Flowers may be fried as fritters. |
| Buckeye, horsechestnut | Sprouts, nuts | Digestive upset and nervous symptoms (confusion, etc.). Have killed children but because of unpleasant taste are not usually consumed in quantity necessary to produce symptoms. |
| Chinaberry tree | Berries | Nausea, vomiting, excitement or depression, symptoms of suffocation if eaten in quantity. |
| Elderberry | Roots, stems | Children have been poisoned by eating roots or using pithy stems as blowguns. Berries are least toxic part but may cause nausea if too many are eaten raw. Proper cooking destroys toxic principle. |
| Jatropha (purge nut, curcas bean, peregrina, psychic nut) | Seeds, oil | Nausea, violent vomiting, abdominal pain. Three seeds caused severe symptoms in one person. However, in others as many as 50 have resulted in relatively mild symptoms. |
| Oaks | All parts | Eating large quantities of any raw part, including acorns, may cause slow damage to kidneys. However, a few acorns probably have little effect. Tannin may be removed by boiling or roasting, making edible. |
| Wild black cherry, chokecherries | Leaves, pits | Poisoning and death have occurred in children who ate large amounts of berries without removing stones. Pits or seeds, foliage or bark contain HCN (prussic acid or cyanide). Others to beware of: several wild and cultivated cherries, peach, apricot and some almonds. But pits and leaves usually not eaten in enough quantity to do serious harm. |

**TABLE 14-2 Continued**

| PLANT | TOXIC PART | SYMPTOMS AND COMMENT |
|-------|-----------|----------------------|
| Yellow oleander (be-still tree) | All parts, especially kernels of the fruit | In Oahu, Hawaii, still rated as most frequent source of serious or lethal poisoning in man. One or two fruits may be fatal. Symptoms similar to fatal digitalis poisoning. |

FLOWER GARDEN PLANTS

| PLANT | TOXIC PART | SYMPTOMS AND COMMENT |
|-------|-----------|----------------------|
| Aconite, monkshood | Roots, flowers leaves | Restlessness, salivation, nausea, vomiting, vertigo. Although people have died after eating small amounts of garden aconite, poisoning from it is not common. |
| Autumn crocus | All parts, especially bulbs | Burning pain in mouth, gastrointestinal irritation. Children have been poisoned by eating flowers. |
| Dutchman's breeches (bleeding heart) | Foliage, roots | No human poisoning or deaths, but a record of toxicity for livestock is warning that garden species may be dangerous. |
| Foxglove | All parts, especially leaves, flowers, seeds | One of the sources of the drug digitalis. May cause dangerously irregular heartbeat, digestive upset and mental confusion. Convulsions and death are possible. |
| Larkspur, delphinium | Seeds, young plant | Livestock losses are second only to locoweed in western United States. Therefore, garden larkspur should at least be held suspect. |
| Lily-of-the-valley | Leaves, flowers, fruit (red berries) | Produces glycoside like digitalis, used in medicine to strengthen the beat of a weakened heart. In moderate amounts, can cause irregular heartbeat, digestive upset and mental confusion. |
| Nicotiana, wild and cultivated | Leaves | Nervous and gastric symptoms. Poisonous or lethal amounts can be obtained from ingestion of cured smoking or chewing tobacco, from foliage of field-grown tobacco or from foliage of garden variety (flowering tobacco or nicotiana). |

WILD PLANTS

| PLANT | TOXIC PART | SYMPTOMS AND COMMENT |
|-------|-----------|----------------------|
| Baneberry (doll's eyes) | Red or white berries, roots, foliage | Acute stomach cramps, headache, vomiting, dizziness, delirium. Although no loss of life in United States, European children have died after ingesting berries. |
| Death camas | Bulbs | Depression, digestive upset, abdominal pain, vomiting, diarrhea. American Indians and early settlers were killed when they mistook it for edible bulbs. Occasional cases still occur. One case of poisoning from flower reported. |
| Jack-in-the-pulpit, skunk cabbage | All parts, especially roots | Contains small needle-like crystals of calcium oxalate and causes burning and severe irritation of mouth and tongue. |

**TABLE 14-2 Continued**

| PLANT | TOXIC PART | SYMPTOMS AND COMMENT |
|-------|-----------|----------------------|
| Jimsonweed (thornapple) | All parts, especially seeds and leaves | Thirst, hyper-irritability of nervous system disturbed vision, delirium. Four to five grams of crude leaf or seed approximates fatal dose for a child. Poisonings have occurred from sucking nectar from tube of flower or eating fruits containing poisonous seeds. |
| Mayapple (mandrake) | Roots, foliage, unripe fruit | Large doses may cause gastroenteritis and vomiting. Ripe fruit is least toxic part and has been eaten by children—occasionally catharsis results. Cooked mayapples can be made into marmalade. |
| Nightshades, European bittersweet, horse nettle (solanum) | All parts, especially unripe berry | Children have been poisoned by ingesting a moderate amount of unripe berries. Digestive upset, stupefication and loss of sensation. Death due to paralysis can occur. Ripe berries, however, are much less toxic. |
| Poison hemlock | Roots, foliage, seeds | Root resembles wild carrot. Seeds have been mistaken for anise. Causes gradual weakening of muscular power and death from paralysis of lungs. Caused Socrates' death. |
| Pokeweed (pigeonberry) | Roots, berries foliage | Burning sensation in mouth and throat, digestive upset and cramps. Produces abnormalities in the blood when eaten raw. |
| Water hemlock (cowbane, snakeroot) | Roots, young foliage | Salivation, tremors, delirium, violent convulsions. One mouthful of root may kill a man. Many persons, especially children, have died in United States after eating this plant. Roots are mistaken for wild parsnip or artichoke. |

Source: National Safety Council, *Family Safety,* Spring 1979, pp. 18–19.

### Child-Resistant Packaging

Many household products and medications in particular are now available in child-resistant packaging. This type of packaging consists primarily of specially designed caps that most young children cannot open, but that can be opened by adults by following simple directions. Other child-resistant packaging includes hard-to-tear strip packaging for pills and specially operated propellant sprays. Child-resistant packaging is one of the foremost factors in the drastic reduction of poisoning accidents in recent years.

### Education

With most of the poisonings occurring in young children, education programs are aimed at the parents, even though it is difficult to test how effective they are. By the time children reach school, they have passed the most dangerous poisoning

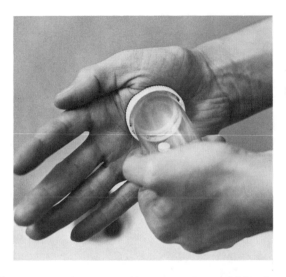

**FIGURE 14-1** Child-proof safety caps. Photo courtesy of the National Safety Council, *Family Safety*.

time. Television would do well to stress poison prevention concepts on children's programs and advertising. Physicians, elementary school programs, and booklets provide other forms of education.

There have been very few evaluations of educational programs, and they have generally been poorly designed. Nevertheless, several studies indicate that behavior toward poison prevention can be influenced by appropriate educational techniques.

Rules to help make a home "poison-proof".

1. Keep household products and medicines out of the reach and out of sight of children, preferably in a locked cabinet or closet—even a fishing tackle box or suitcase can be used. If you must leave the room for even an instant, remove the container to a safe spot or take the child and/or container(s) with you.
2. Store medicines separately from other household products and keep these items in their original containers—never in cups or soft drink bottles.
3. Be sure that all products are properly labeled, and read the label before administering. In a dark room, turn the light on to do so.
4. Since children tend to imitate adults, avoid taking medications in their presence.
5. Refer to medicines by their proper names. Never encourage children to take any medicine by calling it "candy," for later they may be tempted to eat it as a treat.
6. Clean out your medicine cabinet periodically. Get rid of old medicines by flushing them down the drain, rinsing the containers in water, and then discarding them. Do not put any container with its contents into a refuse can.

### Poison Control Centers

There are about six hundred poison control centers across the United States. Their purpose is both to give information regarding household products people have questions about, and, even more important, to give instructions for treatment when

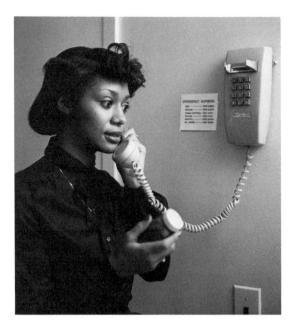

FIGURE 14-2 The telephone number of the nearest poison control center can be found by calling directory assistance or consulting a telephone directory. Photo courtesy of the National Safety Council, *Family Safety*.

someone calls in about a poisoning. The telephone number of the nearest poison control center may be found by calling directory assistance or consulting a telephone directory. That number, as well as that of the local rescue squad, hospital, and physician, should be kept posted on or near the telephone in case of an emergency.

There are differing philosophies about the use of poison control centers. Some centers discourage calls directly from the public—preferring to deal with or through physicians. Other centers will handle calls from the public without hesitation and without involving a physician. Most of these centers are manned twenty-four hours every day of the year to provide emergency information about poisoning. The better centers engage in prevention programs (e.g., lectures, "Mr. Yuk" and "Officer Ugh" symbol distribution).

## POISONING BY INHALATION

The rate of death from poisoning by gases and vapors is increasing. These fatalities are due chiefly to poisoning by carbon monoxide produced by the incomplete combustion of fuels used by motor vehicles, cooking stoves, and heating equipment.

Carbon monoxide is a gas by-product of burning fuel. It is given off from automobiles; campfires; coal, oil, and gas furnaces; and charcoal and kerosene heaters. The smoke from cigarettes also contains carbon monoxide. Because it is colorless, odorless, and tasteless, people may not be aware of its presence. About fourteen hundred people are killed annually.

### Effects

When air is inhaled into the lungs, oxygen is transferred from the air to the blood. Oxygen attaches to a component of blood called hemoglobin; the hemoglobin carries the oxygen to the body's tissues. Carbon monoxide is also capable of attaching to the hemoglobin in the blood. If the air contains carbon monoxide, it attaches to the hemoglobin in place of oxygen.

In low levels, carbon monoxide can cause such symptoms as headache, nausea, and tiredness. As the blood level increases, the person may experience poor vision, dizziness, vomiting. He or she may be in a stupor or experience convulsions. Eventually, he or she will lose consciousness and stop breathing. Refer to Table 14-3.

**TABLE 14-3  Symptoms of Carbon Monoxide Poisoning**

| PERCENT CARBOXY-HEMOGLOBIN | SYMPTOMS |
| --- | --- |
| 10% | Shortness of breath on mild exertion, headache with throbbing temples |
| 20% | Shortness of breath on mild exertion, headache with throbbing temples, nausea, vomiting |
| 30% | Severe headache, irritability, impaired judgment, dizziness, nausea, vomiting |
| 40–50% | Severe headache, confusion, collapse, nausea, vomiting |
| 60–70% | Loss of consciousness, convulsions, respiratory failure. Death if exposure continued. |
| 80% or greater | Rapid death |

Source: Anthony S. Manoguerra, "Carbon Monoxide Poisoning," *Emergency: The Journal of Emergency Services,* January, 1980. Reprinted with permission.

### Human Factors

In the United States, males account for over 70 percent of all deaths. While death occurs at all ages, the death rate is very low in childhood and increases with age.

Children usually fare less well than adults with CO poisoning. Women, because they are usually comparatively anemic, tend to fare less well than men. Exercise or hard labor can cause higher levels of carbon monoxide in the blood quite rapidly during short exposures.

### Environmental Factors

The risk of carbon monoxide poisoning is greatest in the winter: People spend more time indoors with tightly closed windows and doors. Furnaces are turned on, and kerosene burners are brought out.

The automobile is probably the most potent producer of carbon monoxide in the environment. People who drive long distances in older, often poorly maintained cars, such as college students on their winter vacations or migrant farm workers, are at increased risk. Rust is a major factor in damaging the exhaust system and creating holes in the body of the car through which carbon monoxide can enter. Usually these holes are in the muffler and the floor of the car. Even a two-year-old car can have significant rust damage.

Parking inside a garage with the engine running produces many deaths. Many deaths involve persons who are sleeping inside a car, often because of previous drinking. Sleeping may be caused by a combination of alcohol and carbon monoxide, without real intent to fall asleep. Many deaths also involve parking in remote areas for romantic purposes. In addition to parking deaths, drivers also have been overcome by carbon monoxide while the vehicles were in motion.

### Carbon Monoxide Poisoning Prevention

Risk of carbon monoxide poisoning can be lessened by following the guidelines listed below:

1. Keep motor vehicle exhaust systems maintained by regular examination and replacement when needed.
2. Have furnaces serviced by a qualified person once a year.
3. If working indoors with a gasoline-powered vehicle, maintain safe, well-ventilated working conditions.
4. If using a kerosene heater, be sure to follow the instructions provided by the manufacturer.
5. Keep motor vehicles properly tuned up to reduce the amount of carbon monoxide produced.
6. Have good circulation around and under the car if running the engine while the car is standing still.

## POISONING BY CONTACT

### Poison Ivy, Oak, and Sumac

Two million Americans will suffer allergic contact dermatitis from poison ivy, poison oak, or poison sumac this year. Young people are more susceptible than the elderly, and dark-skinned people seem somewhat less susceptible to the dermatitis than others. It is estimated that at least 70 percent of the population of the U.S. would acquire the dermatitis if casually exposed to the plants.

Resistance, or immunity, varies greatly from one person to another and even in the same person at different times, but probably no one is completely immune. Most people thought to be immune have just not been exposed under the right conditions.

### Identification of Poison Ivy, Oak, and Sumac

Perhaps the most neglected area of the prevention of poison ivy, oak, and sumac dermatitis is in teaching people to recognize these plants. Most individuals are unable to pick out these plants in the winter. Many cannot even identify them in their typical summer form but are too embarrassed to admit this to others. Such people are easily taught by using good color pictures.

These poisonous plants are common enough (found in every state but Alaska

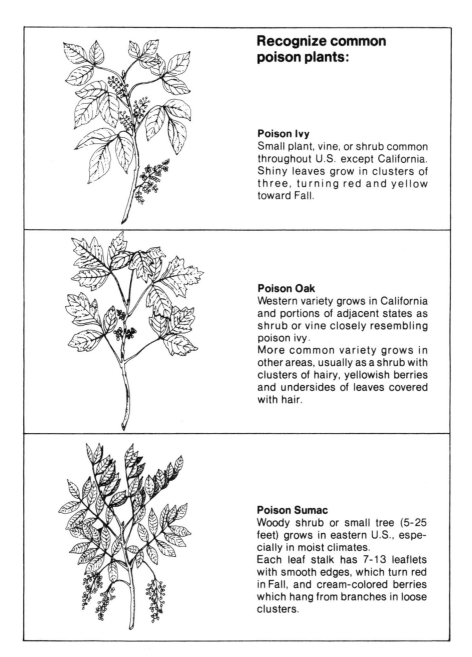

# Recognize common poison plants:

**Poison Ivy**
Small plant, vine, or shrub common throughout U.S. except California. Shiny leaves grow in clusters of three, turning red and yellow toward Fall.

**Poison Oak**
Western variety grows in California and portions of adjacent states as shrub or vine closely resembling poison ivy.
More common variety grows in other areas, usually as a shrub with clusters of hairy, yellowish berries and undersides of leaves covered with hair.

**Poison Sumac**
Woody shrub or small tree (5-25 feet) grows in eastern U.S., especially in moist climates.
Each leaf stalk has 7-13 leaflets with smooth edges, which turn red in Fall, and cream-colored berries which hang from branches in loose clusters.

**FIGURE 14-3** Poisonous Contact Plants in the United States. From *Emergency Medical Procedures for the Backpacker*. Copyright 1979, Logical Communications Inc., Darien, CT.

BOX 14-1

> Leaflets three—let it be.
> Berries white—poisonous sight!
>
> — *Old first-aid axiom*
>
> Poison ivy has three light green, shiny leaflets. In the fall, poison ivy has clusters of white berries and its leaves take on bright colors. Poison oak looks like poison ivy, but its leaflets resemble oak leaves.

and Hawaii) to identify them. Avoidance of trouble is far better than the treatment of it.

*Poison Ivy.* "Leaflets three, let it be" is the first step in identifying poison ivy. To differentiate between poison ivy and other three-leaved plants, remember that the stem of the central leaflet of poison ivy is always longer than the stem of either of the two side leaflets. Poison ivy usually: (1) grows as a low plant, shrub, or climbing vine; (2) has yellow-green flowers and whitish berries; (3) produces green leaves that are shiny when they first come out, turn red and yellow toward late fall, and then drop off.

*Poison Oak.*   Neither of the two poison oak varieties growing in the U.S. are actually oak plants, although their leaves are similar to those of their namesake. Western poison oak also closely resembles poison ivy. This variety is found only on the West Coast below five-thousand foot elevation levels and in low areas and wooded slopes. The more common variety also has three leaves but is found in New Jersey, Maryland, Tennessee, southern Missouri, Kansas, and south to northern Florida and Texas. It grows as a shrub, identifiable by clusters of hairy, yellowish berries. The undersides of the leaves are dense with hair.

*Poison Sumac.*   This plant is never found in land that is dry all year round; it prefers marshes or bogs. Each leaf stalk of the poison sumac has seven to thirteen leaflets, while harmless sumacs may have up to twenty-five leaflets per stalk. The leaflets of the poison sumac have smooth edges; those of its harmless relatives have saw-toothed edges. Poison sumac has cream colored berries that hang from the branches in loose clusters, while harmless sumac have dull red berries in tight clusters that stand upright at the twig's end. Poison sumac is generally found east of the Mississippi River.

An oily resin is present in all of these plants and contains a complex active ingredient, urushiol. Urushiol is distributed widely in the roots, stems, leaves, and fruit of the plant, but not in the flower, pollen, or epidermis. It is this urushiol which produces the contact dermatitis.

### Effects

Although the limbs, face, and neck are common sites of the dermatitis, all areas of the skin that come in contact with the sensitizing substance can be affected. However, different parts of the body may not have the same sensitivity.

Thus, the dermatitis may appear first in one area and later in another. The phenomenon is often called "spreading," but this description is inaccurate. Often, parts of the body that may sustain a heavy concentration of the allergen and exhibit more severe reactions will remain "hypersensitive" for several years.

The characteristic burning, itching, rash, and swelling resulting from poison ivy, oak, or sumac contact may not follow for as long as ten days after exposure. A day or two is the usual interval between exposure and onset of signs and symptoms.

The rash first consists of streaks or patches of red discoloration of the skin associated with itching. Later, blisters develop which break down, resulting in oozing and crusting from the surface. Usually swelling of the tissue, burning, and itching are present. Scratching should be avoided because it can introduce infection or cause scarring. Scratching does not spread the rash. The blisters are filled with serum, not the urushiol which causes the dermatitis.

### Prevention

It is best to stay away from the plants. But they will grow almost anywhere, so this may be difficult. The following are suggested as ways of preventing poison ivy, oak, or sumac:

1. Be able to identify poison ivy, oak, and sumac.
2. Be able to protect yourself when in an area where these plants grow. Long shirt sleeves, long pant legs, and gloves will help guard against possible irritation. Urushiol has been known to remain on clothing for as long as a year. Clothing should be machine laundered or dry cleaned.
3. Never burn poison ivy, oak, or sumac, even though the plants are dead and dry. Smoke from the burning plants may contain droplets of urushiol and cause severe irritation to the skin.
4. Never handle pets that have been running out of doors, especially in wooded or weed areas. If the pet is suspected of having had contact with these plants, it is suggested that a bath be given. The pet itself is in no danger of the urushiol poisoning.
5. Barrier creams designed to keep urushiol from touching the skin are generally considered useless.

## POISONING BY INJECTION

### Insect Stings

The venom of Hymenoptera (bees, wasps, hornets) kills more people than that of snakebites. The number of deaths definitely known to have resulted from such stings averages about forty a year. However, a lot of deaths identified as "natural causes" or "heart attack" may actually have been from insect stings.

It has been estimated that eight in a thousand people are allergic to stinging insects, and four of these eight are severely sensitive. For a severely allergic person, a single sting may be fatal within fifteen minutes.

Emergency first responders need to know more about this important subject. A knowledge of emergency care procedures as well as preventive measures is essential. Having an emergency insect sting kit and knowing how to use it is a must for people in public places such as recreational areas, summer camps, and swimming clubs.

*Description of stinging insects.* Yellow jackets sometimes also bite before stinging. Wasps can inflict multiple stings since their lancet is unbarbed. In contrast, the bee can generally sting a human victim only once before its barbed lancet becomes embedded in the skin.

After a honeybee stings, it is unable to withdraw the barbed stinger from its human victim. As the bee tries to remove the stinger, a portion of the abdomen and venom sac remain in the victim, and the bee dies. This remaining stinger is a sign of a honeybee sting.

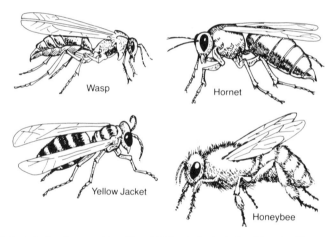

**FIGURE 14-4** Stinging insects. *The First Aid Book*, 2nd ed., by Alton L. Thygerson, © 1986. Reprinted by permission of Prentice-Hall, Inc., Englewood Cliffs, N.J.

The true incidence of serious hypersensitive reactions from stinging insects is not known. However, it is probably much greater than reported because of those victims who never live to report a sting. Fatalities from Hymenoptera most frequently occur in the months of July and August, when exposure is at a maximum. Most stings are on the head, neck, or feet. Statistically, most deaths have occurred in men over the age of thirty.

BOX 14-2

> While there are accounts of individuals who have survived some 2,000 bee stings, generally 500 or more will bring about death. If a person is severely allergic, a single bee sting can kill.

Sixty-five percent of those who die from Hymenoptera stings die within one hour, which stresses the importance and the need for immediate medical treatment.

### Effects

*Types of reactions.* Dr. Claude A. Frazier, a noted authority, classifies the symptoms of most stings as:

- a normal reaction to a single sting,
- a local reaction occurring in proximity to the sting site,
- a generalized reaction which may culminate in true anaphylaxis,
- a toxic reaction resulting from multiple stings, and
- a delayed reaction which closely resembles serum sickness.

*Local reactions.* Itching and pain followed by some redness and swelling at the sting site are the immediate local symptoms of a normal reaction to a single sting. The sting site is gradually surrounded by a whitish zone and a reddish flare, whereupon a wheal forms (about the size of a quarter or half dollar) which subsides after a few hours.

If the sting occurs around the eyes, nose, or throat the local reaction may cause more than the common amount of distress. Stings about the eyes are especially dangerous since they can injure the eye.

*Generalized reactions.* When generalized reactions occur after an encounter with an insect, medical help must be sought swiftly. These reactions may first be indicated by a dry, hacking cough, a sense of constriction in the throat or chest, swelling and itching about the eyes, massive hives, sneezing and wheezing, a rapid pulse, blush of the skin, and a sense of uneasiness.

*Toxic reactions.* Toxic reactions result from innumerable insect stings to a single victim, as when a colony of bees or wasps is disturbed. Even when no sensitivity exists, the amount of venom injected from multiple stings may lead to death. The main symptoms are gastrointestinal (including diarrhea and vomiting), as well as faintness and unconsciousness. These are accompanied by edema without hives, headache, fever, drowsiness, involuntary muscle spasms, and sometimes convulsions.

*Delayed reactions.* Some victims experience delayed reactions to stings. In this case, symptoms of fever, headache, and hives occur as late as ten to fourteen days after the actual sting. If such a victim is stung again, the response may be immediate and anaphylactic. This delay is due to the fact that antibodies have to be formed with the first sting; therefore, they are in production. Thus, a single sting may produce both an immediate and a delayed reaction.

*Prevention of stings.* Insect avoidance is most important. Although it would appear that the likelihood of serious reactions decreases with time if no further stings take place, fatal reactions have been reported in sensitive people stung many years after the previous sting. Sting-sensitive people should be made aware of the following simple avoidance measures. Emergency medical identification should be worn by all those who are sting sensitive. Insect repellents are thought to be of little benefit with sting insects.

1.  Avoid scented cosmetics, soaps, perfumes, lotions, etc.
2.  Avoid wearing floral-colored or dark coarse clothing (white, tan, grey, or light green clothing is best). Bright colors attract bees.
3.  Wear shoes at all times—do not wear sandals.
4.  Avoid loose-fitting garments which may allow insects to become trapped inside and thus become maddened.
5.  Avoid insect feeding grounds such as flower beds, garbage areas, and orchards.
6.  Have insect nests in the vicinity of the home exterminated.
7.  Keep auto windows closed when driving.
8.  Wear long pants, long-sleeved shirts, and gloves if working among flowers or fruits. Cover up.
9.  Avoid wearing anything bright such as jewelry or buckles.
10. Be cautious while eating outdoors—insects are attracted to food.
11. If Hymenoptera are encountered, do not swat at them. Retreat slowly. If retreat is impossible, lie face down and cover head with arms or at least stand still while covering the head with arms. Perhaps the best thing to do is just to let the insect settle—it probably will not find anything of interest and will eventually disappear.

The allergic person's plight is not hopeless; desensitization injections with Hymenoptera venom provide long-term protection. This vaccine is 97 percent effective. After taking the vaccine, if a person is stung again by the same insect, there is virtually no chance of a severe reaction. People who have already had a severe generalized reaction involving the whole body and who are found to be allergic to one or more of the venoms on a skin test should receive this vaccine.

### Arthropods

*The black widow spider.* Black widows are easily recognized—they have coal-black bodies with a distinct red hour-glass-shaped spot on their abdomens. They range in size from ¾ to 1½ inches. They are found throughout the continental United States. By volume, their venom is more deadly than the rattlesnake's, but fortunately is injected in much smaller amounts. The venom is neurotoxic, which means the toxin attacks the junctions between the nerves, and the muscles they control. Death can occur.

*The brown recluse spider.*   The brown recluse spider is now generally believed to be more numerous than originally thought. Having a light brown body about a quarter of an inch long, it is more difficult to recognize than the black widow. It has a dark brown, possibly purplish, violin-shaped figure on its back. Ordinary house spiders may have dark areas on their backs, but they will not have the violin configuration.

*Tarantula spider.*   The tarantula is far more ominous looking than the other two poisonous spiders discussed, but its bite rarely produces symptoms other than mild to moderate pain.

*Scorpions.*   Only the scorpions found in the southwestern United States and Mexico are dangerous to humans. They inflict venom with a stinger located at the tip of the tail, and they are especially dangerous to young children. The deadly scorpion is smaller than the nondeadly variety, with a straw-colored, slender body of about two inches.

*Human and environmental factors.*   In the United States the peak incidence of stings and bites occurs in summer, especially in August for spiders and the spring months for insects. Stinging by bees is most likely on bright, warm days. The proportion of males getting bites and stings exceeds that of females.

### Snakebite

It is estimated that eight thousand people in the United States are bitten by venomous snakes annually. Of these, fourteen to twenty persons die each year, a mortality of less than 1 percent. But the large number of permanent deformities and amputations are also of major concern. Much misinformation exists regarding poisonous snakes.

The only poisonous snakes native to the United States are the rattlesnake, cottonmouth, copperhead, and coral snake. No other native snake can cause anything worse than a small infected laceration.

BOX 14-3

Red and yellow
Kill a fellow
Red and black,
Venom lack. (*or* Friend of Jack)

This is a description of the coral snake, the most toxic of any poisonous snake in the United States, which accounts for 1 percent to 2 percent of snakebites in the United States. Red and yellow bands touching each other identify the coral snake.

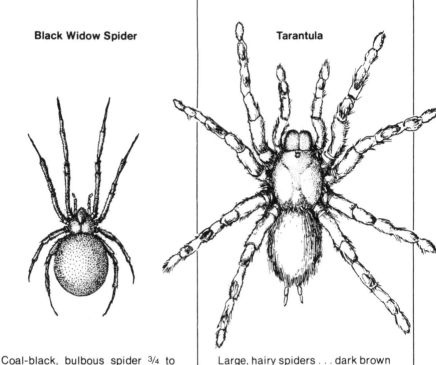

**Black Widow Spider**

**Tarantula**

Coal-black, bulbous spider ¾ to 1½ in. long. Bright red hourglass on abdomen. (Be especially cautious in latrines, where these spiders inhabit underside of seats.)

Possible Signs & Symptoms
- sensation of pinprick or minor burning at time of bite
- appearance of small punctures (but sometimes none)
- within 15 to 60 minutes, intense pain at site spreading quickly
- profuse sweating
- rigid abdominal muscles without abdominal tenderness
- other muscle spasms
- breathing difficulty
- slurred speech, poor coordination
- dilated pupils
- generalized swelling of face and extremities

Large, hairy spiders . . . dark brown to black. Up to 7 in. long.

Possible Signs & Symptoms
- may be similar to Black Widow Spider; however, tarantula bites are generally no worse than a bee sting.

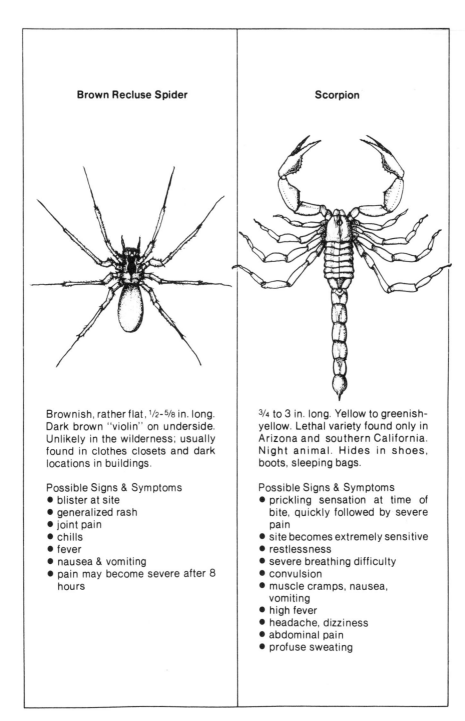

**Brown Recluse Spider**

**Scorpion**

Brownish, rather flat, 1/2-5/8 in. long. Dark brown "violin" on underside. Unlikely in the wilderness; usually found in clothes closets and dark locations in buildings.

Possible Signs & Symptoms
- blister at site
- generalized rash
- joint pain
- chills
- fever
- nausea & vomiting
- pain may become severe after 8 hours

3/4 to 3 in. long. Yellow to greenish-yellow. Lethal variety found only in Arizona and southern California. Night animal. Hides in shoes, boots, sleeping bags.

Possible Signs & Symptoms
- prickling sensation at time of bite, quickly followed by severe pain
- site becomes extremely sensitive
- restlessness
- severe breathing difficulty
- convulsion
- muscle cramps, nausea, vomiting
- high fever
- headache, dizziness
- abdominal pain
- profuse sweating

**FIGURE 14-5** Poisonous spiders. From *Emergency Medical Procedures for the Backpacker*, Copyright 1979, Logical Communications, Inc., Darien, CT.

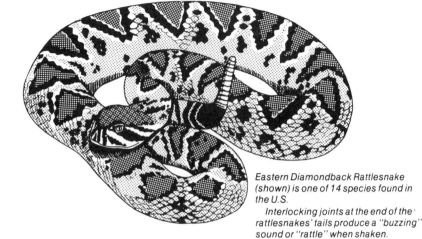

Eastern Diamondback Rattlesnake (shown) is one of 14 species found in the U.S.

Interlocking joints at the end of the rattlesnakes' tails produce a "buzzing" sound or "rattle" when shaken.

### Eastern Diamondback Rattlesnake

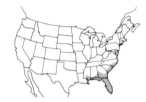

**Description** Dark diamonds with light borders along a tan or light brown background. Diamonds gradually changing to bands in tail. Diagonal brown lines on the sides of face, vertical on snout.
**Habitat** Lowland thickets, palmettos, flatwoods.

### Canebrake and Timber Rattlesnake

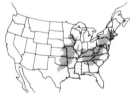

**Description** South: Dark streak from canebrake snake's eye to mouth; dark chevrons and rusty stripe along midline. Pink to tan ground color darker toward tail, which is black in adults. North: timber rattlesnake has yellowish ground color and a dark phase in part of its range
**Habitat** Canebrake: lowland brush, and stream borders. Timber rattlesnake: rocky wooded hills.

### Western Diamondback Rattlesnake

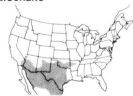

**Description** Light brown to black diamond-shaped blotches along light grey, tan, and, in some localities, pink background. Black and white bands of about equal width around tail and black basal rattle.
**Habitat** Diverse terrain: dry, sparsely wooded, rocky hills, flat desert and coastal sand dunes. Often found in agricultural land and near towns.

## Copperhead

*Northern Copperhead (shown here) and other Copperheads in the U.S. vibrate their tails rapidly when alarmed.*

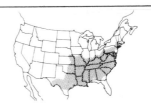

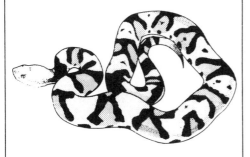

**Description** Large chestnut brown cross bands on a pale pinkish or reddish-brown surface; and coppery tinge of head.
**Habitat** North: wooded mountains; hills; wild, damp meadows; along stone walls; in slab or sawdust piles. South: Lowland swamps and uplands; sometimes found in wooded suburbs.

## Coral Snakes

*Eastern Coral (below) and Texas Coral are dangerously poisonous although their small mouths and short fangs make it difficult to bite most parts of the body.*

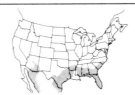

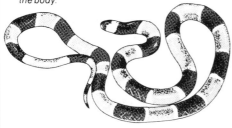

**Description** Red and black rings, wider than the interspaced yellow rings. Black snout, round pupils; no facial pits.
**Habitat** East: grassland; dry, open woods; and frequently suburban areas. West: (much less dangerous), desert and semidesert where there is loose soil and rocks.

## Cottonmouth (water moccasin)

*Eastern Cottonmouth (below), Florida and Western Cottonmouths, are frequently confused with several nonpoisonous water snakes.*

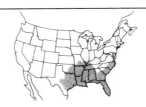

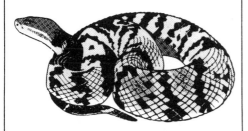

**Description** Dark blotches on brown or olive body. Heavy body and broad flat head.
**Habitat** Semiaquatic.

**FIGURE 14-6** Common poisonous snakes. From *Emergency Medical Procedures for the Backpacker*, Copyright 1979, Logical Communications, Inc., Darien, CT.

The first three of the above are pit vipers, and each has three common characteristics:

1. A vertically slit pupil like the eye of a cat.
2. A triangular, flat head wider than its neck.
3. An infrared heat-sensitive "pit" between each eye and nostril.

The coral snake has a black snout and yellow rings that always separate the black and red rings.

The two most dangerous pit vipers are the eastern diamondback and the western diamondback rattlesnakes. The eastern diamondback is the most dangerous (kills the most people) in the U.S., but of the two, snakebites from the western diamondback occur most often. Rattlesnakes are venomous at birth. Snake habitats range from altitudes of ten thousand feet to sea level or below. They may be found above the timberline, especially in the summer.

*Effects.* The severity of a snakebite will vary in relation to the kind and size of the snake, the amount of venom it injects, the location, depth, and number of bites, the age and size of the victim, and the kind of first aid and medical care received. Venom from some snakes is more toxic than from others, and some inject more venom.

Venom from pit vipers (rattlesnakes, moccasins, copperheads) affects the victim's circulatory system (chemotoxin). Venom from a coral snake affects the nervous system (neurotoxin) of the victim. The coral snake's venom is more toxic than that of the pit vipers, but because it has a small mouth and short fangs, and because of the size and frequency of the eastern diamondback rattlesnake, it is considered more dangerous than the coral snake.

BOX 14-4  *SNAKES: WHICH ARE MOST DANGEROUS?*

Any effort to judge the venomous native snakes according to lethality is unrealistic, because of many factors. Some snakes have highly toxic venom but inefficient "delivery systems." The coral snake is an example. Coral snake venom is among the most toxic of the native venoms, but the small size of the reptile, its blunt head and jaw, and small fangs usually limit venom delivery to a small quantity.

As a rule, only the eastern and western diamondback, canebrake, timber, and Mojave rattlesnakes—and some other subspecies—can be considered life-threatening. They account for about 95 percent of the national death toll from snakebite. Diamondbacks inject the largest quantity of venom.

Less dangerous are the cottonmouth (water moccasin) and rattlesnakes not already mentioned; even less dangerous are the pigmy rattler and copperhead. The copperhead delivers more bites than any other native venomous snake, despite its unaggressiveness, because its habitat often overlaps that of humans —dwellings, farmlands, barns, etc.—increasing the likelihood of provocation.

– *Patient Care*, Patient Care Publications, Inc.

*Human factors.* The incidence of snakebite accidents is higher for males than for females. Over half the bites happen to persons less than 20 years of age. Children less than 5 years of age do not have an excessive bite rate as compared to young people aged 5 through 19 years of age. The lowest bite rate is for people 70 or more years of age. A popular myth is that children have excessively high fatality rates from snakebite accidents. This is not true. The greatest number of deaths from snakebites are found in adults aged 60 to 69 years.

The following are activities being participated in at the time of the bite: playing in own yards and elsewhere, working on a farm or ranch, handling a poisonous snake, hunting or fishing, and recreation other than hunting or fishing.

*Environmental factors.* Most of the states having the highest bite rates per 100,000 population per year are in the southeast and southwest regions of the United States. States east of the Mississippi River with the highest rates are North Carolina, Georgia, West Virginia, Mississippi, and South Carolina. The states west of the Mississippi River with the highest rates are Arkansas, Texas, Louisiana, Oklahoma, and Arizona.

The most widely distributed poisonous snake in the United States is the rattlesnake, with fifteen species. One or more species of poisonous snakes are found in every state except Alaska, Maine, and Hawaii. (There are no snakes of any kind in Hawaii.) Large rattlesnakes are the most dangerous venomous snakes in the United States.

BOX 14-5  *UNUSUAL BUT TRUE*

> Dianne Stilles, eighteen months old, was discovered teething on a venomous —but dead—snake in the yard of her family's home in Melbourne, Australia. "The snake had a few teeth marks on the back of its head," reported her father. "I think Dianne crunched down on its head with her teeth and killed it. She'd bite through your finger if you gave her a chance."
>
> — National Safety Council, *Family Safety*

Copperheads inhabit the eastern United States from Massachusetts to Kansas southward to northern Florida and west to Texas. Cottonmouths or water moccasins are found in aquatic habitats from southeastern Virginia through the southern lowlands up the Mississippi Valley to southern Illinois and west to central Texas. They can bite a person while under water.

The American coral snakes are a group of some forty to fifty species that attain their greatest number and variety in Mexico and northern South America, although they range from the southern United States to Uruguay. The better known United States coral snake is the North American coral snake, which occurs from southeastern North Carolina through Florida and the Gulf States to central Texas and southward into Mexico. The smaller Arizona coral snake inhabits a limited region in southern Arizona, New Mexico, and Sonora.

Snakebites are infrequent during the colder months of the year—November through March—when snakes generally are inactive or hibernating. Most bites (over 90 percent) occur from April through October. The peak months for snakebite accidents in the United States are July and August. This striking seasonal distribution of bites coincides with the period when snakes are most abundant and active and when people have greater exposure because of outdoor occupations or recreation.

The majority of snakebite incidences occur between 6:00 A.M. and 9:00 P.M., which is the period when people are most active outdoors. Many species of poisonous snakes are nocturnal feeders, but people simply do not have as much exposure to the possibility of a bite during the hours after dark.

Most snakebite cases occur in the victim's own yards. Farm or ranch, near a lake, river, or other body of water, in the woods, and in a field away from the house are the other main locations of snakebite occurrences.

BOX 14-6  *UNUSUAL BUT TRUE*

> Deputy Sheriff Bob Alexander of Naples, Florida shot a rattlesnake, and Flash, his dog, moved in to finish it off. The snake's head, snapped off by the violent shaking of the dog, sailed through the air with jaws open. The fangs imbedded themselves in Alexander's hand and sent him to a hospital for treatment.
>
> — National Safety Council, *Family Safety*

*Prevention.*   The following are suggested procedures when in the outdoors:

1. Do not move when you hear a snake rattle. Snakes usually strike at moving objects.
2. In snake-infested areas wear shoes and other types of protection over legs (baggy pants) because more than half of all bites are on the lower part of the leg.
3. Avoid walking at night or in grass and underbrush. Do not climb rocky ledges without visual inspection.
4. Avoid the unnecessary handling of snakes and do not frighten others with snakes. A recently killed snake can strike and the separated head can inject venom even fifteen minutes after the snake's death.
5. Do not sleep on the ground.
6. Be cautious around discarded lumber, debris, and firewood. Keep debris cleaned up. Do not attract mice and rats with garbage; they are the principal food supply for snakes.
7. When walking, be alert as to the intended path. Use a stick to poke clumps of grass and brush before walking through them.
8. Keep the grass, weeds, and brush cut so snakes cannot hide.

# 15

# Firearm Accidents

Guns are abundant in the United States. It is estimated that about one half of all American homes have a firearm. It also has been estimated that the ratio of serious, nonfatal gunshot wounds to accidental gunshot deaths is 13:1.

In a typical recent year, guns were involved in nearly two thousand fatal accidents.

BOX 15-1  *UNUSUAL BUT TRUE*

> In Chicago, John Markiano blew $120 in a big Fourth of July blast. All he did was fire his shotgun once.
>
> When the smoke had cleared, tiny shreads of money were spread all over. Markiano fired his shotgun to celebrate Independence Day without remembering he had stashed $120 in cash down the gun barrel. In fact, he had stuffed $50 down the barrel only that morning.
>
> — National Safety Council, *Family Safety*

## EFFECTS

The seriousness of gunshot wounds is often thought to be caused directly by the bullet. However, the wounding potential of bullets is exceedingly complex and is related to both velocity and bullet mass.

By greatly increasing the velocity, a bullet—despite its small size—contains very lethal amounts of energy. The speed of sound is the measure to which the speed of bullets is compared. Those which are slower than this are described as "low velocity." They are fired from hand guns and tend to be relatively large and round-nosed. "High-velocity" bullets travel faster than sound and can travel three miles. Even a .22-caliber bullet can go a mile or more. They are lighter, more slender, with more pointed noses, and are usually fired from rifles or magnum handguns. The impact velocity will depend on the ballistics of the ammunition and the distance of the victim from the muzzle.

A bullet causes injury in the following ways, depending on its velocity:

*Laceration and crushing.* When the bullet penetrates, the tissue is crushed and forced apart. This is the main effect of low-velocity bullets. The crushing and laceration caused by the passage of the bullet is not usually serious, unless vital organs or major blood vessels are directly injured. The bullet only damages tissues with which it comes into direct contact and the wound is comparable to those caused by weapons such as knives.

BOX 15-2  *UNUSUAL BUT TRUE*

A New Jersey hunter's life was probably saved when his glass eye deflected a shotgun pellet. Charles Wright of Andover, New Jersey, was hit in the left eye by another hunter's errant pellet. His shattered glass eye—which Wright received after a childhood bow and arrow accident—had to be replaced.

— National Safety Council, *Family Safety*

*Shock waves and temporary cavitation.* When a bullet penetrates, a shock wave exerts outward pressure from the bullet's path. This pushes tissues away. This has been described as a "blowing-out" resulting in bursting of tissue. A temporary cavity is created which can be as much as thirty times the diameter of the bullet. As the cavity is formed, a negative pressure develops inside creating a vacuum. This vacuum draws debris in with it.

This temporary cavitation occurs only with high-velocity bullets and is the main reason for their immensely destructive effect. The cavitation lasts for only milliseconds but can damage muscles, nerves, blood vessels, and bone.

In a penetrating wound, there is an entry of the bullet but no exit. In a perforating wound, there is both an entry and exit point. The exit wound of a high velocity bullet is larger than the entrance wound, while the exit wound from a low-velocity bullet is about the same size of the entry wound. In a bullet wound at very close range, the entrance wound may be larger than the exit because the gases in the blast contribute to the surface tissue damage.

Bullets sometimes hit hard tissue (e.g., bone) and may bounce around in the body cavities and cause a great deal of damage to tissue and organs. Also, bone chips can be forced to other body areas, resulting in damage. A split or misshapen

BOX 15-3 *UNUSUAL BUT TRUE*

> George Adams was a 16-year-old Albanian immigrant celebrating his first Fourth of July in Philadelphia when a stray bullet hit him in the chest.
>
> Doctors said the bullet was too close to his heart and lungs to remove, so they left it there. Sixty-nine years later Adams coughed up the bullet.
>
> The retired Detroit resident was having lunch at the Southfield Rehabilitation Center, where he was recuperating from an auto accident, when something caught in his throat.
>
> "I coughed and my throat felt scratchy," he said. "I thought it was a capsule or pill that didn't dissolve, so then I coughed harder. I looked in my hand and saw the bullet. Everyone said it was impossible, but there it was!"
>
> Doctors were puzzled as to why the bullet finally worked its way out after so many years, but Adams thinks it was knocked loose by a combination of the impact of his car crash and the use of a respirator during recovery.

bullet does greater damage because it tumbles, exerting its force over a greater diameter than a smooth bullet going in a straight line.

### Shotgun Wounds

Shotguns are smooth-bore, long-barrelled guns that are designed primarily for killing game birds and small animals. A shotgun wound is caused by many small pellets. Injury is determined by the type and amount of powder charge, the size of pellets, the constriction at the muzzle end of the barrel (choke), and especially the distance from the victim. At a range of ten yards, about 95 percent of these pellets will be within a pattern nine inches in diameter when fired from a full-choke bore. At twenty yards, these wound diameters are doubled. Effective shotgun range is about forty yards, but pellets can travel five hundred yards. Shotguns become ineffective at producing severe wounds at long ranges from loss of velocity and dispersion of the pellets.

## HUMAN FACTORS

A profile of the typical hunting accident indicates that the victim is a male between ten and twenty-nine years of age. Small-game hunters have more accidents (rabbit and squirrel vs. deer hunters). The victim has had one to five years of hunting experience.

While men are the primary victims in hunting accidents, it is women and children who are getting shot in the home. More than 30 percent of firearm deaths in the home happen to children under fifteen years of age.

Cultural factors such as hunting opportunities, violence seen on television, and increased availability of firearms are related to increased incidence of firearm accidents.

## ENVIRONMENTAL FACTORS

Roughly half of the accidental firearm deaths occur in the home. This is a frightening aspect of the firearm accident problem, since these accidents occurred in a situation where there was no intention of doing any shooting at all. Most people think of hunting or target shooting when firearm accidents are mentioned. Most hunters spend just a few days a year in the field and the target shooters a day or two a month on the range, but the guns are kept in the home all year. Without question there is more firearm handling in the home than on the range and in the hunting field combined, yet the emphasis continues to be placed on range and hunter safety.

The problem of firearm safety in the home becomes more complex when the number of untrained people who have access to firearms is considered.

Fatal home firearm accidents appear to have little or no seasonal variation. Hunting fatalities are, of course, definitely related to the hunting seasons (usually the fall months).

The regions with the highest rates are generally the south and the northern mountain states. The Rocky Mountain region has high rates, and this might be partially explained by the hunting opportunities along with a "pro-gun" attitude. The West was won with the gun, and guns have been noted to be very much a part of the western states' culture (e.g., rifles carried in racks in many trucks).

Hunting accidents most often occur between 6:00 A.M. and 9:00 A.M. on a Saturday, Sunday, Monday, or Tuesday.

Shotguns are involved in far more accidents than rifles. This is probably because there is more small-game hunting done with shotguns.

## PREVENTION

An old phrase, "It's always the unloaded gun which does the harm" has often been quoted. This statement may mislead some into thinking that there really is no way to make a gun safe. The saying should suggest instead that people often assume a gun to be unloaded and discover only after an accident happens that it was indeed loaded.

Hunting accidents involving firearms fall into two types: (1) those in which the gun is fired deliberately and (2) those in which the gun fires accidentally.

Accidents stemming from a deliberately fired gun occur in different ways: the hunter shoots another person when he is firing at a moving target; the hunter mistakes another person for game; the hunter fires in the direction of a sound or movement without first identifying the source; a bullet ricochets; a bullet goes beyond the target and strikes an unseen person; the hunter fails to make certain that the gun was unloaded; the hunter uses the wrong ammunition or a faulty gun.

The gun can fire accidentally also in a variety of circumstances: the gun is faulty and fires when dropped or bumped; the hunter slips or falls and fires the gun unintentionally; the hunter has the gun completely ready to fire and the trigger is caught on a limb, barbed wire, or other similar object.

### Safety Rules

1.  Treat every gun as if it were loaded. There is never any excuse for failing to know whether a gun is loaded. Guns should be unloaded when the shooting or hunting is finished, and then checked again before being put away. Leaning on the muzzle of an empty gun, or placing the muzzle on a foot and leaning on the butt, is a dangerous practice. Soon the habit becomes established and the gun is used as a prop when it is loaded. Leaning a loaded or unloaded gun against a tree or other insecure support is unwise.
2.  Always point the muzzle in a safe direction. Even the empty gun should not be pointed toward another person. The safe hunter always knows where his gun is pointing, even when he cannot see the muzzle. The gun must become so much a part of him that it becomes almost a physical extension of himself.

    Much bad gun handling takes place when several hunters begin loading their guns in preparation for the hunt. Often they stand in a group, talking

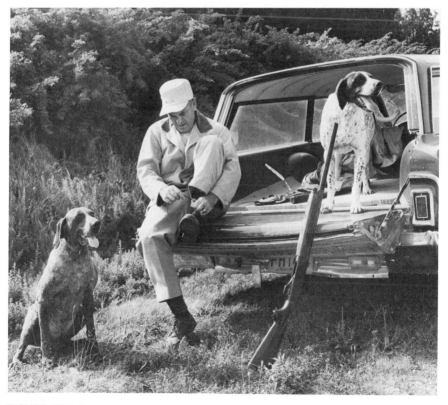

**FIGURE 15-1** Leaning of a gun can be a dangerous practice. Photo courtesy of the National Safety Council, *Family Safety*.

while loading their guns. Nearly everyone has one or more guns pointed at him. Out of respect for safety, each hunter should face away from the circle while loading his gun. He must then carry it so that it does not point at anyone.

3. Be sure of your target—and what is beyond. The shooter should know exactly what he is shooting at. If hunting, he should see the whole animal clearly enough to identify it positively. The gun should be used as if it were a camera. Like the nature photographer, the hunter should have a clear, unmistakable picture of the whole animal before he shoots. He should also anticipate where the shot will go if it fails to hit the game or passes completely through it.

*Zones of Fire.*   When parties hunt together the areas to be covered should be decided in advance. It should be obvious that all hunters cannot shoot at every deer they see without endangering each other. In a group of three, the center hunter takes the game going straight away from him. The hunters at the sides take those on their respective side of the line.

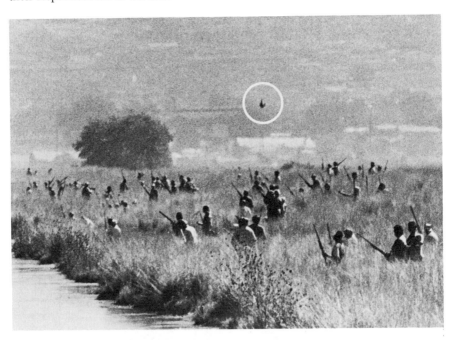

**FIGURE 15-2**  The circle identifies a falling duck. Who shot it? It should be obvious that all hunters cannot shoot at every thing they see without endangering each other. Photo courtesy of the *Deseret News.*

A group of hunters should always try to walk in a side-by-side formation and point their muzzles downward and forward. However, if the hunters must walk in a formation that has some hunters in front of others, the lead hunter should point his muzzle downward and forward, and the other hunters should point their muzzles downward and to the side.

*Self-Protection.*   A bad practice is carrying deer skins or antlers in such a way that they could be mistaken for a live deer. Clothing color can help in avoiding identification mistakes.

*Hunting.*   Remember, most big game is actually killed at ranges under sixty yards. Attempts to kill game by shooting over a hundred yards are usually fruitless.

If the barrel is obstructed by mud, snow, or any foreign substance, clean it out before shooting. Never try to shoot out an obstruction. The barrel will burst.

Almost two-thirds of gunshot wounds are inflicted by the victim's hunting companions. Choosing hunting companions who are responsible and careful is essential. Whenever a hunting companion acts in a dangerous manner, the hunter should immediately reprimand him. If the companion continues to act dangerously, the hunter should stop his activity for the day and refuse to hunt with the individual again.

The National Rifle Association sponsors two firearm safety courses: Home Firearm Safety and Hunter Safety. In hunting safety, the course is primarily trying to reach the new or young hunter. In some states it is a requirement that a young hunter take this course before he can qualify for a hunting license. In home firearm safety, the course is directed entirely to the adult (even those with no recreational interest in firearms).

Most children will be subjected to the handling of firearms whether or not they are doing the handling, so it is necessary that they too know the correct methods. They could be shot even though they are not handling the firearm. They must be able to detect a hazardous situation in order to be able to do something about it, or to know when to leave the area. The NRA Home Firearm Safety Course is not intended to interest children in firearms or shooting; its aim is to impress upon them that firearms do exist and that they should know the hazards that are involved.

The wearing of bright, prominently colored clothing while hunting does avert being shot, but it is interesting that a sizable number of hunting accidents still befall those wearing such apparel.

Guns should be stored completely unloaded (breech and magazine). The action should be closed and the gun uncocked. Storage of guns should be under lock and key with the ammunition stored separately and safely away from the gun(s) (see Figures 15-3 and 15-4).

Basic gun safety practices should be followed. Safe practices include: knowing the gun (determining if it is loaded, how the safety works, etc.), handling the gun properly (treating it as if it were loaded, always pointing the muzzle in a safe

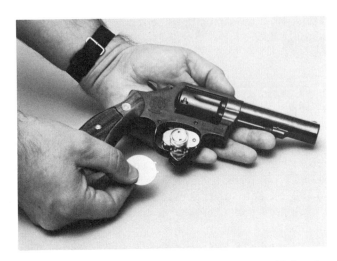

**FIGURE 15-3** Trigger lock. Photo courtesy of the National Safety Council.

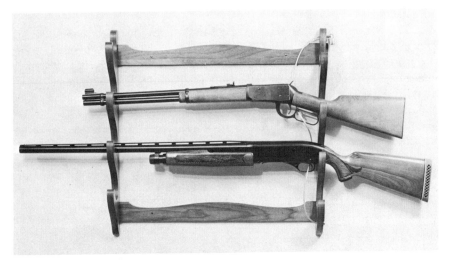

**FIGURE 15-4** Guns secured by a lock. Photo courtesy of the National Safety Council.

direction, keeping the finger outside the trigger guard, and keeping the action open when handling the gun), and accepting responsibility for observing safety rules (exercising self-control, not being a showoff, etc.)

Early training should include an awareness of what a firearm can do. A technique used to demonstrate the effects of a bullet is to fire a .22 hollow-point cartridge through a bar of soap. The effects are dramatic and leave the impression that the firearm can and does do damage.

# 16

# Cold and Heat Injuries

## FROSTBITE

Frostbite is a condition in which tissues of a part of the body—usually an extremity, ear, nose, or cheek—become frozen or partially frozen as a result of exposure to cold.

To most people, frostbite may seem like a remote risk. Yet as more and more people venture outdoors in winter—skiing, hiking, hunting, snowmobiling—it has become an increasing health hazard.

### Effects

As the body tries to conserve heat for vital internal organs in bitter cold, it reduces the flow of warming blood to the extremities. Eventually, if the temperature in the tissue drops low enough, tiny ice crystals begin to form in the watery spaces between the cells. Expanding outward in all directions, the ice ruptures cell membranes and kills the tissue. Also, the reduced blood flow due to sludging and clotting of blood inside small blood vessels raises the possibility of gangrene.

### Types of Frostbite

The extent of injury is not usually known when first seen. At one time, some effort was made to describe frostbite injury in terms of degrees, as presently done with burns (e.g., first-, second-, third-degree). Frostbite injuries are now classified as either superficial or deep.[1]

*Superficial.* Fingers, cheeks, ears, and nose are the most commonly affected body parts. Ice crystals in the skin and other tissues cause the area to appear a white or greyish-yellow color. Pain may occur early and subside. Often the part will feel only very cold and numb, or there may be a tingling, stinging, or aching sensation. The victim may not be aware of frostbite until someone mentions it. When the damage is superficial, the surface will feel hard and underlying tissue soft when depressed gently and firmly.

*Deep.* In a deep, unthawed frostbite, the area (mainly the hands and feet) will feel hard, solid, and cannot be depressed. It will be cold, pale, and numb, and blisters will appear on the surface and in the underlying tissues in twelve to thirty-six hours. Time alone will reveal the kind of frostbite that has occurred.

### Human Factors

The following are factors predisposing a person to frostbite:

- Nutrition. Poorly nourished individuals are more susceptible because of inadequate metabolic heat production.
- State of health. Injuries, disease, and alcohol and drug use can make individuals more susceptible by modifying their heat production and perception, thus altering their ability to take care of themselves in a cold environment.
- Fatigue.
- Tobacco. Nicotine causes constriction of small blood vessels in the extremities, reducing blood flow and allowing rapid cooling.
- Other factors. Age (with the elderly most susceptible) and history of previous cold injuries are less important but also affect susceptibility to frostbite.

### Environmental Factors

When the tissue temperature drops to −2°F, frostbite occurs. There are two other factors—not just cold—that increase body heat loss: moisture and wind.

Moisture—whether from rain, snow, or perspiration—speeds the conduction of heat away from the body.

Wind has a marked effect on heat loss. If the thermometer reads 20°F and the wind speed is 20 mph, the exposure is comparable to −10°F. This is called the wind-chill factor. A rough measure of wind speed is: If you feel the wind on your face, the speed is about 10 mph; if small branches move or dust or snow is raised, 20 mph; if large branches are moving, 30 mph; and if a whole tree bends, about 40 mph. To obtain an idea of the relative degrees of danger according to combinations of wind speed and themometer reading, refer to the wind-chill factor chart in Table 16-1. Table 16-2 may be used to estimate wind speeds.

## TABLE 16-1  Wind-Chill Factor

| ESTIMATED WIND SPEED (IN MPH) | ACTUAL THERMOMETER READING (°F.) | | | | | | | | | | | |
|---|---|---|---|---|---|---|---|---|---|---|---|---|
| | 50 | 40 | 30 | 20 | 10 | 0 | −10 | −20 | −30 | −40 | −50 | −60 |
| | EQUIVALENT TEMPERATURE (°F.) | | | | | | | | | | | |
| calm | 50 | 40 | 30 | 20 | 10 | 0 | −10 | −20 | −30 | −40 | −50 | −60 |
| 5 | 40 | 37 | 27 | 16 | 6 | −5 | −15 | −26 | −36 | −47 | −57 | −68 |
| 10 | 40 | 28 | 16 | 4 | −9 | −24 | −33 | −46 | −58 | −70 | −83 | −95 |
| 15 | 36 | 22 | 9 | −5 | −18 | −32 | −45 | −58 | −72 | −85 | −99 | −112 |
| 20 | 32 | 18 | 4 | −10 | −25 | −39 | −53 | −67 | −82 | −96 | −110 | −124 |
| 25 | 30 | 16 | 0 | −15 | −29 | −44 | −59 | −74 | −88 | −104 | −118 | −133 |
| 30 | 25 | 13 | −2 | −18 | −33 | −48 | −63 | −79 | −94 | −109 | −125 | −140 |
| 35 | 27 | 11 | −4 | −20 | −35 | −51 | −67 | −82 | −98 | −113 | −129 | −145 |
| 40 | 26 | 10 | −6 | −21 | −37 | −53 | −69 | −85 | −100 | −116 | −132 | −148 |

(Wind speeds greater than 40 mph have little additional effect.)

(Little Danger (for properly clothed person.) Maximum danger of false sense of security.

Increasing Danger (Flesh may freeze within 1 minute.)

Great Danger (Flesh may freeze within 30 seconds.)

## TABLE 16-2  Estimating Wind Velocity from Simple Observations

| IF YOU SEE . . . | THE WIND IS PROBABLY BLOWING |
|---|---|
| Flags or pennants hanging limp from their staffs; smoke rising vertically from chimneys and open fires | 0–1 mph |
| Flags and pennants barely moving; leaves moving slightly on tress; smoke drifting lazily with the wind | 0–3 mph |
| Flags and pennants moving slightly out from their staffs; leaves rustling in trees; if you feel wind on your face | 4–7 mph |
| Flags and pennants standing out from their staffs at an angle of 30 to 40°; or leaves and twigs in constant motion | 8–12 mph |
| Small branches moving in tress; dust and paper being blown about | 13–18 mph |
| Flags and pennants flying at 90° angle; small trees swaying | 19–24 mph |
| Flags and pennants standing straight out from their staffs and fluttering vigorously; large tree branches in motion; or if you hear whistling in power lines | 25–31 mph |
| Flags and pennants whipping about wildly on the staffs; whole trees in motion; loose objects being picked up and blown about; or if you find it somewhat difficult to walk when facing the wind | 32–38 mph |
| Twigs being broken from trees; drivers having a problem in controlling their vehicles; or if you hear power lines whining loudly | 39–46 mph |
| Trees bending sharply; structural damage occurring in buildings; the progress of vehicles and pedestrians alike being seriously impeded | 47–54 mph |
| Trees being uprooted; considered structural damage occurring | 55–63 mph |
| Buildings suffering severe damage | 63–72 mph |
| Widespread destruction; or if walking is virtually impossible | more than 72 mph |

## HYPOTHERMIA

Hypothermia is a condition in which a person's internal body temperature has fallen below normal. It occurs when the body loses more heat than it produces, often as a result of being exposed to cold temperatures. Subfreezing temperatures are not necessarily needed for hypothermia to develop. Even in the summer, a tired hiker exposed to wind and rain may develop hypothermia.

### Effects

Two of the body's initial reactions to cold are goose pimples and shivering. If the heat produced by shivering does not keep up with the heat being lost, the body's temperature will fall. If the cooling process is not stopped, mental and physical changes will occur. The victim will appear discouraged or depressed. Movements will become slow and labored, even uncoordinated. Simple tasks such as fastening a zipper will be difficult. He will lose memory and judgment will fail completely. Also appearing is sleepiness and confusion. Hallucinations may occur. Loss of consciousness can happen; muscles can become stiff.

BOX 16-1

There are two recorded cases of victims surviving body temperatures as low as 60.8°F. Dorothy Mae Stevens (1929–74) was found in an alley in Chicago on February 1, 1951, and Vickie Mary Davis of Milwaukee, Wisconsin, at age 2 years 1 month was admitted to an Iowa hospital, in 1956, each with a temperature of 60.8°F. The little girl had been found unconscious on the floor of an unheated house and the air temperature had dropped to −24°F. Her temperature returned to normal after 12 hours and may have been as low as 59°F when she was first found.

— *Guinness Book of World Records*

*Types of exposure.* There are three types of exposure[2].

1. Acute or rapid onset most often results with cold water immersion. Cold water is defined as 70°F or lower. Acute exposure is six hours or less in duration.
2. Subacute exposure is defined as longer than six hours but less than twenty-four hours and involves a land-based experience or immersion in water warmer than 70°F. An example would be a person lying exposed much of the night to snow or rain and cold with clothing or shelter insufficient to maintain body core temperature.
3. Chronic or long-onset exposure happens after exposure to cold temperatures for more than twenty-four hours on land. This is how elderly people die in their homes or apartments.

*Water immersion hypothermia.* There are three basic types of water immersion experiences:[3]

Unprotected individuals. This is where there is a rapid disappearance of an unprotected (no flotation device) individual who either falls through ice or plunges into water below 70°F. Immersion of the face in cold water initiates the mammalian diving reflex, which reduces blood flow to all organs except the heart and brain. An individual may be protected from a drowning death for an extended period of time (thirty to forty-five minutes).

The second type of water immersion occurs when an individual enters cold water with no flotation device,but is able to struggle and swim or tread water to stay afloat for a short time, usually twenty minutes or less. These victims experience "shell" hypothermia in which the muscles become cold and lose their ability to contract and relax.

The third type of water immersion occurs when an individual enters cold water with a flotation device or survival suit or both. Often these individuals are in the water for an extended period of time, frequently many hours.

### Types of Hypothermia[4]

Hypothermia victims may be divided into those with mild hypothermia and those with severe hypothermia, with 90°F core body temperature being the dividing line. A clinical thermometer (one going below 90°F) is needed to measure this.

*Mild hypothermia.* For persons with a temperature above 90°F, shivering is likely. Muscles may be stiff and uncoordinated. They can usually walk, but frequently have a stumbling, staggering walk.

BOX 16-2

---

Chances of recovery from hypothermia:
- 91°F—Chances of normal recovery good
- 80-90°F—Victim will recover but there will be some sort of lasting damage
- Less than 80°F—Most will not survive

---

*Severe hypothermia.* At temperatures below 90°F, the mental and physical changes become marked. Mental derangement is present which includes confusion and disorientation proceeding to stupor and unconsciousness as the temperature continues to drop. Shivering usually stops and the victim cannot perform manual tasks. Muscles may become stiff and rigid, even simulating rigor mortis.

### Human Factors

Under certain circumstances, any individual can become hypothermic, but certain groups are especially susceptible to accidental hypothermia.

*Elderly.* The body's ability to adapt to temperature changes declines with advancing age. Accidental hypothermia is more common and more often fatal in the aged. One study estimated the mortality rate from hypothermia in the elderly at about 80 percent compared to 10 percent in the young. Often victims are found in houses or apartments where thermostats have been lowered due to economic reasons. The aged person living alone without attention from relatives or friends is especially vulnerable.

Many deaths attributed to heart attacks may actually be caused by hypothermia. Experts believe that the condition occurs much more often than is generally recognized. Dr. Richard W. Besdine of the Harvard Medical School estimates that 25,000 people over the age of 65 die each year from accidental hypothermia. A House Select Committee on Aging says that at least 60,000 senior citizens die annually because of cold weather. British researchers have found that an estimated 10 percent of the older population in Great Britain are affected. Health problems play a major role in making the elderly susceptible to hypothermia.

*Campers, hikers, and mountaineers (nonimmersion exposure).* These hypothermia victims generally are healthy and have no predisposing conditions other than external environmental exposure. Exposure accidents involve one or more of the following:

Bad weather, especially freezing temperatures, wind, and precipitation or moisture
Wetness
Physical exhaustion
Inadequate clothing, most frequently inadequate wind protection
Isolation from help
Inexperience and lack of training
Little subcutaneous fat

When clothing offers inadequate protection against the cold, heat loss due to nonimmersion hypothermia must be countered by exercise and thus, heat production. If one overworks, endurance time will be reduced but if one underexercises, hypothermia will result.

*Swimmers, divers, seamen, airmen, etc. (immersion hypothermia).* Water temperature is the most important factor contributing to immersion hypothermia. Body heat loss in water is about 25 times more than heat loss in air of the same temperature. The amount of heat loss will vary from individual to individual, depending on the amount of body fat, the clothing worn, and the extent of exercise.

Movement in cold water increases heat loss and is not recommended as it is for nonimmersion hypothermia. Movement increases blood flow to the extremities. Even a good swimmer should not attempt to swim to shore in cold water unless it is a short distance.

As little effort as possible should be expended in keeping afloat—a lifejacket or other floating aid is critical to survival. The U.S. Coast Guard has recommended that two or more persons huddle together facing each other. Persons alone should remain still and assume the fetal position, also known as HELP (Heat Escape Lessening Posture). Estimates on survival time showing the influence of flotation devices and level of activity are:

| SITUATION (50° WATER) | PREDICTED SURVIVAL TIME (HOURS) |
|---|---|
| NO FLOTATION | |
| Drownproofing | 1.5 |
| Treading water | 2.0 |
| WITH FLOTATION | |
| Swimming | 2.0 |
| Holding still | 2.7 |
| H.E.L.P. | 4.0 |
| Huddle | 4.0 |

In the absence of a flotation aid, treading water is preferable to utilizing the "drownproofing" technique in which one relaxes in the water and allows the head to submerge between breaths, since up to 50 percent of heat loss occurs through the head. Submerging the head in cold water hastens the loss of body heat.

Paradoxically, Dr. Martin Nemiroff, a noted expert on cold water drowning, in his work on resuscitation of near drowning victims, has shown that some individuals can be resuscitated after extended periods of time in cold water. Dr. Nemiroff states that the "mammalian diving reflex" is a major factor in such survivals. Immersion of the face in cold water initiates the diving reflex, which reduces blood flow to all organs except the heart and brain. If this effect is combined with hypothermia, which causes the metabolic demand of the brain to suddenly decline, an individual may be protected from a drowning death for an extended period, if aspiration of water has not been large. However, this is an unusual circumstance; the rule of treading water rather than drownproofing should be followed.

### Cold Injury Prevention

Proper clothing for cold weather provides insulation from cold, ventilation so that perspiration can evaporate, and protection against wind, rain, or snow. Avoid one bulky, heavy, or constricting garment. Instead, wear several layers of light, loose clothing that will trap air and provide adequate ventilation. Wool and polyester down substitutes retain some protective value when wet; cotton and goose or duck down do not.

For ideal protection, wear underclothing made of wool or polypropylene, a synthetic material. Wear layers of wool or synthetic down between underwear and the outer layer of a water-repellent and windproof covering. Waterproof clothing is *not* recommended since it holds in the moisture produced by the body. Protect the head and neck with a scarf and a hat or hood and the face with a mask. Wear two pairs of socks—both wool or one cotton and the other wool—and well-fitting boots high enough to protect the ankles. Inner soles made of a reflective material that retains heat normally lost to the ground are available.

BOX 16-3  *SAFE ICE THICKNESS MINIMUMS*

| | |
|---|---|
| Less than 2 inches | Stay off |
| 2 inches | One man on foot |
| 3 inches | Maximum of two men |
| 4 inches | Ice fishing station |
| 5 inches | Snowmobiles/all terrain vehicles |
| 8–12 inches | Passenger cars, light trucks |
| 24 inches | Commercial trucks, heavy equipment |

Hands are better protected by mittens than gloves. If you need to remove them frequently, wear lightweight gloves under the mittens to protect against heat loss if removing the mittens.

Clothing should not be too tight. Anything that hampers blood flow will increase the risk of frostbite. Do not remain in a sitting position for long periods since circulation of the blood can be impaired.

### Prevention of hypothermia among the elderly:

- Keep room temperature at a minimum of 65°F. A thermometer should be kept in the house and checked daily.
- Have an energy audit to identify ways to prevent heat loss from a home. These are often a free service of local electric companies.
- Advise against using fireplaces in extremely cold weather. If it is used, dampers should be closed soon after a fire is completely extinguished since heat will be lost up the chimney.
- Suggest that extra clothing be worn. Clothing should be worn in several loose-fitting layers. Hands and feet should be covered and a night cap or loose knitted hat worn during the day and night since half of all body heat is lost through the head.
- Make sure that someone checks in daily on elderly persons who live alone.

### Precautions to take when venturing into the out-of-doors:

- Be aware of hypothermia.
- Know your body and its limits. Get into condition before taking a trip into the wilderness.
- Know where you are going. Avoid becoming lost.
- Wear proper clothing. Cotton provides little protection against the cold, and when wet it allows the body to lose heat rapidly. It is best to dress in thin layers which trap air and thus provide good insulation. Wool is better than cotton. The outer layer should be wind and water resistant.
- Eat properly before any outdoor activity and take adquate food along. Avoid alcohol since it increases heat loss.

### Injury Control

Many people suffer frostbite and/or hypothermia when their cars break down in freezing weather. Keep protective clothing in the car if there is any risk of breakdown in an isolated area. When working on a car or snowmobile in the cold, avoid getting gasoline on the hands. While it does not freeze, it takes on the temperature of the surrounding area and cools the skin by evaporation. Avoid contacting metal with bare skin; try not to make repairs without gloves.

Avoid walking through the snow in low shoes. As a rule, stay in or close to the car since rescue teams are more likely to find the car because of size and location.

If the car breaks down and you are stranded in the cold, use the auto heater with a window open slightly to guard against carbon monoxide poisoning or, if possible, build a fire outside. Protect from the wind as much as possible. Avoid becoming wet from perspiration.

## HEAT INJURIES

During recent summer heat waves, deaths in the United States due to the heat were annually estimated at over twelve hundred. Add to that number the individuals who die not during a heat wave, and the problem grows even more serious. Moreover, many thousands of people suffer from one of the three heat-related injuries, but their accounts are never recorded.

BOX 16-4

> The highest dry-air temperature endured by naked men in U.S. Air Force experiments in 1960 was $400°F$ and for heavily clothed men $500°F$. (Steaks require only $325°F$ for cooking.) Temperatures of $284°F$ have been found quite bearable in sauna baths.
>
> *— Guiness Book of World Records*

BOX 16-5

> A temperature of $116°F$ was recorded for Willie Jones, age 51, of Atlanta, Georgia, on July 10, 1980 during a record-breaking heat wave. The $116°F$ was recorded after he had been immersed for 25 minutes in cold water. The attending physician said that his body temperature may have exceeded $120°F$ when first arriving at the hospital.
>
> *— UPI release*

### Effects

When exposed to excessive heat, the healthy person responds by sweating; the evaporation of sweat actually serves as our major cooling system. In addition, the blood vessels near the surface of the body automatically dilate to allow increased blood flow where surplus heat can be radiated to the outside world. Both of these events—sweating plus diversion of blood to skin vessels—can result in circulatory problems. Loss of salt and water through excessive sweating reduces overall blood volume. This, along with diversion of blood from vital organs (heart, brain, and kidneys) to the skin, can allow the body to withstand very high temperatures.

Two important factors—increased air humidity and decreased sweat amount and rate—can upset the balance of the body's cooling mechanism and heighten an individual's risk for one of the heat-related injuries. Air humidity limits and even may prevent the evaporation of sweat. Effective sweat evaporation diminishes rapidly at 60 percent relative humidity or higher and ceases at 75 percent. The mechanism is as severely impaired if sweat amount and rate decrease. A normal person can sweat about a quart an hour for two hours and lose up to 5 percent of body weight without overtaxing the mechanism. A 7 percent loss of body weight is definitely dangerous. The sweating mechanism may shut down to conserve water.

### Types of Heat Injuries

There are three types of heat-related injuries: heat cramps, heat exhaustion, and heat stroke.

*Heat cramps.* These are intermittent, painful contractions of muscles. These cramps often occur in individuals who replace the fluid lost in sweat by drinking water, but do not replace sodium. The sodium depletion is believed to be responsible for the cramps. Heat cramps usually occur in muscles that have been involved in strenuous activity—most often those of the legs. The cramps last a few minutes and generally disappear spontaneously.

*Heat exhaustion.* This is the most common heat-related injury. Excessive salt and/or water loss due to sweating account for the headache, dizziness, weakness, nausea, and vomiting. There is profuse sweating.

*Heat stroke.* This is the most serious of the heat-related injuries. It is characterized by a body temperature of at least 105°F and usually a lack of sweating because the body's heat regulatory activities are not functional, and the main avenue of heat loss (evaporation of sweat) is blocked. There are two basic kinds of heat stroke:

1. Exertional heat stroke can affect a healthy individual when the person works or plays with intensity. These victims may have moist, cool skin rather than the more expected hot and dry feel. Nevertheless, the body temperature will be elevated to 105°F or higher. High school athletes and military recruits are stricken most frequently.

2. Classic heat stroke is more apt to involve fluid and salt loss; it need not be associated with exertion at all. During periods of hot, humid weather, this disorder commonly affects the aged, the debilitated, the chronically ill, the obese, alcoholics, diabetics, and people with circulatory problems. Medications and drugs can increase the likelihood of heat stroke.

### Human Factors

Certain groups of people can be identified as high risk in relation to heat-related injuries.

*Age.* Heat afflicts people of all ages. However, the severity of the reaction tends to increase with age—heat cramps in a 17-year-old may be heat exhaustion in someone forty years old, and heat stroke in a person over sixty.

Advanced age is a characteristic strongly associated with risk of heat-related injuries. Infants under one year of age have also been reported to be at high risk.

Certain groups of young adults may also be at high risk. For example, military recruits, athletes, and those in certain occupations exposed to high temperatures are vulnerable since they are exposed to rigorous training and conditioning in hot, humid weather.

*Insufficient acclimatization.* An unacclimatized person working or exercising in hot weather develops higher core and skin temperatures and a higher heart rate.

*Lack of conditioning.* Less conditioned individuals seem to be less heat tolerant and take longer to acclimatize to heat.

*Dehydration.* Progressive dehydration can occur during a long work period or while running long distances, even though the person drinks ample water during his exertion. The important thing is the water level prior to the work or run period. Those who start exercising while dehydrated reach a higher core body temperature than they would if fully hydrated prior to working or exercising.

*Obesity.* Overweight people are less heat tolerant than people of normal weight. Obese people who do strenuous exercise are at much higher risk for heat-related injuries, especially fatal heat stroke.

*Prior heat stroke.* Several reports indicate that people who have a history of heat stroke have a deficient thermoregulatory capacity. It is not known whether such people inherit this tendency or whether their thermoregulatory capacity was affected during a heat stroke episode. However, other reports indicate that susceptibility to heat strokes due to prior experiences has not been medically substantiated.

*Health problems.* Individuals with such health problems as cardiovascular disease, kidney disease, diabetes, malnutrition, or alcoholism are vulnerable to heat-related injuries.

*Medications.* Those taking any of the three classes of medication that reduce the ability to sweat—diuretics ("water pills"); phenothiazines (the major tranquilizers); and anticholinergics (usually used for gastrointestinal disorders)—are in a high-risk group.

*Occupations.* Already mentioned are athletes and military personnel who are undergoing rigorous training and conditioning in hot, humid weather. Farmers are also in this high-risk group, especially during the harvest season when temperatures usually are high, and prolonged exposure may be necessary to gather the crops.

Table 16-3 shows the apparent temperature (how hot the weather feels) at various combinations of temperature and humidity. When the apparent temperature rises above 130°F, heatstroke may be imminent. Between 105°F and 130°F, heat cramps or heat exhaustion are possible. So is heatstroke, with prolonged exposure and physical activity. Between 90°F and 105°F, heat cramps and heat exhaustion are possible with lengthy exposure and activity. Heat stress varies with age, health, and body characteristics.

**TABLE 16-3   Apparent Temperature**

| RELATIVE HUMIDITY | AIR TEMPERATURE | | | | | | | | | | |
|---|---|---|---|---|---|---|---|---|---|---|---|
| | 70 | 75 | 80 | 85 | 90 | 95 | 100 | 105 | 110 | 115 | 120 |
| | APPARENT TEMPERATURE* | | | | | | | | | | |
| 0% | 64 | 69 | 73 | 78 | 83 | 87 | 91 | 95 | 99 | 103 | 107 |
| 10% | 65 | 70 | 75 | 80 | 85 | 90 | 95 | 100 | 105 | 111 | 116 |
| 20% | 66 | 72 | 77 | 82 | 87 | 93 | 99 | 105 | 112 | 120 | 130 |
| 30% | 67 | 73 | 78 | 84 | 90 | 96 | 104 | 113 | 123 | 135 | 148 |
| 40% | 68 | 74 | 79 | 86 | 93 | 101 | 110 | 123 | 137 | 151 | |
| 50% | 69 | 75 | 81 | 88 | 96 | 107 | 120 | 135 | 150 | | |
| 60% | 70 | 76 | 82 | 90 | 100 | 114 | 132 | 149 | | | |
| 70% | 70 | 77 | 85 | 93 | 106 | 124 | 144 | | | | |
| 80% | 71 | 78 | 86 | 97 | 113 | 136 | | | | | |
| 90% | 71 | 79 | 88 | 102 | 122 | | | | | | |
| 100% | 72 | 80 | 91 | 108 | | | | | | | |

*Degrees Fahrenheit.
Source: National Weather Service.

## Heat-Related Injury Prevention

Simple preventive measures that have been shown to be effective include:

1. Keep as cool as possible:
   a. Avoid direct sunlight.
   b. Stay in the coolest available location (it will usually be indoors).
   c. Use air-conditioning, if available.
   d. Use electric fans to promote cooling.
   e. Place wet towels or ice bags on the body or dampen clothing.
   f. Take cool baths or showers.
2. Wear lightweight, loose-fitting clothing.
3. Avoid strenuous physical activity, especially in the sun and during the hottest part of the day.
4. Increase intake of fluids, such as water and fruit or vegetable juices. Thirst is not always a good indicator of adequacy of fluid intake. Some studies indicate

that fluid intake in hot weather should be $1\frac{1}{2}$ times the amount that quenches thirst. Persons who are overweight or large in build or who are engaged in strenuous activities, such as sports, may require more than a gallon of fluid intake daily in very hot weather. Persons for whom salt or fluid is restricted should consult their physicians for instructions on appropriate fluid and salt intake.

5. Do not take salt tablets unless so instructed by a physician.
6. Avoid alcoholic beverages (beer, wine, and liquor).
7. Stay in at least daily contact with other people.

### Dehydration

Water is one of the first and most important needs. You may get along for weeks without food, but you cannot live long without water, especially in hot areas where you lose large quantities of water through sweating.

Many people do not realize how vital water is to the human body. While the average adult male body is about 63 percent water by weight, the average adult female body is only about 52 percent water. This difference is related to the fact that adipose tissue has a relatively low water content, and generally, females have greater proportions of adipose tissue. Also, obese people of either sex contain proportionally less body water than do lean people.

The importance of water cannot be overemphasized, since death occurs when water loss amounts to about 15 percent of the body weight, which can happen in about seven to ten days after complete deprivation of water.

A person can survive by drinking as little as one quart of fluid per day under the most ideal conditions, but one and one-half to two quarts of fluid is preferable, even in cold areas. If the climate is hot, the amount should be increased to three or four quarts. In very hot and/or humid conditions involving considerable sweating, four or five quarts of water might be necessary to prevent dehydration.

Infants, children, nursing mothers, the ill, and persons doing heavy physical work usually need more water.

In a healthy person, there is a balance between the intake and the output of water by the body as well as a normal distribution and balance of the body fluids and their electrolytes. Water intake from fluids and foods occurs by way of the gastrointestinal tract. Water is eliminated by the kidneys, gastrointestinal tract, skin, and lungs.

*Thirst.* Maintenance of an adequate intake of water is largely regulated by thirst when there is free access to water. Painful thirst has been experienced by very few Americans.

Water intake is under voluntary control; we can, of course, drink at will. There is, however, an unconscious control mechanism that tells us when we are thirsty. When water loss has reached 1 percent of the body weight, the sensation of thirst is experienced. In the hypothalamus of the brain is a region of nerve cells called the thirst center. When this area is stimulated by the presence of high salt concentrations in the body fluids, a reflex is started that produces the sensation of thirst. This stimulates us to drink and prompts the kidneys to conserve water. Thirst symptoms develop because the mouth and pharynx become dry (parched) as a result of declining saliva production. This produces discomfort in swallowing, and relief is obtained only by drinking (wetting the mouth does not work). The thirst reflex is much stronger than that of hunger, and the limit of endurance for thirst is a matter of days, whereas hunger can go on for weeks. When water loss reaches 5 percent of the body weight, a state of collapse ensues; when the water loss is over 10 percent of an individual's body weight, death is likely to occur (refer to Table 16-4).

While the thirst sensation provides helpful clues, it is far from an accurate indicator of the body's fluid needs. For example, regardless of the availability of water, most athletes do not consume enough to prevent a water deficit on hot, humid days. It has been shown that male athletes who are acclimated to the heat rarely drink more than two-thirds the fluids lost in sweat. It seems that fluid balance can only be maintained by taking frequent drinks, whether thirsty or not, prior to and during exercise, without reaching the point of discomfort. More than nine quarts of sweat can be lost in a hard day's work in hot weather. Clearly, then, the individual needs water replacement hour by hour.

There is an archaic practice of restricting fluids to athletes as a means of discipline, prevention of stomach cramps, or increasing performance. This has no scientific basis, and it leads to poor performance, early fatigue, and occasionally, serious illness and death. Fluids and salt loss through sweating must be replaced to keep the body in balance. Loss of salt encourages fluid loss and can lead to dehydration over a period of a few days or even hours. Experiments with subjects walking in the desert show that a person can lose as much as one quart of water per hour (two per hour is possible during exercise or while working under hot, humid conditions).

Fluid loss through sweating should be replaced as rapidly as possible. But water alone will not replace the minerals lost in sweat. To provide efficient replacement of lost minerals, pleasant-tasting drinks were developed. The three minerals lost in sweat—sodium, potassium, and chlorine—are called "electrolytes" due to

**TABLE 16-4   Signs and Symptoms of Dehydration**

| 1%-5% OF BODY WEIGHT | 6%-10% OF BODY WEIGHT | 11%-20% OF BODY WEIGHT |
| --- | --- | --- |
| Thirst | Dizziness | Delirium |
| Vague discomfort | Headache | Spasticity |
| Economy of movement | Dyspnea (labored breathing) | Swollen tongue |
| Anorexia (no appetite) | Tingling in limbs | Inability to swallow |
| Flushed skin | Decreased blood volume | Deafness |
| Impatience | Increased blood concentration | Dim vision |
| Sleepiness | Absence of salivation | Shriveled skin |
| Increased pulse rate | Cyanosis (blue skin) | Painful urination |
| Increased rectal temp. | Indistinct speech | Numbness of the skin |
| Nausea | Inability to walk | Anuria (decreased or deficient urination) |

their presence in the body as electrically charged particles (ions). Electrolytes control and maintain fluid exchange throughout the body to permit the constant flow of dissolved nutrients into the cell and remove waste products. The maintenance of body fluid and electrolyte balance is critical.

BOX 16–6

> "Water, water everywhere nor any drop to drink" (from *Rime of the Ancient Mariner* by Samuel T. Coleridge). A man adrift in the ocean with only seawater available cannot fulfill his thirst. Drinking salt water will not quench his thirst because the salt content of seawater is three times that of the blood. The excess ingested salt has to be excreted, and this requires more water than was consumed in the seawater. It is a losing battle, and the result is accelerated water loss and a quicker death.

### What is Dehydration?

Dehydration is the result of water imbalance in which the output exceeds the intake, causing a reduction of body water below normal. In other words, dehydration results when the body loses more fluid than it takes in.

People of any age can become dehydrated, but it develops more quickly and is most dangerous in small children. The kidneys of infants are less able to consume water than those of adults. Consequently, infants are more likely to become dehydrated than adults. Elderly persons also are more susceptible to developing water imbalances, because the sensitivity of their thirst mechanisms tends to decrease with age, and physical disabilities may make it difficult to obtain adequate fluids.

Therefore, dehydration can occur as a result of two basic situations: decreased intake or increased output.

*Decreased intake.*    Restriction of water intake can occur under many conditions. Examples are: mental patients who refuse to drink water, persons in an unconscious state or coma, those who find themselves in a hazardous situation with no drinking water (e.g., lost in the desert or adrift on the ocean), and paralyzed or physically handicapped people, who may find consumption of water difficult.

*Increased output.*    Reasons for abnormal water loss include: increased perspiration due to fever, warm environments, or increased physical activity (especially in warm, humid conditions).

### Signs and Symptoms of Dehydration

Military survival manuals describe three levels of dehydration based on the percentage of loss of body weight. The signs and symptoms resulting from these differing degrees of dehydration are listed in Table 16–4 in their usual order of appearance.

There are several good ways to test for dehydration:

- Little or no urine; the urine is dark yellow
- Sunken, tearless eyes
- Dry, sticky saliva
- Sunken "soft spot" on an infant's head
- Loss of elasticity of skin. Pinch a small amount of skin and hold it up for a second, like a little tent of flesh, and then release it. Normally, the skin pops down instantly to its previous position. If a person is dehydrated, their skin will remain raised and then *slowly* return to its previous position.

### Desert Survival

In the United States, a lot of people find crossing a desert almost unavoidable. Anyone who wants to get from Las Vegas to Los Angeles must cross the Mojave Desert. Anyone who wants to get from Salt Lake City to Reno must cross the Great Salt Lake Desert.

Most travelers cross American deserts in the comfort of their air conditioned cars. There are good highways right through the deserts, and as long as the traveler does not leave them, nothing much can really happen; regular patrols can bring assistance in case of trouble.

Tragedies in the desert usually occur only when inexperienced desert travelers leave the paved road despite the many warning notices.

Cases about desert tragedies make one thing clear: for anyone who has to survive in the desert, the heat of the day is the chief danger and can both cause and affect the lack of water. Temperatures reach amazing levels. In July 1913, the temperature was recorded at 134°F in the shade in the Great Salt Lake Desert. The temperature goes up to 176°F when the thermometer is put in the sand at noon during the summer. On the side of Interstate 15, which goes through the Mojave Desert, it has sometimes been 140°F in the shade at noon.

Everyone knows that people sweat in heat, but not everyone knows the reason for this. It is because human skin works like an air conditioning system in keeping the body temperature at about 98.6°F.

If the external temperature is extremely high, as in the desert, the sweat mechanism is utilized. The skin's millions of sweat glands secrete tiny drops of water which they take from the body cells and tissues. These drops evaporate leading to a cooling of the body.

The best-known work dealing with survival without water was carried out by Dr. E. F. Adolph and was based on experiments with volunteers and analyses of desert survivors' reports.

A man's capacity for survival depends on three related factors: the temperature of his surroundings, his physical activity during the survival period, and the amount of water he can get. For example, during the building of the Hoover Dam in the desert between Nevada and Arizona, there were workers who drank up to six and a half gallons a day. It has been reported that rangers in Death Valley consume three to five gallons of water daily.

Dr. Adolph constructed Table 16-5 showing how long a man can live with various temperatures (in the shade) assuming he is not physically active.

**TABLE 16-5  How Long Can a Man Survive in the Shade?**

| MAX. DAILY TEMP. SHADE DEGREES FAHRENHEIT: | WITH NO WATER | 1 qt. | 2 qt. | 4 qt. | 10 qt. | 20 qt. |
|---|---|---|---|---|---|---|
| | EXPECTED DAYS OF SURVIVAL | | | | | |
| 120 | 2 | 2 | 2 | 2.5 | 3 | 4.5 |
| 110 | 3 | 3 | 3.5 | 4 | 5 | 7 |
| 100 | 5 | 5.5 | 6 | 7 | 9.5 | 13.5 |
| 90 | 7 | 8 | 9 | 10.5 | 15 | 23 |
| 80 | 9 | 10 | 11 | 13 | 19 | 29 |
| 70 | 10 | 11 | 12 | 14 | 20.5 | 32 |
| 65 | 10 | 11 | 12 | 14 | 21 | 32 |
| 50 | 10 | 11 | 12 | 14.5 | 21 | 32 |

Source: E. F. Adolph's *Physiology of Man in the Desert.*

This table refutes the idea that people stranded in the desert can increase their survival chances by dividing up their water supplies so as to stretch the water supply over a longer period of time. The recommendation is to drink whenever you are thirsty, no matter how large or small your water supply is.

The information given by Dr. Adolph and other scientists shows that anyone standing in the hot sun needs three times as much water as those in the shade.

Anyone who keeps these few basic rules can greatly increase the chance of survival in the desert.

BOX 16-7

---

The *Guinness Book of World Records* reports the longest case of survival without food and water as being 18 days by an 18-year-old Austrian man who was put in a holding cell on April 1, 1979, but was totally forgotten by the police. On April 18, 1979, he was discovered close to death, having had neither food nor water.

---

### Small Children in Hot Cars

A study produced interesting facts about the hazard of a parked car in relation to heat stress. The highest temperatures were recorded in both cars with windows closed and cars parked in the direct sun. Small cars seemed to be worse in this regard. The inside car temperature rose faster, in the hotter part of the day, under direct sun exposure.

Ventilation is even more important than direct sunlight. Contrary to common belief, it has been found that partially open windows do not provide adequate ventilation.

The practice of leaving small children in cars and of elderly adults waiting in a parked car in the hot sun with inadequate ventilation is more widespread than recognized.

### Sunburn

Sunburn is one of the most common injuries to the human skin. A sunburn is caused by overexposure to ultraviolet rays, causing damage to the tissues of the skin. The nerves become inflamed, causing pain, and the small blood vessels become injured, causing redness, swelling, and leakage of plasma, which result in blister formation.

It is difficult for any individual to gauge accurately the amount of ultraviolet light the skin has received. It is not until after exposure that the redness, tenderness, and discomfort of sunburned skin confirm the person's error of judgment.

Most persons with normal skin can be adequately protected against burning by using a commercial sunscreen. However, certain individuals are so sensitive to the sun that they cannot be sufficiently protected by such preparations. The best "sunscreen" for these people is probably four walls and a roof. Opaque clothing provides better protection than the best chemical sunscreens.

To help individuals select an effective sunscreen, the system of rating products by the "skin protection factor" (SPF) has been developed. The higher the SPF number, the greater the protectiveness against sunburn. Individuals who usually burn easily and severely require a sunscreen with an SPF of eight or higher.

Choosing a sunscreen should be guided by the person's skin type and prior sun exposure. The likelihood for sunburning lessens during the summer, since the normal tanning response of the skin provides protection during subsequent exposures. Sunscreen effectiveness also is determined by how much is applied—the more the better. These products wash off through swimming or sweating.

Suntanning can create a sense of well being in most people, and the skin produces vitamin D after sun exposure. However, these benefits must be weighed against the negative effects—wrinkling, pigmented spots, atrophy, elastic tissue damage, etc. In short, sunlight is hazardous to the skin, especially in the development of skin cancer.

The public should be educated about the danger of ultraviolet light, and encouraged to be wise in outdoor activities. The regular use of hats and sunscreens also should be encouraged, especially for sun-sensitive, fair-skinned individuals.

Simple guidelines for suntanning without burning are:

1. *Midday exposure.* Avoid exposure at least from 10 A.M. until 2 P.M. solar time when the sun's short ultraviolet rays—the burning rays—are at their peak. Though the sun may seem as bright at 4 P.M. as it does at noon, the burning rays are reduced. Remember to adjust one hour for daylight saving time.

2. *Acclimating.* Limit exposure on the first day to fifteen minutes. If you do not burn, you can increase fifteen minutes a day to thirty to forty-five minutes per day. When you can tolerate forty-five minutes a day, extended time in the sun will usually not adversely cause a burn.

3. *Sunscreens.* These do not keep you from getting a tan; they only lessen the likelihood of burning.

4. *Cloudy day burns.* Some of the worst burns occur on days when the sun is not shining brightly.

5. *Temperature tricks.* You may feel cool because of the cooling effect of the water and lake breeze and still get a bad burn.

6. *Water.* Ultraviolet rays penetrate water. A burn can still result even if you spend the day immersed in water.

7. *Medications.* Some drugs cause an increased sun sensitivity.

8. *Vacations.* If you have not been exposed to the sun and are going into sunny climate, try to get two to three weeks of gradual exposure before you leave.

## NOTES

1. Alton L. Thygerson, *The First Aid Book,* 2nd ed. (Englewood Cliffs, N.J.: Prentice-Hall, Inc., 1986).

2. Cameron Bangs and Murray Hamlet, "Out in the Cold—Management of Hypothermia, Immersion, and Frostbite," *Topics in Emergency Medicine*, 2, no. 3 (October 1980), 20.

3. *Ibid.,* p. 21.

4. *Ibid.,* p. 25.

# 17

# Electric Current Injuries

## ELECTRICAL BURNS

Electrical burns are always worse than they seem. Electric current passing through tissues generates extreme heat. The wound can be very deceptive, with intact skin hiding massive tissue damage. Three to five percent of the admissions to major burn centers are victims of electrical burns.

Severe electrical burns occur when an individual makes contact with an electrical source in activities such as:

- linemen contacting "hot" wires
- persons contacting high tension lines through machinery
- persons installing television, CB, or other antennas
- parachutists and hang gliders falling into power lines
- children climbing power line poles
- others include being struck by lightning, children chewing through electrical cord insulation, children sticking pins or other metal objects into electrical outlets, among others

### Effects

There are six factors influencing the effects of electricity on the human body: (1) the type of current; (2) the value or intensity of the current; (3) the voltage or force of the current; (4) the resistance of the body; (5) the pathway of the current; (6) and the duration of contact.

There are two types of electrical current—alternating and direct. Alternating is more dangerous than direct current because of the severe muscular spasms that result. The victim is unable to let go of the energized object and consequently suffers a more serious injury. Direct current does not produce these strong muscular contractions.

The value or intensity of the current is measured in milliamperes. As the value of the current increases, so does the severity of the electrical injury. The effects of various current values range from a tingling sensation (1 milliampere) to painful sensation (5 milliamperes) to muscular contractions (15 milliamperes) to asphyxia (30 milliamperes) to ventricular fibrillation (60 milliamperes). Fifteen milliamperes is also known as the "let-go 'current'" or the maximum value of current from which a victim can manage to release his grip on the energized object. Beyond this, the current causes severe spasms of the muscles and prevents the victim from letting go of the source of electricity.

The force of the current is called the voltage. It is divided into two categories—low tension (currents of ten thousand volts or less) and high tension (currents of more than ten thousand volts). In general, the greater the voltage, the more extensive the injury.

Resistance of the body to electricity consists of both the resistance offered by the skin at the point of contact and internal resistance. After an electric current has penetrated the skin, it travels through the body along the lines of least resistance—usually the nerves and the blood vessels. As a rule, the greater the skin resistance, the more severe the local burn, whereas the lesser the skin resistance, the greater the systemic effort of the current.

The pathway of the current determines the severity of the injury as well. If the pathway does not include any of the vital organs—heart, lung, brain, kidney—the resulting injury is less likely to be fatal.

BOX 17–1

The only living man in the world to be struck by lightning 7 times is former Shenandoah Park Ranger Roy C. Sullivan (US), the human lightning-conductor of Virginia. His attraction for lightning began in 1942 (lost big toenail) and was resumed in July 1969 (lost eyebrows), in July 1970 (left shoulder seared), on Apr 16, 1972 (hair set on fire) and, *finally*, he hoped, on Aug 7, 1973: as he was driving along a bolt came out of a small, low-lying cloud, hit him on the head through his hat, set his hair on fire again, knocked him 10 feet out of his car, went through both legs, and knocked his left shoe off. He had to pour a pail of water over his head to cool off. Then, on June 5, 1976, he was struck again for the sixth time, his ankle injured. When he was struck for the *seventh* time on June 15, 1977, while fishing, he was sent to Waynesboro Hospital with chest and stomach burns.

— *Guinness Book of World Records*

The duration of contact also affects the outcome of the injury. The longer the duration of contact, the greater the damage.

### Human Factors

Death rates are highest among young adult males. The overall male:female ratio of 17:1 is one of the highest for all accidental deaths. Exposure of males to potentially dangerous situations is the logical explanation for their higher death rate.

### Environmental Factors

In rural areas the death rate from electric current is three times the rate in cities.

Deaths from electric current occur mainly in the summer. This may be partly related to seasonal patterns in construction and farm work. Also greater use of outdoor electrical equipment could be a factor during the summer.

### Prevention

Electrical injuries constitute nearly twelve hundred fatalities in the United States each year which could be prevented if safety guidelines were followed.

Houses should be checked to see if they are wired correctly. Inadequate wiring is indicated by any of these observations:

1. Lights dim when an appliance goes on
2. Fuses blow or circuit breakers trip out frequently
3. Toasters and irons fail to heat properly
4. TV picture shrinks
5. Motors slow down

One of the most common hazards in the home is misuse of electrical cords. The type of cord should be appropriate for the equipment used. Cords should be inspected for signs of wear, especially at plugs and connections (wear can cause shocks, shorts, or fires). Cords should be placed where they will not be tripped over or be exposed to excessive wear (examples: under rugs, through doorways). They should not be twisted, crushed or placed near heat or in water. When disconnecting the cord from the wall outlet, the plug itself should be pulled.

Safety principles should be used around electrical appliances as well. An electrical appliance should never be turned on by a person standing on a wet floor and should not be immersed in water. Touching a metal object and an appliance at the same time or touching appliances with wet hands is dangerous. An appliance should be unplugged before cleaning and disconnected if it sparks or stalls. Electrical outlets and extension cords should not be overloaded.

Those who work outdoors should also be cautious. Ladders, aluminum siding, and other equipment should not be placed near or against power lines. Antennas are unwieldy and difficult to handle and can easily fall against power lines, causing injury or death. Therefore, antenna installations should be left to experts. Before digging or planting, one should know the location of underground wires.

Safety must be stressed for children. Children should not play in trees that have wires running through them. Flying kites or model airplanes is best done in open fields—away from electrical wires. If the toy becomes entangled with overhead wires, children should be told not to attempt to get it down and not to touch any dangling wires or strings. Youngsters should not climb supporting structures for power lines or enter substations and transformer vaults.

## LIGHTNING INJURIES

Lightning is responsible for more deaths than any other type of stormy weather phenomenon. The general lack of respect for lightning may be attributed to the fact that limited publicity is given to deaths by lightning and that most reported incidents involve only one or two persons. Floods and tornadoes are more likely to make headlines because they affect larger areas and often cause multiple deaths, injuries, and widespread damage. Nevertheless, the average annual death toll for lightning is greater than for tornadoes or hurricanes.

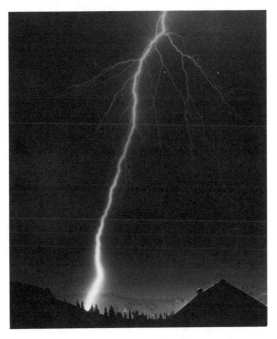

**FIGURE 17-1** Lightning is responsible for more deaths than any other type of stormy weather. Photo courtesy of the National Oceanic and Atmospheric Administration.

**TABLE 17-1  Electrical Trouble Shooting Guide**

| SYMPTOM | POSSIBLE CAUSES | CORRECTIVE ACTION |
|---|---|---|
| Fuse blows or circuit breaker trips frequently | Fuses only: temporary overload caused by starting current in motors. | Replace fuses with dual-element time-delay type. |
| | Overloaded circuit | Check wattage of lights and appliances on circuit (1800 watts maximum for 15 amp circuit and 2400 watts maximum for 20 amp). |
| | Short Circuit | Turn off all lights and unplug all appliances. If fuses still blow or circuit breakers trip, the trouble is in the wiring, a switch, receptacle or other built-in device. A qualified electrician is needed. Check all plugs for evidence of burning or sparking. Repair or replace. If trouble is still not found, turn on lights and plug in appliances one by one. When defective device is found, disconnect until repaired or replaced. |
| | Circuit breaker only: possibly defective | Replace breaker. |
| Lights flicker or dim periodically | Temporary overload caused by motor starting | Not harmful; put motor on separate circuit if trouble is annoying. |
| | Wiring inadequate | Install heavy-duty wiring for high-amperage appliances; use No. 10 or No. 12 wiring to outlying buildings. |
| | Inadequate electric service | Add wattage of all lights, appliances and motors you use at the same time. If they exceed the rating of the electrical service into your home, a larger service must be installed. |
| | Loose connections with aluminum wiring | See last item. |
| | Power supply or service entrance problems | Contact your power company. |

228

**TABLE 17-1 Continued**

| SYMPTOM | POSSIBLE CAUSES | CORRECTIVE ACTION |
|---|---|---|
| Air conditioner runs slowly | Excessive voltage drop in home wiring, or | Have new separate circuit installed for air conditioner. |
| | Use of improper extension cord. | Put in new circuit or use an extension cord with 14 gauge wire. |
| Odor of burning insulation | Defective ballast in fluorescent light. | Replace ballast. |
| | Overloaded or defective extension cord or power cord. | Replace with proper size cord. |
| | High resistance fault in electrical appliance or lighting assembly. | Check each appliance or light assembly for odor or excessive heat. Replace or repair. |
| | Loose connection and high resistance fault at receptacle, switch or fixture. | Shut off power and tighten connections. See last item, this page. |
| Shock from electrical appliance | Defective wiring or loose connection | Unplug until repaired. |
| TV picture shrinks | Refrigerator or other motor starting. | Switch appliance to another circuit. |
| Cover plates over outlets, switch receptacles or lighting assemblies hot, particularly when not in use | Loose wiring connection. | Shut off power and tighten connections. Refer to Underwriters' Laboratories Bulletin 48, Aluminum Building Wires & Connectors, available from UL, 207 E. Ohio St., Chicago 60611, or consult your electrician. |

**WARNING:** NEVER MAKE REPAIRS TO ANY ELECTRICAL WIRING UNLESS THE POWER IS DISCONNECTED BY OPENING THE CIRCUIT BREAKER OR REMOVING THE FUSES.

TABLE 17–2   Location of Lightning Deaths and Injuries

| LOCATIONS | DEATHS | INJURIES |
|---|---|---|
| Open fields, ball fields, etc. | 27% | 28% |
| Under trees | 17% | 14% |
| Boating, fishing and water related | 13% | 5% |
| Tractors, heavy road equipment, etc. | 6% | 3% |
| Golf courses | 4% | 4% |
| Telephones | 1% | 3% |
| Various other and unknown locations | 32% | 43% |

Source: H. N. Vigansky, *Storm Data*, 1983.

Between January 1940 and December 1976, lightning is reported to have killed more than 7,500 Americans and injured more than 20,000 others. This means annual averages of about 200 killed and 550 injured. But because incomplete reporting has produced conservative numbers, the actual death toll is probably double the reported number.

One interesting fact is that 80 percent or more of both deaths and injuries from lightning occur to males. This is undoubtedly because the situations in which large groups are most often struck are quite frequently male oriented: football and baseball games, fairs, golf matches, camping, picnicking, outdoor work, and outdoor military training.

Proximity to water appears to be an important factor. Farmers, ranchers, and others in outdoor occupational groups are especially vulnerable to lightning strikes. Furthermore, use of the telephone and of CB and other radio equipment is related to lightning incidents.

BOX 17–2

> Excluding lightning bolts, the highest reported voltage electric shock survived was one of 230,000 volts by Brian Latasa, 17, on the tower of an ultrahigh voltage power line in Griffith Park, Los Angeles, November 9, 1967.
>
> — *Guinness Book of World Records*

The risk of being struck by lightning is greater than we tend to think. It is estimated that some eighteen hundred thunderstorms are in progress over the earth's surface at any given moment, and that lightning strikes the earth one hundred times each second.

Some portions of the globe are far more vulnerable to lightning than others. The greatest frequency of lightning is on the island of Java, where thunderstorms occur on the average of 223 days of the year. Within the United States, lightning occurs most frequently in Florida. Florida has an average of ten or more reported lightning deaths annually. There is an ample supply of moisture in Florida from the surrounding water, and the solar heating of the land lifts the moist air. The result-ing cumulonimbus clouds extend to several miles in height and produce regions in Florida that have about ninety days of thunderstorm a year.

### How Lightning Works

Lightning is an electrical charge which flashes not from cloud to earth—as it sometimes appears—but from earth to cloud. When storm clouds gather, the wild turbulence inside them results in a separation of electrical charges. Usually, negative charges accumulate in the lower part of the cloud, while positive charges build up in the earth and in the upper part of the cloud. Lightning occurs when the attraction between these opposite charges becomes strong enough to bridge the gap separating them.

An imperceptible stroke "leader" advances from the cloud step by step toward the ground, establishing the path the stroke will take. When it nears the ground, an avalanche of charges rushes upward through the conducting path, re-uniting positive and negative charges (or ions). This return stroke produces the brilliant flash and the clap of thunder. The leader will follow the path of least re-sistance. It may seek out a tree, a chimney, or a human—or whatever provides the shortest gap and the best conductor.

Lightning may contain as much as half a million amperes. The intense heat generated when lightning strikes directly often causes all the sap in a tree to boil instantaneously and evaporate.

The average bolt is about ½ to ¾ inch thick. It is surrounded by a four-inch-thick channel of super-heated air. The length of a stroke may vary from two thousand to fifteen thousand feet or more.

### Effects

When lightning strikes the human body, it sometimes only causes burns and tissue destruction, injuries that do not necessarily cause death. Far more serious effects are the loss of respiration and interference with the rhythmic beat of the heart (ventricular fibrillation).

Most victims are not struck directly. People hit while standing under a tree,

BOX 17-3 *UNUSUAL BUT TRUE*

Shoe salesman Ernie Ramos wore a pair of old tennis shoes on his last fish-ing trip, and his choice of wardrobe apparently saved his life.

Ramos, 26, said from his hospital room the rubber soles on his sneakers acted as insulation when he was struck by a bolt of lightning during a fishing trip. He said doctors expect he will regain full use of his right arm and hand, which were burned when he was struck by the "bright blue flash" at Calavaras Lake.

— *San Antonio, Texas (UPI)*

for example, usually get only a small part of the current that passes through the tree and onto the surface of the ground. But the human body cannot tolerate more than a very small amount of electricity. A fraction of an ampere for one or two seconds can easily cause death.

When a victim is struck by lightning, he sustains a high voltage injury from an electrical charge far more intense than the so-called high tension wires carrying electricity to man's machinery.

After the lightning bolt strikes the skin, there will be a charred and depressed entrance and exit wound. The entrance wound may be surrounded by a spider-like or zigzag burn. The burned area will be red, hot, sensitive and swollen with a varying number of blisters eventually forming in the area.

### Prevention

Some parts of the day are riskier than others. According to studies, about 70 percent of lightning injuries and deaths occur in the afternoon, 20 percent between 6:00 P.M. and midnight, 10 percent between 7 A.M. and noon, and fewer than 1 percent from midnight to 6:00 A.M. Lightning is also far more common from May through September than in other months.

Armed with these facts, protect yourself when a thunderstorm threatens. Get inside a home or large building, or inside an all-metal (not convertible) vehicle. Inside a home, avoid using the telephone, except for emergencies. If you are outside, with no time to reach a safe building or an automobile, follow these rules:

Do not stand underneath a natural lightning rod such as a tall, isolated tree in an open area.

Avoid projecting above the surrounding landscape, as you would do if you were standing on a hilltop, in an open field, on the beach, or fishing from a small boat.

Get out of and away from open water.

Get away from tractors and other metal farm equipment.

Get off and away from motorcycles, scooters, golf carts, and bicycles. Put down golf clubs.

Stay away from wire fences, clotheslines, metal pipes, rails, and other metallic paths which could carry lightning to you from some distance away.

Avoid standing in small, isolated sheds or other small structures in open areas.

In a forest, seek shelter in a low area under a thick growth of small trees. In open areas, go to a low place such as a ravine or valley. Be alert for flash floods.

If you are hopelessly isolated in a level field or prairie and you feel your hair stand on end—indicating lightning is about to strike—drop to your knees. Do *not* lie flat on the ground. This will ensure that as small an area as possible is touching the ground and will minimize the danger of your body acting as a conductor.

# 18

# Disasters

Disaster is a fact of life. Each year thousands of disasters, large and small, natural and man-made, strike somewhere in the United States. These catastrophes range from airplane crashes involving just a few casualties to hurricanes, tornadoes, and earthquakes with massive destruction.

BOX 18-1

We fear things in proportion to our ignorance of them.

*— Livy*

Strangely enough, most people survive emergency disaster situations. Good luck and sheer willpower often have a lot to do with survival. Training about disasters needs to be modified from a "nice-to-know" to a "must-know" requirement.

Numerous, valuable facts about disasters are discussed in this chapter. For example:

- What kinds of disasters are to be expected?
- What will be their characteristics?
- When can disasters be expected?

## RIVER FLOODS

In popular usage "river flood" simply describes an overflow of water from a river onto normally dry land. Professionally speaking, a river is "in flood" when its waters have risen to a height at which damage from the force of currents and inundation can occur in the absence of protective works.

Devastating floods occur in almost every part of the United States. For the United States in recent years, the average yearly death toll as a result of floods has been eighty-three, with annual losses in property damage totaling $1 billion.

Certain areas such as the Pacific Northwest, the Rocky Mountain and Great Basin areas, and part of Southern California experience floods only during well-defined seasons. On the other hand, along the southeastern and Gulf coasts, floods occur without any pronounced seasonal pattern. There are yet other areas—the Northeast and in the basins of the Ohio and Mississippi rivers—where a great flood may occur at any time of the year but where most floods occur during a fairly well-defined flooding season.

By analyzing records of stream flow and other data, the probable frequency of floods for a given river can be estimated. For example, a flood might be referred to as a "ten-year flood," meaning that a flood of this size occurs about once in ten years. However, it is impossible to predict accurately that such a flood will occur in any particular year.

The immediate effects of floods are brought by inundation and the force of currents. Flood damage can lead to costly deprivations. Many people are left homeless. Forced evacuations can separate family members. Transportation, communica-

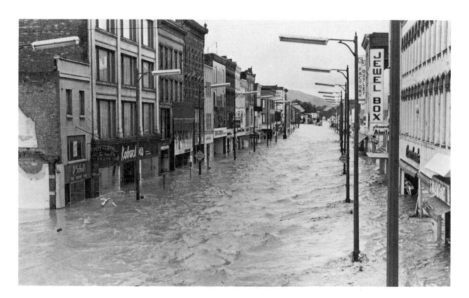

**FIGURE 18-1**  Flood waters. Photo courtesy of FEMA.

tion, and rescue services can be seriously disrupted—when medical emergencies are at a peak. Water may be contaminated through broken water and sanitary systems.

Although floods are notoriously unpredictable—some providing ample warning, others taking the countryside by surprise—conditions that give rise to flooding are generally well known.

The primary sources of this excess water are abnormally heavy rainfall and runoff from large accumulations of packed snow. Flooding from snowpack is caused by rising temperatures, sometimes accompanied by rainfall, that melt the snow rapidly. Other causes of flood include ice jams blocking the river flow, dam failures, and destroyed watersheds.

## FLASH FLOODS

In flash floods, swift currents can be especially vicious, and the potential for devastation is compounded by the fact that flash floods often occur with little or no warning. Overtaken suddenly by a wall of churning water and debris, people and animals are swept downstream, injured, and drowned. In recent years, flash floods have taken an average of more than one hundred lives a year and have been reported in almost every region of the United States.

Most flash floods occur in mountainous areas, where torrential thunderstorms can change trickling brooks into raging torrents. On small streams, especially near the headwaters of river basins, water levels may rise quickly in heavy rainstorms, and flash floods can begin before the rain stops falling.

Rainfall of more than four inches in a few hours is recorded many times each year; in the United States, the record rainfall for one hour exceeds ten inches. Under such conditions, there is little time between detection of flood conditions and the arrival of the flood crest.

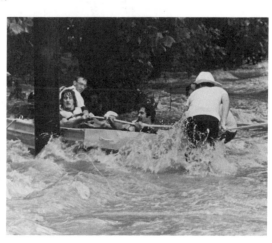

**FIGURE 18-2** Flash-flood rescue operations. Photo courtesy of the National Oceanic and Atmospheric Administration.

## TORNADOES

The tornado is a violent local storm with whirling winds of tremendous speed. It appears as a rotating, whirlpool-shaped cloud that extends toward the ground from the base of a thundercloud—the familiar and frightening tornado funnel. It is from the twisting spiral updraft that tornadoes have been dubbed "twisters." These small, short-lived storms are the most violent of all storms and, over a small area, the most destructive.

Tornadoes do their destructive work through the combined action of strong rotary winds, flying debris, and the partial vacuum in the center of the vortex. As a tornado passes over a building, the winds twist and rip at the outside walls, while the reduced pressure in the tornado's "eye" causes an explosive pressure difference between the inside and outside of the building.

People are highly vulnerable. Often, with little or no warning and in a matter of seconds, a tornado can transform a thriving street into a ruin. Death and injury result from the disintegration or collapse of buildings, debris driven by the high winds, flash flooding caused by the accompanying downpour, and electrocution from fallen utility lines.

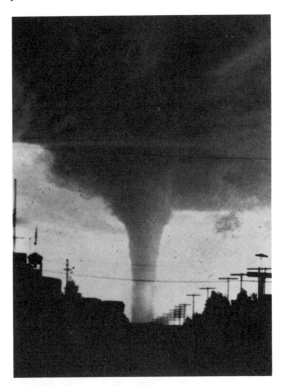

**FIGURE 18-3** Tornadoes are most likely to be killers when they are least expected. Photo courtesy of the National Oceanic and Atmospheric Administration.

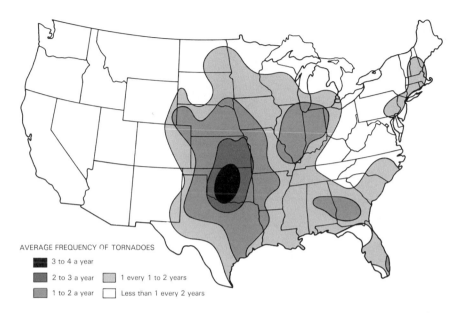

AVERAGE FREQUENCY OF TORNADOES

■ 3 to 4 a year

■ 2 to 3 a year    ▨ 1 every 1 to 2 years

▨ 1 to 2 a year    ☐ Less than 1 every 2 years

**FIGURE 18–4** Where U.S. tornadoes occur most often. Source: National Oceanic and Atmospheric Administration.

Tornadoes are almost exclusively an American problem; they have been reported in areas outside the United States, but not often. In the United States, they have occurred in all fifty states, in every season of the year.

Normally, the number of tornadoes is lowest during December and January and highest in May.

Reliable statistical records on tornadoes date back only to 1953. An average of 622 tornadoes occur each year in the United States, about half of them during April, May, and June. Average annual frequency by states for this period ranges from 104 tornadoes in Texas to fewer than three in most of the northeastern and far western states.

Tornadoes may occur at any hour of the day or night, but they form most readily during the warmest hours of the day. Most tornadoes (82 percent) occur between noon and midnight, and the greatest single concentration (23 percent) falls between 4:00 P.M. and 6:00 P.M.

Tornadoes typically form during warm, humid, unsettled weather, when there is a squall line of severe thunderstorms. Sometimes two or more tornadoes are associated with a parent thunderstorm. As the thunderstorm moves, tornadoes may form at intervals along its path, travel for a few miles, and then dissipate.

The forward speed of tornadoes has been observed to range from almost no motion to 70 mph. On the average, tornado paths are only an eighth of a mile wide and are seldom more than ten miles long. However, there have been spectacular in-

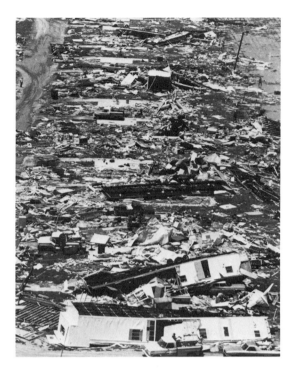

**FIGURE 18-5** Tornado destruction of mobile homes. Photo courtesy of NOAA.

stances in which tornadoes have caused heavy destruction along paths more than a mile wide and almost three hundred miles long.

## HURRICANES

A hurricane is a large spiral of winds blowing at speeds of 74 mph or higher around a relatively calm center—the "eye."

The practice of naming hurricanes with female names began during World War II and was the official National Weather Service policy from 1953 to 1978. Now, however, the practice is to use male and female names alternately. The first tropical storm of a season is given a name beginning with the letter A, then the second storm's name begins with a B, and so on.

Usually people are most vulnerable to the ravages of hurricanes during the initial phase. Death and injury usually result from drowning, flying debris, and electrocution from downed utility lines.

On the average, the area that contains winds with speeds of at least 74 mph covers some 100 miles in diameter, while gale-force winds—exceeding 40 mph—extend over an area 400 miles in diameter. Its spiral—counterclockwise in the Northern Hemisphere and clockwise in the Southern Hemisphere—is marked by heavy cloud bands.

Over the years, the toll in lives exacted by hurricanes has diminished. In the United States, this reduction has resulted primarily from timely warnings. Most death and destruction is caused by wind, floods, and—most lethal of all—storm surges.

Along the Atlantic and Gulf Coasts, the normal hurricane season extends from June through November. The record number of Atlantic hurricanes in a single season is twenty-one.

Because the amount of energy associated with hurricanes is so immense, there is as yet no satisfactory way of modifying or controlling them. Our best hope is that with early warning and other precautionary measures, we can minimize losses in human life and property.

## FOREST, BRUSH, AND GRASS FIRES

Man is responsible for 65 percent of the thirty thousand forest, brush, and grass fires that annually occur throughout the United States. Arsonists and debris burners are responsible for about 21 percent and 16 percent, respectively. Lightning, which accounts for about 35 percent of the fires over the entire United States, is the leading cause of forest fires in the western part of the country.

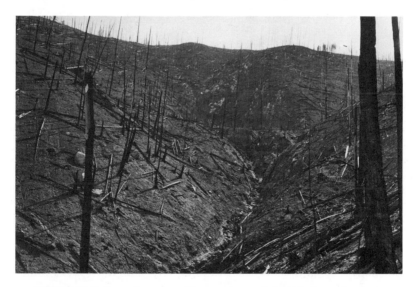

**FIGURE 18-6**  Burned over area. Photo courtesy of the U.S. Forest Service.

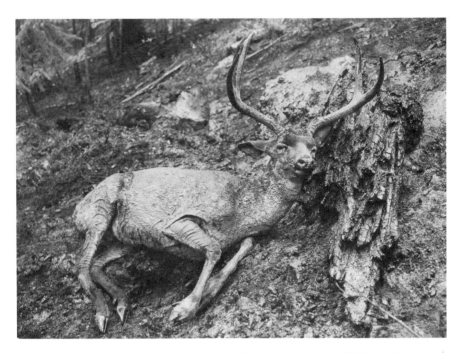

**FIGURE 18-7**   Forest fires destroy wildlife. Photo courtesy of the U.S. Forest Service.

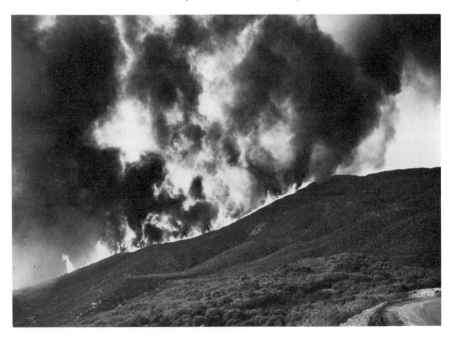

**FIGURE 18-8**   Brush fire. Photo courtesy of the U.S. Forest Service.

Loss of life, although not usually as high as in other disasters, is a too-frequent tragedy in fire disasters.

In the East, the normal fire seasons are spring and fall, while severe weather conditions may cause them to extend through the summer and winter months. In the West, the normal fire danger period develops during the dry summer months. This whole pattern can be materially altered by changes in weather and forest fuels and by the carelessness of man. A drought or a prolonged dry spell threatens with a continuous fire potential until sufficient precipitation occurs.

## EARTHQUAKES

The actual earth movement of an earthquake is seldom a direct cause of death or injury. However, this movement causes the collapse of buildings and other structures. Most casualties result from: (1) falling bricks and plaster; (2) splintering glass; (3) toppling furniture, collapsing walls, falling pictures and mirrors; (4) sea waves generated by earthquakes; and (5) fire caused by broken gas lines and spillage of gasoline and other flammables.

Several million earthquakes occur annually throughout the world. They range from barely perceptible tremors to catastrophic shocks. Most earthquakes originate beneath the sea, where they cause little concern—unless they create tsunamis. About seven hundred shocks each year may be classed as strong—that is, capable of causing considerable damage where they occur.

There are well-defined seismic belts stretching over large areas of the world. Earthquakes in these well-defined belts are to be expected; but great shocks also

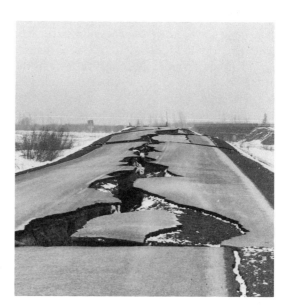

**FIGURE 18-9** Earthquake damage. Photo courtesy of the U.S. Army.

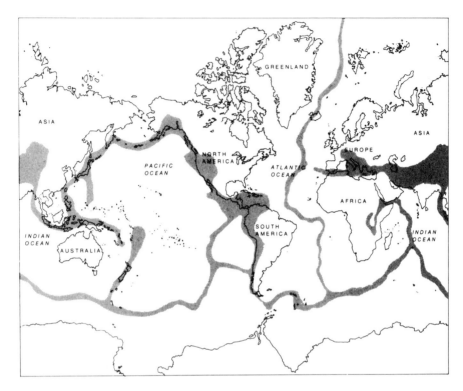

**FIGURE 18-10**  Major seismic belts of the world. Source: NOAA.

occur occasionally outside these belts. The cities of the Pacific Coast are therefore not alone in their vulnerability to earthquakes, for the threat also exists in many areas ordinarily considered only moderately seismic. As a matter of fact, there is seismic activity in all regions of the United States.

Earthquake-prone areas include some of the most densely populated regions of the world, such as Japan, the western United States, and the shores of the Mediterranean Sea.

The loss of life in the United States has been relatively light, considering the number of destructive earthquakes that have occurred. This is explained partially by better-than-usual construction practices, but more by fortuitous circumstances, such as the majority of the people being in relatively safe places at the time of earthquakes.

## TSUNAMI

A tsunami (pronounced soo-'nah-mee) is a train of ocean waves created by disturbances—usually earthquakes—in the ocean floor. The term tidal wave is sometimes used, but this is inaccurate, because tsunamis have almost nothing to do with tides.

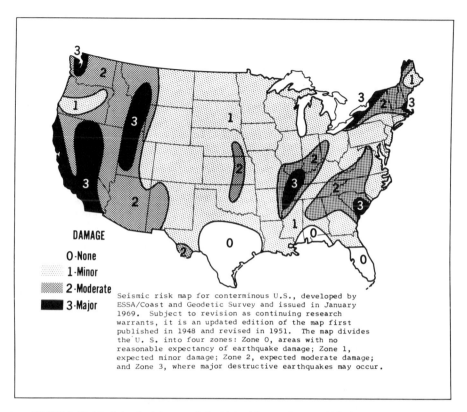

Seismic risk map for conterminous U.S., developed by
ESSA/Coast and Geodetic Survey and issued in January
1969. Subject to revision as continuing research
warrants, it is an updated edition of the map first
published in 1948 and revised in 1951. The map divides
the U. S. into four zones: Zone 0, areas with no
reasonable expectancy of earthquake damage; Zone 1,
expected minor damage; Zone 2, expected moderate damage;
and Zone 3, where major destructive earthquakes may occur.

**FIGURE 18-11** Seismic risk map of the United States. Source: U.S. Geological Survey.

Tsunami waves are enormously destructive to life and property and have been responsible for some of the worst disasters in history.

Tsunamis generally occur only in and around the Pacific Ocean. Since 1900, more than 180 tsunamis have been recorded in the Pacific. Of these, 34 caused damage near the source only, and 9 were destructive both locally and distantly. Japan is the most frequent victim; but other areas such as the Aleutian Islands, Hawaii, and Chile are especially susceptible. Historically, a tsunami of major proportions has struck the United States or its Pacific possessions on the average of once every eight years.

Once waves are generated, they speed silently across the open ocean at velocities approaching 600 mph. The wave may be only two feet high in mid-ocean, but its tremendous energy is revealed in the long period between crests—from fifteen minutes to two hours. When the waves enter shallow water along a coast, they are slowed to less than 40 mph. Then the tsunami waves become roaring monsters of a hundred feet or more.

Current standards tentatively define hazard areas on Pacific coasts as follows: areas within one mile of the coast and lower than fifty feet above sea level are danger areas for tsunamis of distant origin; and areas within one mile of the coast and lower than a hundred feet above sea level are danger areas for tsunamis of local origin. Tsunamis cause such devastation that the affected areas are generally left devoid of all housing and vital services.

Early warning and well-organized evacuation procedures are the best short-term measures. If warning is received early enough (two to five hours), people can be evacuated.

## LANDSLIDES

The United States was, until recently, considered less susceptible to disasters from landslides because most of its mountainous areas are not heavily populated. However, growth in populated areas has begun to push steadily into marginal areas.

Landslides involve great amounts of material which move with tremendous force and often at startling velocity. Everything in the path of a large slide is destroyed.

Available data indicate that slides are not common on slopes of less than five degrees or where the mean annual precipitation is less than ten inches.

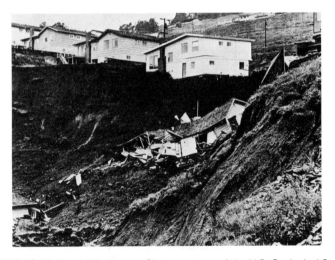

**FIGURE 18-12**   Landslide damage. Photo courtesy of the U.S. Geological Survey.

## WINTER STORMS

Winter storms are generated, as many summer thunderstorms, along the boundaries called "fronts," between polar and tropical air masses.

Nearly everyone east of the Pacific coastal ranges remembers significant winter storms—days of heavy snow, interminable blizzards, inconvenience, economic loss, and sometimes, personal tragedy. Winter brings them all.

Every winter is probably a bad year for some portion of the country—and winter storms can kill without breaking weather records. The danger is persistent, year after year. Of reported deaths from winter storms, more than a third are attributed to automobile and other accidents; just under one-third to overexertion, exhaustion, and consequent fatal heart attack; fewer than one-quarter to exposure and fatal freezing; and the remainder to such causes as home fires, carbon monoxide poisoning in stalled cars, falls on slippery walks, electrocution from downed wires, and building collapse.

## AVALANCHES

Avalanches are steadily becoming more of a hazard to reckon with in the United States, as logging and mining operations, resorts, and recreational homesites move into mountain areas and as Americans spend more time skiing, snowshoeing, snowmobiling, and doing other winter activities. Every year, more and more people are caught by avalanches.

Although avalanches kill people in many ways, the great majority of fatalities are caused by suffocation. In a typical avalanche burial, little air is trapped in the space around the victim, and it is only a matter of time until he loses consciousness and dies. The weight of snow bears down on the victim's throat and chest and fur-

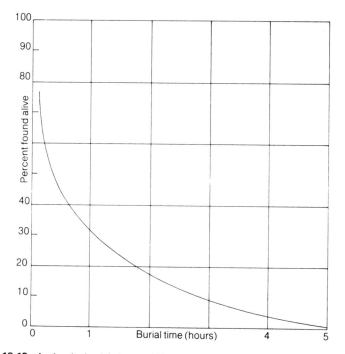

**FIGURE 18-13** Avalanche burial time and likelihood for survival. Source: U.S. Forest Service.

ther accelerates respiratory failure. The snow usually packs so tightly that the victim is immobilized and must helplessly await his fate.

Some victims are killed outright or severely injured by the moving avalanche. The victim may be dashed into a tree or building or hit by flying debris. Head injuries, abdominal injuries, and broken necks, backs, and legs are common. Some victims die of hypothermia, exhaustion, or shock. Fewer than 20 percent of those who are buried with no trace showing above the snow are recovered alive.

Statistics compiled in Switzerland and in the United States show that the victim's chance of survival diminishes rapidly with burial time and depth of burial. Statistically, after half an hour of burial, the victim's chance of surviving is about 50 percent. A victim often cannot survive a fifteen-minute burial in an unfavorable position (snow packed tightly around mouth and nose). This is understandable, since a person usually loses consciousness about 45 to 120 seconds after breathing stops. Nevertheless, if the victim is buried in a favorable position, without snow packed tightly around his mouth and nose, he may survive for hours.

## HEAT WAVES

Most people survive heat waves, and they tend to remember them only as periods of sweltering discomfort; seldom are we impressed by death tolls resulting from heat waves. However, in a "normal" year, about 175 Americans die from summer heat and too much sun. Among natural hazards, only winter storms and lightning—not hurricanes, tornadoes, floods, or earthquakes—take a greater average toll.

Studies show that heat waves afflict people of all ages. However, the severity of the reaction tends to increase with age.

## VOLCANOES

The U.S. Geological Survey has issued a study that shows that other volcanoes in the United States could, in the near future, follow Mount St. Helens in erupting and devastating large areas. Though most volcanoes in the U.S. are considered dormant, the threat of volcanic eruptions in the near future has not diminished.

Volcanoes considered most likely to erupt in the future (have cycles of 100 to 200 years) are listed according to their likelihood of erupting in the near future:

1. Mount St. Helens, Washington
2. Mono Inyo Craters, California
3. Lassen Peak, California
4. Mount Shasta, California
5. Mt. Rainier, Washington
6. Mount Baker, Washington
7. Mount Hood, Oregon

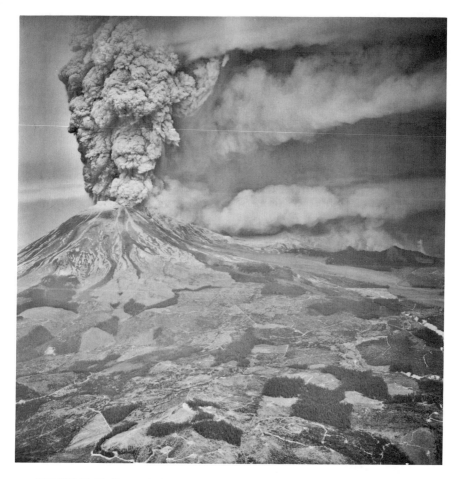

**FIGURE 18-14** Mount St. Helens, Washington, erupting. Photo courtesy of FEMA.

Other volcanoes with longer cycles but that have a good possibility of erupting are in Wyoming, Arizona, and New Mexico.

Mount St. Helens will continue to be a serious threat for at least twenty to thirty years.

## SKILLS FOR DISASTER PREPAREDNESS

Disasters may come about through the forces of nature or through man's manipulations, but that they will come is certain. Where do we turn when these perils occur? The answer is that we should be self-reliant. This is not to say that we have no need of others. Self-reliance means exercising our developed abilities to do for ourselves what is rightly our responsibility.

In order to be better prepared for disasters, every adult should be able to help with the following:

1. Identify the potential emergencies and disasters most likely to occur
   a. Recognize their characteristics (e.g., when, where, etc.)
   b. Recognize their effects upon people and property
   c. Follow suggested procedures before, during, and after a disaster
2. Provide adequate shelter
   a. Within the home
   b. Improvised shelters (in case of evacuation)
3. Extinguish fires and check for safety
   a. Use a fire extinguisher
   b. Check for gas, water, electrical, sewage breaks
   c. Turn off appropriate utilities
4. Provide water
   a. Store water
   b. Locate source of water inside and outside the home
   c. Carry water
   d. Siphon water
   e. Disinfect water
5. Provide food
   a. Store food (both a two-week food supply which requires no heat nor cooking and a long-term food supply
   b. Cook food
   c. Process grains without the use of electricity
6. Provide light
   a. Store and use light sources (candles, matches, flashlights, extra batteries, chemical light)
7. Provide heat
   a. Have a fireplace, stove (camp, charcoal grill, etc.)
   b. Store and select fuels (wood, coal, newspapers)
   c. Start a fire
8. Dispose of human wastes
9. Provide first aid and medical self-help
   a. Select and store first-aid supplies
   b. Render appropriate first aid to the injured and suddenly ill (this includes cardiopulmonary resuscitation)
   c. Store individual medicines
   d. Obtain a good first-aid book. A good example is *The First Aid Book*, 2nd ed. by Alton L. Thygerson, published by Prentice-Hall (1986).
10. Obtain assistance
    a. Signal to aircraft (body signals, ground signals, signal mirror)
    b. Contact community emergency resources

For all of our modern scientific knowledge and technological know-how, we are no match for the violent forces of disasters. More wisdom is necessary. Planning and proper action save lives. If a person can develop the listed skills, that person will be far better prepared and have a greater chance of surviving.

"The farther you are from the last disaster, the closer you are to the next one" is an oft-quoted statement made by emergency preparedness specialists. We do live in an age of catastrophe. Every American will likely be either a victim or witness to at least one natural disaster during his or her lifetime. The tragedy of disasters is that we can all be better prepared than we are.

# 19

# Occupational Safety

About twenty-one million Americans—one of every four workers—are exposed to known health hazards on the job. At least two million workers are injured each year in job-related accidents.

Job safety is a problem which concerns most Americans—either directly or because of hazards faced by family members and friends.

In terms of lost production and wages, medical expenses and disability compensation, the cost is huge. Therefore, the Occupational Safety and Health Administration (OSHA) was created by Congress to help workers and their employers do something about the problem.

During the 1960s, the accident rate in American industry began to climb dramatically, increasing over ten years to rates 30 percent above those of 1958. It was also during this time that new occupational diseases were discovered in alarming numbers.

There are several reasons for this deterioration of job safety and health conditions. One is increased mechanization. Another is the rapid increase in the production and use of industrial chemicals. Whole industries have literally been invented since the 1930s: plastics, petroleum-based chemicals, and synthetic fabrics, among others.

The National Safety Council has estimated that the total cost of workplace injuries is nearly $34 billion per year. Worker's compensation alone costs industry

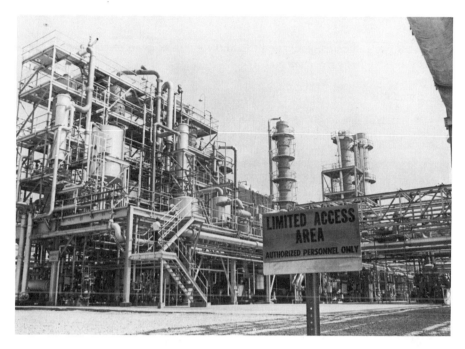

**FIGURE 19-1** One in every four American workers is exposed to known health hazards on the job. Photo courtesy of the Occupational Safety and Health Administration.

an estimated $12 billion per year—a cost which is passed on to the consumer. Production time lost due to on-the job accidents, according to the National Safety Council, amounted to over forty million workdays.

The costs of workplace hazards can be reduced. One trucking firm achieved a 65 percent drop in compensation costs since worker safety laws were passed. Boise Cascade, a large timber and housing company, estimated that in three years, accidents in Boise's operations were reduced by one-third, saving over $12 million per year.

## OSHA'S COVERAGE

In general, OSHA covers all employers and their employees in the United States. The following are not covered by OSHA:

- Self-employed persons;
- Farms at which only immediate members of the farm employer's family are employed; and
- Workplaces already protected by other federal agencies under other federal statutes (e.g., Coal Mine Health and Safety Act and the Federal Metal and Nonmetallic Safety Act).

## HOW OSHA WORKS[1]

OSHA adopts standards and conducts inspections of workplaces to determine whether the standards are being met.

### Standards

A standard is a legally enforceable regulation governing conditions, practices, or operations to assure safe and healthful workplaces.

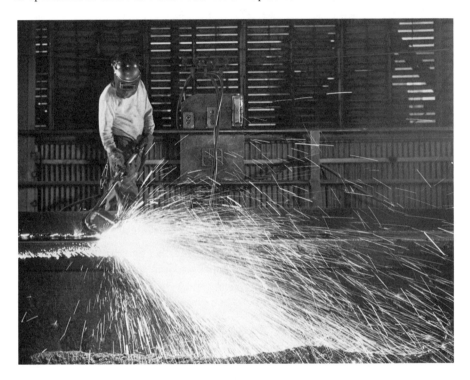

**FIGURE 19-2** Compliance with safety standards. Photo courtesy of the Occupational Safety and Health Administration.

Compliance with national safety and health standards is what an inspector (compliance officer) looks for when he or she inspects a workplace. There is a concern with what standards apply there and whether the employer and employees are complying with them.

The standards are published in the Federal Register. All amendments, corrections, insertions, or deletions involving standards are divided into three major categories: General Industry, Maritime, and Construction. Copies may be obtained from the nearest OSHA regional office or the OSHA Office of Management Services in Washington, D.C.

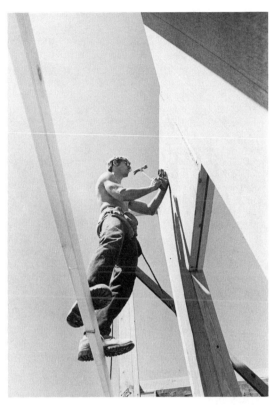

**FIGURE 19-3** Noncompliance with safety standards. Photo courtesy of the Occupational Safety and Health Administration.

*Compliance and inspection.* Of major interest is the OSHA inspection system. Since OSHA began its inspection program, in more than one out of every three workplaces inspected, all the required standards were met, so no citations were issued. That ratio is rising as employers become more familiar with their responsibilities and recognize the positive benefits that accompany compliance with OSHA standards.

Reduced job injury and illness rates, less down time, improved employee morale, and savings in workmen's compensation insurance all demonstrate that "safety pays."

*When will an inspector call?* Obviously, not all five million workplaces covered can or should be inspected immediately. The worst situations need attention first. So a system of priorities has been established:

1. Imminent danger situations are given top priority. An imminent danger is any condition where there is reasonable certainty that a danger exists that can be expected to cause death or serious physical harm immediately, or before the danger can be eliminated through normal enforcement procedures.

   Serious physical harm is any type of harm that could cause permanent or prolonged damage to the body or which, while not damaging the body on

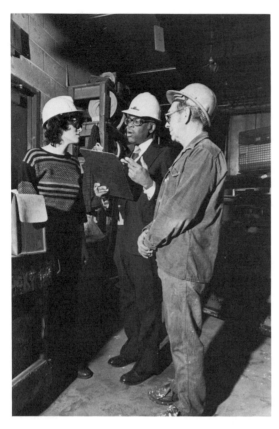

**FIGURE 19-4** An OSHA inspection. Photo courtesy of the Occupational Safety and Health Administration.

a prolonged basis, could cause such temporary disability as to require in-patient hospital treatment. OSHA considers that "permanent or prolonged damage" has occurred when, for example, a part of the body is crushed or severed, an arm, leg, or finger is amputated, or sight in one or both eyes is lost. This kind of damage also includes that which renders a part of the body either functionally useless or substantially reduced in efficiency on or off the job. An example: bones in a limb shattered so severely that mobility or dexterity will be permanently reduced.

Temporary disability requiring in-patient hospital treatment includes injuries such as closed fractures, concussions, burns, or wounds involving substantial loss of blood and requiring extensive suturing or other healing aids.

Employees should inform the supervisor or employer immediately if they detect or even suspect an imminent danger situation in the workplace. If the employer takes no action to eliminate the danger, an employee or the authorized employee representative may notify the nearest OSHA office and request an inspection.

Upon inspection, if an imminent danger situation is found, the inspector will ask the employer to voluntarily abate the hazard and to remove endangered employees from exposure. Notice of the imminent danger also must be posted. Before the OSHA inspector leaves the work-place, he or she will advise all affected employees of the hazard.

2. Catastrophes and Fatal Accidents. Second priority is given to investigation of fatalities and catastrophes resulting in hospitalization of five or more employees. Such situations must be reported to OSHA by the employer. Investigations are made to determine if OSHA standards were violated and to avoid recurrence of similar accidents.

3. Valid Employee Complaints. Third priority is given to employee complaints of alleged violation of standards or of unsafe working conditons.

4. Special Emphasis Programs. Next in priority are programs of inspection aimed at specific high-hazard industries, occupations, or health substances. Industries are selected for inspection on the basis of the death, injury and illness incidence rates, employee exposure to toxic substances, etc. Special emphasis may be regional or national in scope, depending on the distribution of the workplaces involved.

5. Random selection from all types and sizes of workplaces in all sections of the country.

*Inspection tour.* Inspections come under the supervision of the OSHA area director. Assignments are made on the basis of the priorities discussed before.

Before making an inspection, the inspector becomes familiar with as many relevant facts as possible about the workplace and determines which OSHA standards are pertinent. Special equipment for testing for toxic substances in the air, for noise, etc. are taken.

Inspections are conducted during regular working hours of the establishment except in special circumstances. OSHA regulations prohibit advance notice of inspections except in cases where such notice would serve to make the inspection more effective.

To start an inspection, the inspector presents himself at the establishment, displays credentials, and asks to meet the appropriate employer representative. The employer is informed of the reason for the visit, and the inspector outlines, in general terms, the scope of the inspection, including safety and health records desired for review, employee interviews, the walkaround, and the closing conference.

The inspector and the employer and employee representatives then proceed through the establishment, and each work area is inspected for compliance with OSHA standards.

The inspector takes appropriate notes of conditions and discusses them. Photographs of particular situations to record apparent violations or conditions that may change during the inspection or shortly thereafter, and other appropriate investigative techniques may be used.

The inspector also looks at the OSHA records of deaths, injuries, and illnesses, that employers of eight or more employees are required to keep, and determines that the annual summary has been posted.

Numerous apparent violations may be found that can be corrected immediately. These could include blocked aisles, unsafe floor surfaces, hazardous projections, unsanitary conditions, etc.

After the walkaround, the inspector discusses with the employer what has been seen and reviews probable violations. Also discussed is the time the employer believes he will need to abate hazards.

The inspector then returns to his office, writes a report, and discusses it with the area director. The area director or his superiors determine what citations will be issued and what penalities, if any, will be proposed. These are sent to the employer by certified mail.

The inspector may not, on his own, impose or propose a penalty "on the spot" at an inspection, nor can he close down an establishment or process. OSHA can act quickly in the courts to deal with imminent danger situations.

There are various types of violations which may be cited and penalties which may be proposed. Penalties of up to $10,000 may be a possibility. Follow-up inspections ensure that cited violations have been properly abated.

This has been a summary of what the Occupational Safety and Health Administration is all about and how it operates. OSHA's basic policy is to implement the mandate of Congress fully and firmly, yet fairly, and not to harass employers or employees.


## LEADING WORK-RELATED DISEASES AND INJURIES

The National Institute for Occupational Safety and Health has developed a list of the ten leading work-related diseases and injuries (see Table 19-1). A discussion of the second category, musculoskeletal injuries, appears below.

### Musculoskeletal Injuries

Physical demands of many jobs make the body's musculoskeletal system highly vulnerable to a variety of occupational injuries. Manual handling of materials, repetitive motions, and vibration are prime causal factors in the development of the following disorders:

*Injuries associated with the manual handling of materials* (such as unaided lifting and lowering): Low back injuries, often due to improper manual handling of materials, are the largest single subset of musculoskeletal injuries. The Bureau of Labor Statistics recently reported that approximately one million workers sustain back injuries annually and that back injuries account for one out of every five injuries in the workplace. About one-fourth of all workers' compensation indemnity expenditures are for back injuries.

*Repetitive motion-associated trauma:* Repetitive motion can cause "cumulative trauma disorders," including tendinitis and bursitis. These disorders may be caused or aggravated by repeated twisting or by awkward postures, especially when combined with a large amount of force. Workers at risk include those employed in fields such as construction, food preparation, clerical work, product fabrication, and mining.

**TABLE 19-1   The Ten Leading Work-related Diseases and Injuries—United States.**

1. Occupational lung disease; asbestosis, byssinosis, silicosis, coal workers' pneumoconiosis, lung cancer, occupational asthma

2. Musculoskeletal injuries: disorders of the back, trunk, upper extremity, neck, lower extremity; traumatically induced Reynaud's phenomenon

3. Occupational cancers (other than lung): leukemia; mesothelioma; cancers of the bladder, nose, and liver

4. Amputations, fractures, eye loss, lacerations, and traumatic deaths

5. Cardiovascular diseases: hypertension, coronary artery disease, acute myocardial infarction

6. Disorders of reproduction: infertility, spontaneous abortion, teratogenesis

7. Neurotoxic disorders: peripheral neuropathy, toxic encephalitis, psychoses, extreme personality changes (exposure-related)

8. Noise-induced loss of hearing

9. Dermatologic conditions: dermatoses, burns (scaldings), chemical burns, contusions (abrasions)

10. Psychologic disorders: neuroses, personality disorders, alcoholism, drug dependency

*The conditions listed under each category are to be viewed as *selected examples*, not comprehensive definitions of the category.

Source: National Institute for Occupational Safety and Health.

Prevention or reduction of musculoskeletal injuries can be accomplished with measures such as:

1. *Substitution.* Machines such as hoists, cranes, and dollies can substitute for workers in some aspects of the manual handling of materials.
2. *Improved equipment design.* Research has shown that improved design of some vibrating tools virtually eliminates hazardous vibration; suspension or isolation systems which greatly reduce whole-body vibration can be added to vehicles.
3. *Task design.* Manual tasks can be altered to minimize biomechanical stress to the worker.
4. *Worker education.* Injuries due to musculoskeletal stresses may be reduced by preplacement strength testing, training workers in proper ways to perform tasks, and on-site programs of exercise and physical therapy.
5. *Variation of work practices.* Periodic rotation of workers to jobs with different physical demands may reduce physical stress upon the body.

## WORKMEN'S COMPENSATION

Workmen's compensation may be regarded as a form of "no-fault" insurance. The law requires the employer to remunerate an injured employee whether or not negligence can be proved. About 80 percent of all workers in the United States are covered by workmen's compensation laws.

Although the workmen's compensation acts are all different, there are three fundamental conditions that must be satisfied for an injured worker or the worker's dependents to receive benefits: (1) The injury must have resulted from an accident; (2) it must have arisen out of the worker's employment; and (3) it must have occurred during the course of the worker's employment. The costs of workmen's compensation insurance are paid by the employer. Criticism about workmen's compensation centers upon the inadequate amounts an injured worker may be receiving.

## MANAGEMENT RESPONSIBILITIES FOR SAFETY

Without management support any safety efforts will be in a constant state of frustration. Accident prevention and injury control requires a sustained effort by all. However, managers are the only ones who can direct that the safety effort be carried out and the only ones who can provide the authority to ensure it is a positive activity. Unless managers do provide support, accidents will take place. The Occupational Safety and Health Act places the responsibility for employee safety mainly on the employers.

## FARM SAFETY

The National Safety Council reports eighteen hundred deaths in agricultural settings (includes farming, forestry, fishing, and agricultural services).

Beef farms have the highest work injury rate and dairy farms the lowest.

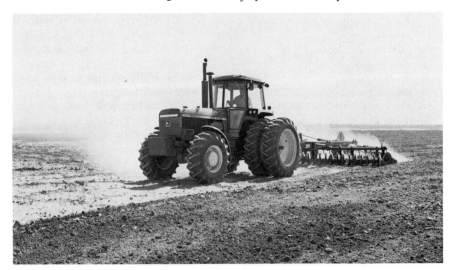

**FIGURE 19-5** The farm tractor, an essential piece of farm equipment, accounts for about half of all farm fatalities. Photo courtesy of Deere and Company.

Those most endangered are: (1) 5- to 14-year-olds; (2) males; and (3) hired workers other than family members.

The tractor is the most essential part of today's farm equipment. Yet this piece of essential farm equipment accounts for about half of all farm fatalities. About half of the tractor fatalities result from overturn. Overturning is usually caused by such things as working on steep slopes, improperly operating front end loaders, hitching loads too high, and going too fast for conditions. Rollover bars are effective in preventing death and injury.

Next in importance in tractor death cases is the victim being run over by the tractor; in over one half of these cases the person first fell from the tractor.

Farm machinery is hazardous because many farm machines are intended to change the size, shape, consistency, or density of agricultural products by cutting, shredding, tearing, or compressing. Rotating parts can snag clothing, trap a hand or foot, or trap a victim around the working parts.

Today's modern farm machines have many safety features built into them to protect their operators. Farm machinery may be made up of such varied components as pulleys, belts, flywheels, pick-up teeth, gears, rotary cutters, and augers. Most of the new machines have metal "guards" to protect operators from entanglements. Still, a number of farmers will remove these guards in order to better facilitate maintenance.

Machinery such as hay balers have pick-up teeth and an auger, and at times the hay may bind up in the auger. The careless operator may attempt to free up the auger with his hands and become entangled, resulting in massive tissue damage and fractures.

Combines have an assortment of pulleys, belts, and gears which require daily greasing. Sometimes a farmer may attempt to grease the machine without shutting it off. A victim may become entangled between a pulley and belt.

### Uniqueness of Farming

Certain circumstances involved in the farm environment are unique compared with other industries, and these should be kept in mind when reading and interpreting farm accident data. Farm business and family living are sometimes erroneously viewed as separate and distinct when, in fact, the division between them is often hazy. This close intermingling makes farming a mode of life rather than strictly an occupation.

Most farm and ranch work is performed by family members not affected by state or federal labor regulations. In the agricultural industry, it is not uncommon for persons under eighteen and over sixty-five years of age to be performing farm-related work. These age groups make up only a small percentage of the workers in other industries.

Workers in agriculture must perform a wide variety of tasks in all kinds of job conditions, while those in conventional industries usually are limited to routine tasks performed under controlled conditions. Farmers often work alone and, if injured, first aid or medical assistance may be delayed. Most workers in other industries have fellow workers at close proximity who can summon assistance immediately if an accident occurs. Workers in conventional industries usually have regular work hours while farmers may work twelve to eighteen hours per day, seven days a week during the busy periods of the year.

Because the agricultural work population is not concentrated, as in most other industries, it is more difficult to reach them with safety programs and information. Job safety training is entirely voluntary on the farm and ranch, and no on-site personnel are responsible for job safety as in most other industries. Protective equipment such as safety shoes, hard hats, and respirators, while more common in other industries, are used by few farmers.

## NOTES

1. This section is adapted from Occupational Safety and Health Administration, *All About OSHA: The Who, What, Where, When, Why, and How of the Occupational Safety and Health Act* (Washington, D.C.: Superintendent of Documents, 1983).

# 20

# School Safety

The school safety program should be a broad and comprehensive one. The term school safety program is used to describe all school activities which promote the safety of school-age youth.

School administrative policy enables the school safety program to function. Without strong administrative support and encouragement, the program is doomed for failure.

Accidents are the leading cause of death among the age group attending school. Because large segments of time are spent in school and because hazards do exist in school programs, teachers, administrators, and parents should place the safety of students high on any priority listing of school needs. Though the vast majority of accidents in the school program result in injuries rather than death, there is a carry-over of safety consciousness into other aspects of life when a student may not be in a school setting. For example, safety attitudes learned at school transfer into out-of-school activities which may be more hazardous.

## SAFETY CURRICULUM

Every school has a legal obligation to provide learning experiences in safety as a part of the regular school curriculum. The emphasis in safety education should be upon practical ways of avoiding accidents through behaving safely.

Specific learning experiences should be provided in such areas as the following: fire prevention, home safety, school safety (e.g., as it pertains to playgrounds, buses, classrooms, school patrols, etc.), pedestrian safety, bicycle safety, motor vehicle safety, water safety, vacation safety, and work safety.

Safety education can be thought of as a part of the broader field of health education and should be integrated as much as possible with the health education curriculum.

The safety curriculum should apply to the entire school program. Obvious areas where safety is a concern involve shops and laboratories, physical education and athletics, and driver education. Emphasis on accident prevention can be included in every subject, however. For example, instead of the English student writing about what the daffodil thinks of spring, he or she might utilize a safety concept that has real practical value; this is where the area of safety lies—that of practicality and usefulness. Students can learn all there is to know about any subject or topic, but failure to learn well certain basic safety principles can lead to disastrous results.

Elementary schools have been most likely to include safety information within their curriculum and the tendency is for safety information to be included less as students progress through the grades. If one were looking for the safety instructor in most American high schools, the driver education teacher would be pointed out. While if one looks for the elementary teacher known for teaching safety, every teacher is cited in all grade levels.

Safety information varies with geographic area. For example, a school in the rural areas might focus on farm safety while the city school may emphasize pedestrian safety. This points out that a safety program for one school may not be appropriate for another. All state departments of education have curriculum guides for teachers which provide guidelines and suggestions for better safety instruction. The National Safety Council and other agencies have curriculum guides available for teacher use.

## FIRE SAFETY

One of the most important safety responsibilities of the schools is to develop an effective fire safety program. This program should include fire safety learning experiences. No school administrator or teacher should ever think of his or her school as being fireproof.

One part of a school fire safety program should include regular inspection of all school buildings for fire hazards. This means school administrators and teachers should become educated on the nature of fire hazards and fire control.

Another part of a school fire safety program is the establishment of a learning type of fire drill under supervision on a regular basis. Most states require such drills on a monthly basis or each school term. Drills should be held in the winter since fires are more likely to occur then. It has been shown that regular drills can remove the sense of panic that sometimes develops at the sound of a fire alarm. Evacuation

should take no longer than two minutes, and all drills should be conducted on the assumption that an actual fire exists.

## DISASTER PREPARATION

Depending upon the geographical locality, disaster drills are periodically conducted. During the 1950s, drills for nuclear attack were often held. Today, more and more schools conduct tornado drills and hurricane drills. Areas to be considered in planning for emergency drills include: bomb threats, school bus emergencies, nuclear attack, crowd control at school events, chemical spills, power failure, fires, earthquakes, and tornadoes.

## SAFETY INSPECTIONS

In the more hazardous locations (e.g., shops, labs, physical education, etc.) safety inspections are a must. In many places they are required. Teachers can construct their own safety inspection checklist or acquire one prepared by a professional or safety organization. Such listings are useful since many administrators and teachers are not totally aware of all of the potential hazards.

## SAFETY PATROLS

Schools have used older students or adults to protect younger students from the hazards of crossing streets en route to or from school. They have saved lives, and such patrols provide learning experiences for older students which have a positive carry-over into their lives.

The success of a school safety patrol program depends upon the teacher chosen to supervise the group of students working on the safety patrol.

## SCHOOL BUS TRANSPORTATION

School bus transportation accidents kill about 150 children each year. Actually, considering the large number of students carried daily on school buses, the safety record of the school bus program is remarkably good. However, the potential for a major disaster is great. Considering the fact that school buses contain forty, fifty, or more students at one time, if a school bus collides with a train or truck or goes off a highway, numerous deaths and injuries are quite likely. Multiple fatalities have occurred when such events have happened.

Every school district should have written policies, rules, and regulations to

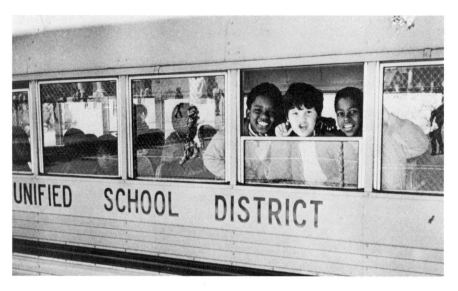

**FIGURE 20-1** The school bus safety record is remarkably good. However, the potential for catastrophe is great. Photo courtesy of the *Deseret News*.

govern the operation of the school bus transportation system. Some of the guidelines include:

1. Driver qualifications
2. Basic driver training programs
3. Maintenance standards
4. Student conduct on the bus
5. Emergency procedures

## ACCIDENT REPORTING

There are several good reasons for the establishment of an accident reporting system in all schools. One obvious reason is that in the event of a lawsuit (which can come years later because of the statute of limitations), an accident report can identify not just who was injured, but who witnessed the accident. The report provides information about the injuries, what first aid was given, and where the student was taken for medical care.

Another reason for keeping accident reports is the usefulness they provide in pinpointing accidental injury problems. For example, are students getting too many sprained ankles in a physical education class, or are students falling off a certain playground apparatus? Corrective measures can be taken when problems are known.

A third use for accident records is the determination of the effectiveness of the school safety program. For instance, since starting measures to reduce sprained ankles in a physical education class (e.g., stretching more and warming up or requiring a certain type of gym shoe) accident reports can indicate whether the incidences of a particular type of accidents is decreasing.

## FIRST AID AND EMERGENCY CARE

Every school should have a policy regarding the handling of any injured or sick student. Although no one policy can fit all situations, some of the following can serve as indicators for an effective policy:

- First aid and emergency care procedures to be taken in the event of a student injury or illness.
- Identification of one or more persons qualified and appointed to render first aid and emergency care.
- Notification of parents or guardians. If parents cannot be reached, identification of other responsible persons.
- Provisions for transporting injured and ill students home or to a hospital.

The school should keep up-to-date emergency information on all students, showing addresses and telephone numbers of parents and others to be called. Any known condition (e.g., allergies to bee stings, drugs, diabetes, heart disease, etc.) should be known.

All administrators and teachers should have the basic first-aid skills by which to save a life. First-aid supplies should also be available for use in emergencies.

# 21

# Sports and Recreational Safety

Modern technology has freed man from daily routines and thus has allowed more time in which to play sports and engage in recreational pursuits. Most sports are relatively safe from injury and death. Others pose great threats to the life and limb of participants.

The National Injury Information Clearinghouse annually issues a listing of injuries caused by various sports activities severe enough to require hospital emergency room treatment (Table 21-1). Some of the figures, no doubt, are too low. The list obviously reports only a limited number of sports injuries since many injured participants do not require emergency room attention. Such data serve to point out the seriousness of the sports injury problem.

## RECREATIONAL SPORTS INJURIES

### Backpacking

Backpacking can be extremely demanding and requires preparation to avoid problems such as heat stroke, dehydration, sunburn, insect bites, blisters, and excessive fatigue. It is wise to learn how to avoid the injuries rather than treating the problem after it has happened.

Dehydration can occur as a result of excessive sweating. Several quarts of body water can be lost while backpacking on a hot day and must be replaced so that sweating can continue to cool the body.

**TABLE 21-1** Sports Injuries

| SPORT | INJURIES (IN THOUSANDS) |
|---|---|
| Baseball | 478 |
| Football | 470 |
| Basketball | 434 |
| Skating (roller, ice) | 225 |
| Swimming | 126 |
| Soccer | 96 |
| Volleyball | 75 |
| Tennis, badminton, and squash | 67 |
| Wrestling | 66 |
| Fishing | 64 |
| Gymnastics | 62 |
| Guns | 60 |
| Hockey (field, ice) | 50 |
| Exercise equipment | 48 |
| Snow skiing (downhill, cross-country) | 45 |
| Track and field | 44 |
| Horseback riding | 44 |
| Boats | 37 |
| Toboggans, sleds, snow disks, and snow tubing | 32 |
| Water skiing, tubing, and surfboarding | 29 |
| Skateboards | 28 |
| Dancing | 26 |
| Golf | 23 |
| Martial arts | 19 |
| Bowling | 19 |
| Lacrosse | 10 |
| Boxing | 10 |
| Snowmobiles | 8 |
| Trampolines | 8 |
| Billiards and pool | 6 |
| Handball | 5 |
| Cheerleading | 5 |

NOTE: Estimated number of injuries associated with consumer products requiring emergency room treatment in the United States, July 1, 1980–June 30, 1981.

Source: National Injury Information Clearinghouse.

Sunburn can be prevented by liberal use of a commercial sunscreen (not suntan oil) that contains para-aminobenzoic acid (usually abbreviated PABA). A hat and protective clothing are also helpful.

The most effective insect repellants contain the chemical N, N-diethylmetatolumide (usually abbreviated DEET). Repellants with a cream or synthetic wax base will last longest.

Foot blisters can be avoided by wearing properly fitted and broken-in hiking boots, two pairs of clean dry socks, and using a drying powder. Friction spots should be covered with moleskin as soon as they become painful.

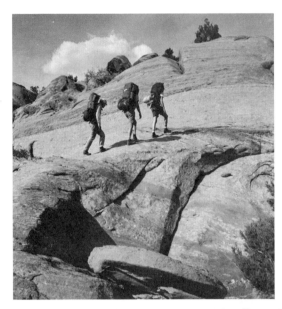

FIGURE 21-1 Backpackers face many hazards. Photo courtesy of the Utah Travel Council.

To decrease fatigue, increase aerobic fitness by starting at least two months before the intended trip. Walking can be the initial starting program for aerobic fitness, then jogging can begin with the goal of at least three miles at a comfortable pace. When training for backpacking, it is better to increase distance rather than intensity.

Light weight training will help prepare for carrying a pack. Barbell exercises specific to backpacking include the curl, partial squats, and shoulder shrugs.

Beyond the jogging and weight training, get some actual experience carrying a backpack while wearing your hiking boots. Load the pack with about thirty-five pounds of sand bags and carry it around for progressively longer periods of time.

### Baseball and Softball

Very few deaths to either players or spectators have resulted directly from baseball or softball. However, serious and minor injuries occur each year, especially among younger and beginning players. Most injuries could be prevented by proper coaching of baserunning, throwing, and hitting. Protective equipment such as face masks, padding, and batting helmets are a must.

BOX 21-1 *UNUSUAL BUT TRUE*

> Len Boyer of the Modesto, California, Reds baseball team hit a towering fly to left field.
>
> San Jose outfielder Mike Prieto moved back to make the catch, but suddenly lost the ball in the lights. The ball bounced off his head and carried another twenty feet over a fifteen-foot fence for a home run.
>
> — National Safety Council, *Family Safety*

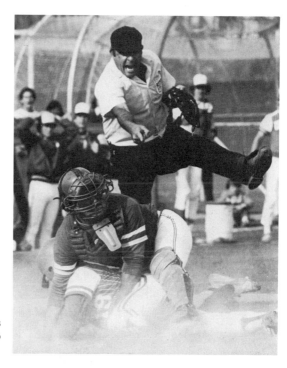

**FIGURE 21-2** Protective gear is a must in many sports. Photo courtesy of Mark A. Philbrick.

BOX 21–2 *UNUSUAL BUT TRUE*

> A pigeon winging along over Fenway Park during a Red Sox-Tiger baseball game was struck by a pop fly off of a batter's bat and fell to the ground only a few feet from home plate. It was the only fowl ball of the game.
>
> — National Safety Council, *Family Safety*

### Basketball

Originally developed as a noncontact sport, the game has lost most of its characteristics of a noncontact sport. There is a great deal of body contact and very little protective equipment to prevent injuries. Though deaths are few, injuries are many.

BOX 21-3 *UNUSUAL BUT TRUE*

> A Mississippi State basketball player in a game against Georgia slam dunked the ball for two points and found himself underneath the basket when the ball came through. It struck him on the head, knocking him unconscious for several minutes.
>
> — National Safety Council, *Family Safety*

### Football

It is said that a high school boy who participates in a full season of football has a 20 percent chance of being injured sometime during the season and an 8 percent chance of sustaining a serious injury.

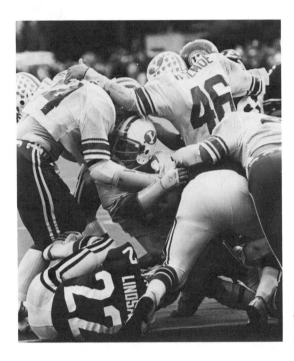

**FIGURE 21-3** All kinds of injuries happen to football players. Photo courtesy of Mark A. Philbrick.

*Injured player evaluation.*    All kinds of injuries happen to football players, from the life-threatening to the run-of-the-mill types.

*Head and neck area injuries.*    Some believe that all football players who play through high school and college suffer at least one concussion during their playing career. Concussions have been categorized into degrees—class I, II, and III. A player does not have to be knocked out to suffer a concussion.

In a class I concussion (mild) there is no loss of consciousness, but the player is momentarily dazed, may have ringing in his ears, memory loss for recent events, or a little dizziness. He usually recovers within a few minutes.

In a class II concussion (moderate), the player is knocked out momentarily (less than five minutes). When he comes to he usually does not know where he is or what has been going on and is a little dizzy and unsteady.

In a class III concussion (severe), there is a loss of consciousness for over five minutes. The player should be immediately evacuated to a hospital for an adequate medical evaluation.

*Fatalities.* The majority of fatalities are sustained in games rather than in practice. In recent years about 90 percent of the direct fatalities have been caused by head and neck injuries. A number of indirect deaths have occurred as the result of heat stroke because of lack of acclimation on the part of the players, practicing under conditions of high air temperature and humidity, not being allowed to drink water freely, and not being given rest periods in the shade.

The number of direct fatalities has dramatically decreased in the last several decades. Improved football equipment has aided this decrease. However, a major rule change eliminating the head as a primary and initial contact area for blocking and tackling ("spearing") has helped reduce the increased number of paralyzing neck injuries and deaths.

The American Football Coaches Association feels that enforcement of the rules prohibiting "spearing," using properly fitted helmets, and excellent physical condition are the factors which will help reduce fatalities and serious head and neck injuries from football.

No figures as to the number of players who are permanently disabled as the result of football injuries could be found, but one report of serious damage to the central nervous system resulting from injuries to the head and neck suggests that this number may be larger than previously suspected.

### Golfing

Golf is the most universal of all outdoor games, and it is played with two potentially lethal weapons—the golf ball and the club. When a ball leaves the club-head, it is apt to be traveling at about 136 mph. The golf club is apt to be swung at a speed of about 110 mph.

*Accidents are rare in golf although they do occur.* Numerous deaths have been recorded when a golf ball strikes someone on the head. There are also reports of death from being hit on the head with a club. Eyes have been damaged and jaws broken. One golfer became so excited after sinking a sixty-foot putt that he threw his club into the air. It came down, struck his partner and knocked him unconscious. One player was killed when the shaft of his club snapped off, rebounded from a tree, plunged into his body and the jagged edge severed an artery.

*Lightning is a hazard on a golf course.* Numerous players, caddies, and course maintenance personnel have been killed by lightning on golf courses. In many cases the victims were taking refuge under a tree during the storm, an unsafe

BOX 21-4  *UNUSUAL BUT TRUE*

Crop-dusting pilot David Hughes of Fresno, California was spraying the fairways of the Fort Washington golf course when a golfer lofted a tee shot that crashed through the plane's windshield and bounced off Hughes' helmet. He was momentarily dazed, but managed to land the plane safely.

— National Safety Council, *Family Safety*

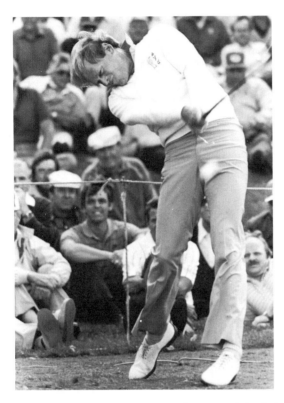

FIGURE 21-4 Accidents are rare in golf, but two potentially lethal weapons are used—the golf ball and the club. Photo courtesy of Mark A. Philbrick, with permission of Johnny Miller.

place to be. Other persons have been struck by lightning while holding an open umbrella or golf club. During an electrical storm on a golf course, trees and shelters should be avoided.

*Miscellaneous hazards on golf courses* include electric golf carts which have sometimes run over players. Water hazards are sometimes just that, when players fall into them. Even bees have attacked some players. Some players have broken an arm or leg because of the force of a golf swing. In some areas ticks pose a problem.

Shots from a sand trap near the green can be among the most dangerous shots in the game. Even the most skilled golfers can shank or skull a shot from a trap, thus playing companions and caddies need to protect themselves.

When a ball is traveling toward a player or group of players, the word *fore* should be shouted loudly so that the people endangered are warned. Unfortunately, shouting *fore* sometimes has the opposite effect of a warning since many golfers do not know how to react correctly. In an attempt to spot the oncoming ball, many golfers look toward the direction of the yell. This exposes a player's face and eyes to the ball. The correct reaction is to turn away from the direction of the sound and lower the head. A player still may be struck, but he is less apt to incur serious injury. Ducking behind a golf cart, golf bag, or tree when possible is suggested when *fore* is heard.

BOX 21-5  *UNUSUAL BUT TRUE*

> As Richard Rocca was passing the Cedar Brook Golf Course near Belle Vernon, Pennsylvania, a golf club (not ball) crashed down on the hood of his car.
>
> An investigation revealed that the No. 9 iron belonged to a golfer who lost his grip on the club as he was trying to blast his way out of a sand trap.
>
> — National Safety Council, *Family Safety*

Golfers must learn how to deal with the sun by wearing a hat and sun screen.

Golf, like many other noncontact sports, is not considered particularly dangerous. Golfers can best protect themselves and others from injury by obeying the rules of etiquette and using common sense.

### Hang Gliding

One of the most spectacular of the new sports is hang gliding, in which man may have come the closest he ever will to "fly like a bird."

Hang glider flying has grown rapidly in popularity in recent years. It is a relatively easy sport to learn and is low in cost. The glider can be flown from locations

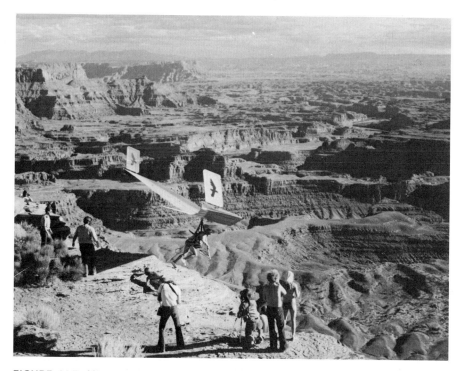

**FIGURE 21-5** Minute for minute, hang gliding is probably the most dangerous sport. Photo courtesy of Gerald Petersen, UDOT.

where most other air vehicles could not be used. To become airborne the "flyer" may run downhill or jump from a very high rock or overhanging cliff.

*Causes.*  Based on the medical literature, hang gliding accidents fall into two groups: (1) errors made before flight and (2) errors made during flight.

Preflight errors include inadequate equipment checks, misinterpreting unsafe weather and wind conditions, and using alcohol or drugs before flying.

In-flight mistakes include being confused by wind changes, attempting turns beyond one's capability (most dangerous maneuver is the 360 degree turn) and being too preoccupied with scenery to remember landing sites or to avoid obstacles. Errors during in-flight maneuvers are the main cause of fatal accidents, according to a study published in the *Journal of Trauma.*

*Effects.*  Inexperience and lack of discipline in flight are the main causes of nonfatal hang gliding accidents.

Hang gliding is dominated primarily by males, thus explaining the reason for male dominance of fatality and injury statistics. Several women, however, have been killed.

A National Safety Council report identified the average fatality age as twenty-five years. Ages of fatality victims have ranged from twelve to sixty-seven years.

The more experienced the pilot, the more likely he is to come to a tragic end. Serious injury seems to be a greater threat to the flyer whose gliding experience permits him to risk higher flying over rough terrain in marginal weather conditions and to risk launches from cliffs rather than the running start from safer and more gradual slopes. Almost 60 percent of the fatal accidents occurred to flyers with more than two hundred flights.

If you hang glide for about three years, your chances of having a serious injury are about one in five. Minute for minute, hang gliding is about as dangerous a sport as any although the hang glider's actual flying time in a day's activity totals only ten to twenty minutes.

*Prevention.*  The following possible preventive safety measures have been suggested:

1. approved schools with minimum hours of instruction before allowing independent flights
2. licensing of flyers
3. licensing and certification of air-worthiness of equipment
4. safety clothing—includes a helmet, gloves, shin pads, long-sleeved shirts and pants, and sturdy ankle-top boots
5. approved areas for flying, with no obstructions or environmental hazards
6. airspeed indicator to aid in speed and height judgment
7. avoidance of alcohol and drugs before flying
8. avoidance of wind conditions that involve sheer conditions, down drafts, and unpredictable conditions (i.e., no flying in some localities between 11:00 A.M. and 3:00 P.M. on hot days, when dangerous currents are likely)

### Horseback Riding

Today there are more horses in many states than during the time of the pioneers when livelihood and transportation depended upon horsepower. Most horses today are used for pleasure and not work.

1. Always speak to a horse as you approach it. A horse's vision is restricted directly in front and to the rear. Failure to speak may startle the horse into kicking.
2. Pet a horse by first placing a hand on its shoulder or neck. The touch should be a rubbing action and not a dab at the end of a horse's nose.
3. While working around horses, stay close to the horse. If it kicks, you will not receive the full impact.
4. Make the horse walk beside you when you lead it. A position even with the horse's head or halfway between the horse's head and its shoulder is considered safest.
5. When saddling, it is safest to keep the unfastened cinches and stirrup secured over the saddle seat. Ease them down when the saddle is on.
6. Pull up slowly to tighten the cinch. Check the cinch three times: after saddling, after walking a few steps, and after mounting and riding a short distance.
7. Never mount or dismount a horse in a barn. Sidestepping and rearing horses have injured riders who failed to take this precaution.
8. Ride abreast or stay at a full horse's length from the horse in front. This avoids the possibility of your being kicked or the horse being kicked.
9. Before a horse kicks or bites, his ears usually lay back flat against his head.
10. Let a horse pick his own way through rough parts of the trail. He can lower his head and get a good look at the ground before stepping. He can see only where he puts his front feet. Usually, he will put his hind feet on or near the spot where his front feet landed.

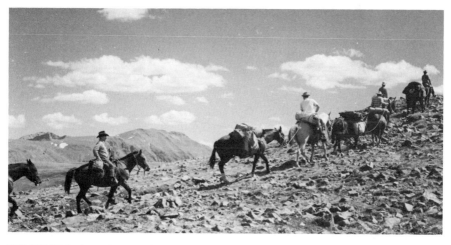

**FIGURE 21-6** Let a horse pick his own way through rough parts of the trail. Photo courtesy of Gerald Petersen, UDOT.

The National Safety Council recommends the following horseback riding rules:

- Beginners should start with competent instruction.
- Approach every horse quietly and never unexpectedly from behind.
- Choose a horse whose disposition and training matches the rider's capabilities.
- Check the tack (harness, bridles, etc.) for wear and cracking.
- Use the correct size stirrup.
- Make sure the girth or cinch is tight.
- Never attach yourself to the horse by any tack or equipment.
- Wear footwear with a deep heel. Never ride in sneakers, sandals, or moccasins.
- Consider wearing protective headgear whenever riding.

### Racquetball

There are three types of racquetball players: those who wear eye guards; those who have little knowledge of the risk to unprotected eyes; and those who resist wearing eye guards because they have not been hurt so far.

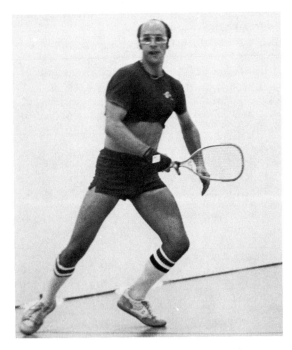

**FIGURE 21-7** There is a risk to unprotected eyes in racquetball. Photo courtesy of the National Safety Council, *Family Safety*.

It is apparent that some type of mandatory eye guard should be required. Many racquetball clubs will not allow a player on the court without an eye guard.

The *Journal of Physical Education and Recreation* recommends the following for preventing all types of racquetball injuries:

1. Avoid looking back to watch an opponent returning the ball. However, if you do, look out of the corner of your eye.
2. Wear good shoes to prevent slipping.
3. Give your opponent plenty of room to swing and follow through.
4. Toward the end of a close game, do not crowd your opponent—you both might be tired, and this is when someone usually gets injured.
5. When your opponent is striking a ball, it is safer to stand diagonally to his rear than directly to his side.
6. Avoid hitting an opponent with the ball or racket—call a hinder (unintentional interference with an opponent or flight of the ball, no penalty is assessed).
7. Give your opponent the opportunity to get to and/or strike at the ball from any position.
8. Hinders should be called without a claim by a player, especially in close plays and on game points.
9. All players should have rackets with a thong that must be securely wrapped on the wrist when playing.

The use of a racquet makes this a very hazardous game because of the danger of being hit by racquet or ball. Yet the nature of the game attracts players of all ages and both sexes to participate in a very competitive sport which can afford positive exercise results.

Players who wear prescription lenses are especially at risk during play because the glasses cannot withstand balls traveling at speeds up to 127 mph.

### Skating

*Prevalence of injuries.* With the increasing popularity of roller skating, ice skating, and skateboarding among Americans of all ages, the U.S. Consumer Product Safety Commission reports that skating has become a significant cause of recreational injuries. Skating injuries treated in hospital emergency departments are over 250,000 each year.

As might be expected, at least half of all skating injuries are suffered by teenagers, and well over two-thirds of the injuries were to girls and women. By contrast, the great majority of skateboard accidents occurred to boys and men.

*Causes.* Skating accidents are associated with these causal factors:

1. Skating too close. Other skaters stopping abruptly in front of the skater or vice versa.
2. Product structural problems, such as improper modification and repairs.
3. Poor skating surface. Environmental hazards such as cracked or uneven cement sidewalks, rocks, tree branches, or other debris can cause tripping.
4. Other causes can include the "human factor"—a) inexperience with the skates or with "trick" skating; b) horseplay and pushing; c) lack of attention; and d) misuse, such as going up and down steps with skates on.

*Prevention.* Protective gear, such as padding on knees and elbows and gloves, may not fully protect skaters from fractures, but it can reduce the number and severity of cuts and scrapes and is therefore recommended. Other protective equipment is also available.

Learning how to fall in case of an accident may help reduce the chance of being seriously injured.

### Snowmobiles

The U.S. Consumer Product Safety Commission estimates that more than eight thousand people receive hospital emergency room treatment each year for injuries associated with snowmobiles.

Some of the major accident patterns associated with snowmobiles include:

1. Collisions with fixed or moving objects, especially when driving on or beside public roads. This reflects the majority of snowmobile accidents. The unusually loud noise of most snowmobiles makes it hard to hear other vehicles, and braking suddenly on snow- or ice-covered roads is dangerous.
2. Excessive speed, unfamiliarity with the machine, and riding in unfamiliar terrain or near bodies of water.
3. Driving while intoxicated, after dark, or too close together.

Some accidents have been caused by product failure, such as a throttle that sticks open, brakes that fail, or skis that fall off. Many accidents also involve human error. Since they are capable of high speed, snowmobiles tempt people to race and to try jumps or other stunts. Snowmobiles can roll over easily when turning corners and go out of control at high speeds.

Snowmobiles can be great fun, but they must be used with good sense. The National Safety Council recommends the following ten points for snowmobile safety:

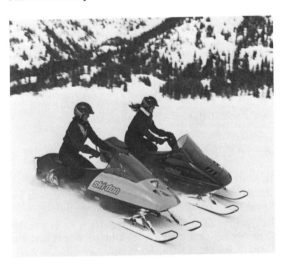

FIGURE 21-8 Snowmobiles can be great fun, but they must be used with good sense. Photo courtesy of Bombardier, Inc.

1. Driving instruction is required for the safe operation of a snowmobile.
2. Treat a snowmobile with the respect and care due any power-driven vehicle, and recognize the limitations of operating ability.
3. Study carefully the operating manuals supplied by the manufacturer of the snowmobile.
4. Know your legal status regarding licensing, traffic regulations, and responsibilities pertaining to public liability and property damage when operating a snowmobile.
5. Avoid public thoroughfares and when necessary cross at right angles using extreme caution.
6. Do not operate a snowmobile on frozen lakes or rivers without first checking ice thickness and having an intimate knowledge of water currents.
7. Wear protective, warm, windproof clothing; insulated footwear and mitts; shatterproof, tinted goggles; and a safety helmet.
8. For casual snowmobiling, within reach of assistance, carry spare drive belt and spark plugs with tools for installation.
9. For a distant safari, the following pieces of equipment should be carried— snowshoes, emergency fuel, map and compass, ax, knife, waterproofed matches, mess kit, emergency rations, first-aid kit, waterproof shelter, survival blanket.
10. Do not attempt distant safaris without an experienced person in charge; use the "buddy system" of two or more snowmobiles.

### Snow Skiing: Cross-Country

Cross-country skiing is rapidly becoming more popular as a winter sport. This growing popularity is due to the sport's many advantages. Cross-country skiing allows the enjoyment of the outdoors without disturbing the environment. Clothing and equipment are reasonably priced. There are no costs for lift passes. It is a vigorous form of exercise with a low injury rate that attracts families and people of all ages.

However, as the sport's popularity increases, so do injuries; and certain injuries are establishing a repeated pattern.

Cross-country skiing does not have accurate statistical data of injury rates because most cross-country skiers ski at unsupervised noncommercial areas. Most injuries are minor, and injured skiers often seek care at a variety of medical care facilities days later and often hundreds of miles away from the injury site.

Because cross-country skiing is among the most strenuous sports, the metabolic rate is greatly increased and heat production is therefore greater. In fact, U.S. ski team members have been shown to sweat regardless of subzero conditions for training and competition. This is a major cause of cold injury. Clothing wet with perspiration greatly increases heat losses. Such heat loss predisposes skiers to frostbite and hypothermia when they stop or become exhausted.

Windchill is another cause of cold injury in skiers, even on calm days. On a long downhill run, skiers produce their own windchill, depending on the speed, and frostbite easily occurs to exposed skin.

The circulation of blood may be constricted in the hands by the pole straps and in the feet by the boot. Most cross-country gloves and boots are poorly insulated, so severe frostbite can occur with longer exposure.

Although the injury rate for cross-country skiing is low, serious injuries sometimes occur. In machine-groomed tracks, skiers can reach speeds of 45 to 50 mph. Icy conditions expose beginning skiers to high speeds on unmaintained trails.

Areas exposed (i.e., nose, ears, and chin) are susceptible to sunburn on sunny days and frostbite in cold weather, especially to the fingers, toes, and feet.

The eyes are subject to injury caused by the extreme brightness of light reflected from the snow, which may result in corneal burns from ultraviolet light. Appropriate protective measures are adequate sunglasses and goggles.

Another hazard associated with this sport is risk of avalanche. Those engaging in cross-country skiing should be well versed in the avoidance of potential avalanche areas.

### Guidelines for safe cross-country skiing

1. Those with a history of heart disease, diabetes, lung disease, high blood pressure, or stroke should be supervised by a medical professional knowledgeable in exercise prescription. Cross-country skiing requires more energy than most sports, and cold weather increases the risk.
2. Become physically fit before the snow falls.
3. Do not ski alone other than on short excursions that are well marked, maintained, and traveled.
4. The best single way to prevent injuries is *not* to fall. If necessary, take off the skis and walk.
5. Do not use heel fixation devices. Cross-country bindings are not safety or release bindings.
6. Wear clothing in layers. As you warm up, shed outer layers to allow water vapor to evaporate. When you rest, put layers back on to avoid chilling. Cross-country skiing is vigorous exercise and sweating can occur even in subzero conditions.
7. Avoid frostbite. Mittens are better than gloves. If a part gets numb, warm it up immediately.
8. Wear a windbreaker. Skiers create their own windchill which produces frostbite sooner.
9. For extended tours, take warm liquids and food to maintain energy and strength.
10. Dress and equip yourself for the activity and not for style.
11. In some areas, use an avalanche cord, take a sectional probe, and use an emergency signaling device.
12. Warm up before beginning skiing hard.
13. Wear adequate sunglasses or goggles.

### Snow Skiing: Downhill

Nine out of ten skiing injuries involve the lower limbs—mainly at three sites: lower leg, ankle, and knee. Most ankle injuries are fractures or sprains. Two types of fractures are common in the lower leg: spiral-oblique fracture of the tibia and fibula,

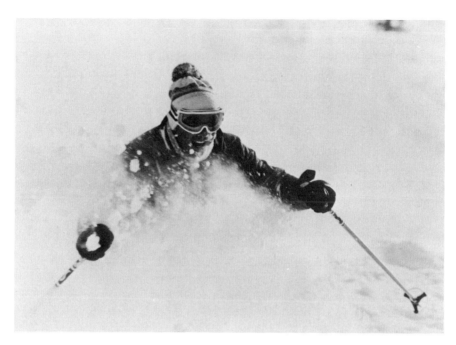

**FIGURE 21-9** The beginning skier is three times more likely to be injured than the expert. Photo courtesy of the Utah Travel Council.

and a transverse fracture of tibia and fibula (boot-top fracture). The knee suffers the most common ski injury—a sprain of the medial collateral ligament. This is usually caused by catching an inside ski edge and having the ski move away from the body.

Almost every type of fracture can occur in skiing. Most fractures occur in the lower extremities; these are also the most severe.

Although the subject of fractures highlights articles on skiing, the rate of occurrence of a ski fracture is about once for every forty-two years of average recreational skiing. Most ski injuries are merely nuisances, forcing the skier to take off a few days from skiing.

*Causal factors.* Many factors have been indicated as causal factors in ski injuries. Two factors are often explored and are discussed in some detail below.

*Skiing ability.* It is not surprising that beginners have far more accidents than veteran skiers. They have less technical knowledge of the sport, they know less about their equipment, and they often sadly misjudge their abilities. And though beginners have the most accidents, they spend considerably less time per day on the slopes than veterans.

The novice is three times more likely to be injured than the expert. Various reasons have been suggested for increased ability leading to a decrease in injuries:

1. The awkward posture assumed by the novice skier in the snowplow position.
2. The inability of the novice to "fall properly."
3. The increased frequency of falling by novices.

Well documented is the decrease in injury rates that comes with experience, and this decrease appears to occur regardless of whether that skiing experience has resulted in an increase in expertise. For example, as a general rule, the beginning skier skis more safely his fifth year than in his first year, regardless of the fact that he still classes himself as a "beginner."

*Sex.* The injury rate for women has been higher than men's rates. Interestingly, as the number of expert women skiers has increased, the rate of injury for women has declined.

Although it is not known for certain why females are more likely to be injured than males, some authorities contend it is due to the lack of conditioning. Others claim the reason is due to a woman having a lighter body structure which is less able to withstand mechanical injury forces.

*Prevention.* Anyone who has broken a leg or suffered a sprain in a skiing mishap can testify that there is nothing very glamorous about the experience. First aiders and the ski patrol can make this unpleasant experience better with proper care and attention to the injured skier.

Skiing can be a safer sport if the following guidelines are followed by individual skiers:

1. Physically conditioning the body to develop endurance. Good conditioning does not mean doing strenuous exercise the week before leaving for skiing. It means a daily regimen of exercise over an extended period of time.
2. Without question, any beginner should get expert instruction. Many experts recommend a minimum of five lessons. These should familiarize the new skier with the basic turns and give him the right amount of confidence. Such instruction will increase skills and not only will aid in preventing injuries, but also make it more enjoyable.
3. Properly fitted, properly adjusted, and properly maintained equipment is a must. For the fitting and adjusting of ski equipment, the beginner should rely on a reputable ski shop. The ski binding is the most critical part of skiing gear. When a skier loses control, he must be released from the skis before he suffers a serious injury. At the same time, the binding should not release too easily, exposing the skier to injury from an unnecessary fall.
4. While skiing, do not ski beyond your ability. The slopes at most ski areas are clearly marked according to their difficulty. Do not stop in the middle of the slope. Look both ways before crossing a trail. After a fall, fill in any depressions made in the snow by the body or equipment. Holes or bumps are very hazardous to skiers who follow down the slopes.

Ski injuries usually are merely nuisances, forcing the skier to take off a few days from skiing. Even the more severe injuries do not deter skiing for more than a week or two for the majority of the skiers.

### Soccer

Soccer does involve bodily contact between participants. Injuries can be expected and do occur. There is little protective equipment other than the option of wearing shin guards. Deaths are few except in world soccer games when riots break out during games and spectators are severely injured or even killed. American soccer has not experienced such rioting.

### Track and Field

Track and field is one of the safest of all sports. Field events (e.g., throwing of the discus, hammer, and javelin) are by far the most dangerous events accounting for the few deaths that have occurred in the sport. Other events such as pole vaulting, hurdles, and relays present special hazards.

### Water Skiing

Serious or fatal accidents in water skiing are infrequent. The accidents which do occur involve either the amateur or the reckless. This includes the untrained boat driver, the beginning skier, and the poor swimmer.

Safe procedures include:

1. Being a good swimmer.
2. Wearing a flotation device.
3. Having a "spotter" (an experienced observer) aboard.
4. Watching the water ahead.
5. Obtaining and maintaining proper equipment.
6. Following standard hand signals and holding aloft a flag when a skier is down in the water.
7. Avoiding skiing after dark.
8. Avoiding busy areas (docks, other boats, fishermen, etc.)

### Wrestling

Actual contact time in a single high school wrestling match approximates that of a football player over an entire football game.

There are certain injuries common in and peculiar to wrestling. For example, the head is often used as a fifth extremity in wrestling, not only for moves, but also as the initial contact area during a swift take-down maneuver. Nosebleeds and lacerations of the head are common even if the proper headgear is worn.

Weight loss has continued to be the wrestler's Achilles' heel. Weekly weight fluctuation of about four pounds can be common. Though many guidelines for safe weight loss have been established, abuses still abound. Some weight-reduction methods used by many wrestlers are dangerous.

Five factors could probably be related to injury prevention: (1) headgear use in practice and competition; (2) improved mat surfaces and mat-surface care; (3)

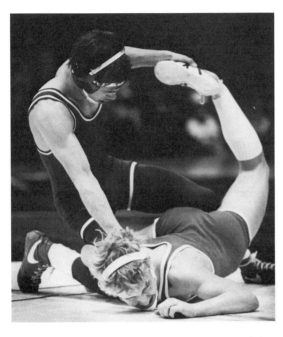

**FIGURE 21-10** Contact time in a single high school wrestling match approximates that of a football player over an entire football game. Photo courtesy of Mark A. Philbrick.

stretching and neck-strengthening exercises; (4) alert, conscientious referees; and (5) an adequate number of coaching and training personnel.

## PREVENTION OF SPORTS INJURIES

There are three main means of preventing sports-related injuries. First is the strengthening of the skeletal muscles. The second is through protective equipment, which either supports or shields parts of the body likely to be damaged. The third method of prevention lies in the game or contest rules.

### Mouth Protectors

Mouth protection has become one of the most successful preventive programs in sports. It is estimated that at least two million athletes have been equipped with mouth protectors, and their numbers grow by the thousands each year. As many as 150,000 injuries may be prevented each year.

There are three types of mouth guards: (1) stock, in which one size fits all; (2) mouth form, which either molds to the teeth during wear or is formed after being heated; and (3) custom, which are made from a dentist's cast of the athlete's mouth.

There are no data showing greater protective qualities in any one of the three types of mouth guards. However, it has been observed that a comfortable mouth guard is most likely to be worn regularly, and custom mouth guards are the most comfortable. A custom mouth guard should be made for an athlete who has braces.

Today mouth guards are used in many sports other than football, including field hockey, wrestling, soccer, basketball, gymnastics, squash, racquetball, lacrosse, karate, judo, surfing, trampolining, skydiving, skiing, weight lifting, the shot put, discus, skateboarding, rugby, parachuting, volleyball, and motocross.

Mouth protection programs are conspicuously absent in women's sports.

The mouth protector is a relatively inexpensive piece of equipment, but one which can aid immeasurably in preventing permanent and disfiguring injuries to the teeth and mouth, as well as fractures and concussions.

Dental injuries still occur, especially when coaches do not rigorously enforce league rules requiring mouth guards during play.

# 22

# Safety Instruction

## WHY SAFETY INSTRUCTION?

The purpose of safety instruction is to create safer behavior. It does so by increasing safety knowledge, skills, and positive attitudes. Safety instruction is an applied science with its own body of knowledge, and it seeks to apply research findings to the realities of daily life.

Unfortunately, safety instruction is often limited to transmitting safety facts, and the relationship between safety facts and safe behavior is weak. Take, for example, drivers who are well informed about the risk of not wearing safety belts, or motorcyclists not wearing helmets who are knowledgeable about injuries resulting from crashes. In other words, knowledge of safety facts does not guarantee safe behavior, nor does ignorance of safety facts prohibit safe behavior. Safety instruction's purpose is to increase our ability to make the intelligent choices that will enhance the quality of life in order to live longer, fuller, happier lives.

Therefore, it is the responsibility of social institutions (e.g., schools, industry, government, etc.) to provide people with the opportunity to learn how to be safer. However, this responsibility is too frequently preempted by other priorities.

If all items of knowledge were of equal value, there would be no question as to the value of safety instruction since it would then be considered on the same level as any other subject offered in the schools or industry.

Unfortunately, this is not the case. No matter how broadly one defines the "usefulness" of knowledge in a particular subject, the problem of priority is still a significant problem. For example, this belief is why the 3Rs (reading, 'riting, 'rithmetic) receive, in most cases, top priority in schools even though other subjects may be considered as essential.

Mankind's achievements are due to education. Education is demonstrably effective in other fields and there is no reason to assume a lack of effectiveness in safety instruction. The effectiveness is, however, difficult to quantify or measure.

In a very simple world one can learn what he or she needs to know through natural daily experience. In former times, such as during the early pioneer days on the frontier, life was fairly simple. The existing hazards were fewer and more easily recognized. Yes, drownings and falls then accounted for death and losses as they do today, but technology had not yet provided this complex world in which we cannot learn the essentials of safe behavior through the slow process of personal discovery. Today there is so much to learn, and what we do not know can harm us.

Throughout the nation and the world—in practically every city, town, and village—in the schools, in civic organizations, in industry—everywhere, safety instruction is taking place. All of these efforts make a common assumption: that children and adults can learn to behave safely and that the multiple and varied activities included in safety instructional programs are effective to this end.

In the schools, the instruction of children in safe behavior has been prescribed by law in some states since 1920. Safety became part of the school curriculum from the kindergarten through the senior year in high school, with specific topics allocated to the levels where they would best meet the needs of the students and be most readily understood by them.

Apart from the schools, safety instruction has long occupied a position of major importance in industry and traffic improvement efforts. Other examples include various agencies and organizations providing safety instruction (e.g., poison control centers' instructional efforts, wildlife resource departments' hunter safety courses). Individuals have provided instruction (e.g., a physician lecturing on the importance of child safety restraints in cars).

Research has shown that the concepts of safety do reach the subjects to whom the programs are directed. But rarely have studies been continued to the point of determining the extent to which such concepts affect behavior.

## PLANNING A LESSON

Lesson planning is sometimes like Mark Twain's statement about the weather: "Everybody talks about it, but nobody does anything about it!" A lesson plan is the instructional blueprint that describes those activities which will enable the student or class to reach that lesson's objectives. Some instructors are criticized for following a lesson plan, but such plans are important. There are many different ways of planning the lesson—what works well for one instructor may not work so well for another. Most important, the instructor must feel comfortable with the lesson plan. However, the instructor who does not plan is planning for failure.

### Steps in Lesson Planning

*Step 1: Identify the objective for the lesson.*   Some lessons may have a single objective, while others may have several related objectives. Most instructional plans lack a clear expression of objectives. Although most instructors believe in objectives, usual past objectives or goals have been based on what the teacher had to accomplish or ambiguously described what the student was expected to achieve. Simply defined, an objective is an instructional goal which requires the student to demonstrate his or her learning of something by performing some observable act (e.g., describe the issues involved with mandatory motorcycle helmets or list solutions for the reduction of drownings). In some way, the learner should know the kind of performance which will be used as an indication that learning has, in fact, been accomplished. Ways of making objectives clear to the learner include:

1.  Say or write the objective and illustrate it if clarification is needed.
2.  Show samples of acceptable work done by other learners.
3.  Give a practice test which is similar to the evaluation test.
4.  Demonstrate how to perform the objective.

The foremost requirement of an objective is that it convey precisely the instructional intent of the instructor. Action verbs such as "know," "understand," "enjoy," and "appreciate" are ambiguous or "fuzzy" terms. Objectives must describe what the learner (not the instructor) will be doing, because only in this way can the learner be assessed. Instructors, parents, employers, and other interested persons cannot look inside people's heads to determine what they have learned. Hence, to say that a person "knows how to swim," or that a person "understands the first aid for snakebite" creates a great deal of ambiguity. What does it mean to "know," or to "understand"? These words are imprecise in that they may be interpreted in a variety of ways. However, to say that a student can "write" or "state orally" or "perform" is much less ambiguous. These actions can be observed and the capabilities a student possesses can be inferred from the achievement the student is able to demonstrate.

An objective describes what the learner will be *doing* when he or she has achieved the objective. There are other components suggested by instructional design experts, but the above suggestion for having the objective student-oriented, specifying instructional outcomes, and using an action verb denoting observability is simple enough and easily mastered.

Verbs denoting action are not difficult to find. Common ones are: writes, draws, states orally, selects, matches, names, collects, applies, solves, compares, contrasts, constructs.

Examples of a variety of objectives are presented below. Notice that each states what the student will be doing as he or she demonstrates that the stated objective has been achieved.

**Example 1.** Using a copy of *Accident Facts*, the student should be able to classify home accidents into one of the eight types of home accidents.

**Example 2.** Given a list of disasters, the student will be able to identify three disasters which took more than twenty-five lives in the United States last year.

**Example 3.** Given a map of the community, the student will pinpoint on the map five hazardous conditions located during a community safety hazard survey.

**Example 4.** Given a list of fires, the student will be able to classify each according to the type of fire and suggested extinguisher.

*Step 2: Identify the concepts and content.* Concepts and content are selected in answer to the question "What does the student need to know to achieve this objective?"

Example of concepts and content include:

**Example 1.** An accident in the home or on home premises to occupants, guests, and trespassers is a home accident, and has nine categories (e.g., falls, firearms, drowning, etc.).

**Example 2.** Risk is something we can measure and safety is something we must judge.

**Example 3.** Accidents produce social and economic consequences of great importance.

**Example 4.** Measures to prevent accidents and reduce injuries have been in existence since ancient times.

*Step 3: Select or develop instructional activities.* Having written an objective and the related content to be learned, instructional or learning activities are selected and/or developed.

All learning begins with perception. Direct personal experience is usually the surest route to accurate learning. There is a psychologically correct learning experience through which content may be learned. This starts by perceiving a referent in the most direct way possible. The referent is an actual physical object or an event or process about a concept. When direct contact with a referent (actual physical object) is not feasible, students can still perceive a referent fairly well if it is vividly portrayed by vicarious means (e.g., pictures, story, etc.).

Next, learning activities that cause the learner to think about the referent are needed. Some examples are class discussions of all sorts—buzz sessions, panels, debates, and question-answer activities.

The next step is application. There are many types of activity which can be used to provide experience with content developed in class. An application activity should be used after the content knowledge has been acquired by the students. Use of the content learned enhances retention and its usefulness. However, time and other constraints may prohibit application for all content.

TABLE 22-1   Learning Activities

| SHOW* | DISCUSS | APPLY |
|---|---|---|
| Show the class what you want them to learn through use of: | Engage the class in discussion to: | Encourage the application of ideas and concepts through: |
| Objects | Raise questions | Assignments |
| Pictures | Cite and elicit examples | In-class activities which require |
| Stories | Pose problems | students to use ideas |
| Charts | Consider various points of | Specific out-of-class projects which |
| Diagrams | · view | challenge students |
| Films | Seek reasons | Follow-up measures to ensure |
| Real experiences (past and present) | | good results |
| Recordings | | |
| Role playing | | |
| Textbook content | | |

*This step should serve as an effective interest arouser and provide a common background experience which can be used later as a reference point for discussion. It is most effective when it is stimulating and eye-catching, although reference to a previous group experience can also be very effective.

Adapted from Asahel D. Woodruff, *Basic Concepts of Teaching* (San Francisco: Chandler Publishing Company, 1961), pp. 93ff.

In summary, providing learning activities for students is a three-fold task. The instructor must first *show* the referent to the students. The only exception to this occurs when the students have already perceived the referent in the past, and are able to discuss something with which they are already familiar. The instructor must then conduct *discussion* to clarify the content. Finally, the instructor must guide the students in *application* of newly acquired knowledge. A partial listing of some of the ways of showing a referent, clarifying it through discussion, and trying it out, is given in Table 22-1.

As tools serving the instructor, lesson plans will vary in format and degree of specificity. For example, some instructors include the exact questions they plan to ask; others write only one or two words as clues.

There are several forms for lesson plans to be developed. A simple form which contains all the necessary items is shown in Table 22-2.

Sample completed lesson plans are provided to aid in understanding the ideas of this section (Tables 22-3 and 22-4).

### Planning a Skill Lesson

The teaching of a skill is also an important task of many safety instructors in various situations (e.g., using a fire extinguisher, carrying a rifle, using a ladder, etc.).

The process of teaching skills involves several steps:

1. Preassessing students' readiness or ability to perform skill.
2. Providing a model of skill for the learner (e.g., film or actual demonstration).

**TABLE 22-2  Sample Lesson Form**

Topic or Title: _____

Objectives:

   1.

   2.

| Concepts/Content to be Taught | Learning Activities |
| --- | --- |
| 1. | 1. Show: |
| |     Discuss: |
| |     Apply: |
| 2. | 2. Show: |
| |     Discuss: |
| |     Apply: |

**TABLE 22-3  Sample Lesson Plan**

Topic: Multiple Cause Concept of Accident Causation

Objectives: After this lesson each class member should be able to define the multiple cause concept, and identify the implications this concept has for safety and the recognition of accident causes and prevention.

| Concept/Content to be Taught | Learning Activities |
| --- | --- |
| 1. Accidents generally result from a combination of human-agent-environmental factors acting in a closely interwoven fashion. This is called the multiple cause concept. | 1. Show: Hand out a newspaper account* of an accident to each student. Have students circle words, phrases, and/or sentences which might describe factors contributing in causing the accident. Write marginal notes if needed. |
| | Discuss: Ask: 1. Which words, phrases, and/or sentences were circled? 2. How did each contribute to the accident? |
| | Apply: For each of the contributing factors identified in the accident account, have students suggest one preventation measure. This is done outside of class and is to be submitted to the instructor. |

Note: As many different accident cases can be evaluated in class as time allows.

*It is recommended that the newspaper account be typed double-spaced and duplicated for each student.

**TABLE 22-4  Sample Lesson Plan**

Topic: Dog Bites

Objectives: The students should be able to:
1. Recite the magnitude of the dog bite problem.
2. Describe dogs most likely to bite.
3. List reasons for dogs biting humans.
4. Name ways of avoiding a dog bite.

| Concepts/Content to be Taught | Learning Activities |
| --- | --- |
| 1. An estimated one million people in the U.S. are bitten by dogs each year and an unknown number die as a result of these attacks. Dog bites compose one of the major public health problems and are one of the main causes of childhood injury. | 1. Show: Write the number "1,000,000" on chalkboard.<br><br>Discuss: Ask:<br>1. How many people are bitten each year?<br>2. How many class members have been bitten?<br>3. What is the risk of being bitten during a year in the U.S.?<br><br>Apply: Survey your neighborhood as to incidences of dog bites. |
| 2. Several types of dogs are known as "biters."<br>  a. German shepherds<br>  b. Doberman pinchers<br>  c. St. Bernards<br>  d. mongrels<br>  e. "packs" of dogs running loose<br>  f. bitch with pups<br>  g. etc. | 2. Show: Pictures of different dogs.<br><br>Discuss: Ask:<br>1. Which appear to be biters?<br>2. Which breed bites the most often?<br>3. Which breed kills the most often (per capita basis)?<br>4. What accounts for a certain type of dog to be dangerous?<br>5. Which type of dogs have bitten class members?<br><br>Apply: Survey your neighborhood for the number and types of dogs most likely to bite. |
| 3. Dogs bite for various reasons:<br>  a. provoked or teased<br>  b. threatened<br>  c. trained<br>  d. environmental conditions<br>  e. etc. | 3. Show: Read or display cases of dog biting episodes.<br><br>Discuss: Buzz groups. Each group will be given one or more cases to analyze in terms of identifying: (a) victim's age, sex, etc.; (b) when? (c) where? (d) reasons.<br>At the conclusion of the analysis, groups will report to the class their results.<br><br>Apply: For each category (who, when, etc.), have students suggest at least one preventative measure. |

**TABLE 22-4 Continued**

| | |
|---|---|
| 4. Things people do innocently are often interpreted by dogs as threats. Likewise, people often mistake dog behavior for aggression when it is not. Ways to avoid dog bites include:<br>a. Never run away from a dog.<br>b. Keep your eyes on a dog.<br>c. Do not startle a dog.<br>d. Do not threaten a dog.<br>e. Be friendly by using dog's name, but do not pet dog.<br>f. etc. | 4. Show: Display an umbrella and say that in case of a dog attack, you could pop-open the umbrella which will startle a dog into retreat.<br><br>Discuss: Brainstorm<br>1. Ways of avoiding a dog bite.<br>2. If you know you are going to get bitten, what should be done? |

3. Helping students identify the movements or parts of the skill to be performed in sequential order.
4. Providing for time when students are coached toward better performance of the skill.
5. Providing for feedback and correction during practice.
6. Providing for adequate repetitive practice. Duration and frequency of practice sessions are important.
7. Evaluating the results.

## TEACHING TECHNIQUES

There is really nothing sacred about teaching methods. There are several reasons for instructors continuing their use of the traditional teaching methods. Perhaps they have never experienced innovative methods, or feel most comfortable replicating the methods to which they themselves have been exposed. This is not meant to imply that traditional methods have no place in the instructional process.

Certainly no single learning method should be labeled as the "best" approach. Each of the various kinds of teaching methods has a place in instruction. Each has certain values and certain limitations.

Presented here is a ready reference of some of the techniques for instruction. A good instructor uses a variety of approaches and adapts his or her teaching methods to the needs of the students and to the unique characteristics of the lesson.

This presentation does not intend to treat all the teaching methods. Neither has an attempt been made to discuss each method fully.

### Use A Variety of Methods

A class should not fall into a monotonous pattern because of insufficient instructor planning and preparation. Lessons may need to have elements of sameness, but here too variety may offer a refreshing change. Change may mean a list of study questions on the chalkboard or a short cassette tape of some expert.

Curriculum guides attempt to give assistance to instructors. However, they cannot tailor each lesson to fit every situation and special circumstance. The instructor can follow the suggested content but must provide the teaching methods. At least three to six methods should be used in each lesson presentation.

Some methods can be used more frequently than others. Discussion, chalkboard, and storytelling could be used in almost every lesson.

Instructors might find a tendency to use the same three or four methods every time. Carefully consider others that you could use for variety. A word of caution. Each method used should be appropriate to the lesson and not used solely for the sake of variety.

The following teaching methods are briefly discussed:

| | | |
|---|---|---|
| agree-disagree statements | debate | panel discussion |
| brainstorming | demonstration | role playing |
| buzz session | guest speaker | special report |
| case study | lecture | storytelling |

*Agree-disagree statements.* A list of statements which are provocative is handed to each class member with the instructions to agree or disagree with each statement. Then the students are formed into small groups of five to six students and instructed that each group is to reach a consensus on the factual information statements. After all the groups have finished, the instructor gives the correct answers and instructs the students to mark those statements on which more elaboration and clarification are needed. This discussion can easily involve many minutes of a class session.

Examples of statements which could be used are found on page 10.

*Brainstorming.* Brainstorming is a way of involving the entire group in finding solutions to a problem. The idea is to invoke a storm of ideas from all the participants. Ideas are accepted without criticism. The object is to have as many ideas as possible suggested regardless of how wild they may seem.

To conduct a brainstorming session:

1. Explain the rules. There should be no criticism, no judgments of any kind. All ideas are acceptable, the more creative the better.
2. Choose a recorder to write quickly all suggestions on the board so everyone can see them, or the instructor can serve as the recorder.
3. Define the problem very specifically. Write it on the chalkboard.
4. Get the group started and keep things relaxed.
5. Stop the brainstorming after a fairly short time—five minutes or so for most topics, fifteen to twenty minutes for real-life problems.
6. Refine the ideas by choosing a solution.
7. Summarize the conclusions. State the original problem and the solution or solutions which have been found.

Brainstorming may be difficult in a large group. Groups of eight to fifteen members are usually best. Brainstorming may be difficult with a group whose ages or backgrounds differ. This teaching method is most effective for short periods of time. Criticism may surface from the students before the session is over if prolonged.

*Buzz sessions.* A buzz session is a short period (about six minutes) during a class when the group is divided into small groups of two to six people to "buzz" (talk quickly and busily) about a specific question. The group should be small so everyone can be involved. Keep the time short to encourage the group not to waste a minute.

Buzz sessions can help warm up a class for a general discussion.

To set up a buzz group:

1. Divide the class into groups of three to six.
2. Make the discussion topic very specific and, if desired, tell the groups that they will be asked to report back to the class. All the groups may discuss the same topic, or you may assign each group a particular aspect of the problem. Make sure each group understands its assignments.
3. Each group needs a chairperson and a recorder. Assign these, or let the group choose.
4. Give them a time limit in advance. Circulate between the groups and give a two-minute warning.
5. Reconvene for reporting. Each group should report.
6. Summarize the results, making sure that the problem is solved, or that the connection with the lesson topic is clear.

If the assignment is not clear, the groups will not be productive. If the instructor does not circulate to keep the groups on the subject, buzz sessions can turn into visiting sessions.

*Case studies.* A case study is a story or problem situation that can lead into a discussion or dramatize an important point in the lesson. It may be a true experience or realistic problem situation that the instructor has made up.

Case studies can be used to help students relate to the lesson, to dramatize the main point, to help class members experience problems vicariously, or to review a past lesson or introduce an upcoming one.

There are at least three kinds of case studies: (1) the lead-in to a discussion, (2) the written assignment, and (3) the pictorial case study. These are explained in more detail below:

1. The discussion lead-in. When the story reaches its climax, ask the students, "What would you do?" Help class members find solutions to the problem through discussion. At the end, summarize and help class members decide what action they plan to take when confronted with similar problems. You might want to tell the class the outcome of a true story after they have arrived at their solution to the problem.

2.  The written assignment. Provide each class member with a written copy of the case. Have students list all the possible solutions to the problem. They individually analyze the solutions and then choose the solution which is best. They should be prepared to discuss the decision they have made.
3.  The pictorial case study. Present the story through a picture of the accident or of the injury. The instructor asks questions of the class.

An example of a case situation follows:

You are the parent of Steve who was apprehended for drunken driving. He was fined and had his license revoked. As Steve's parent, which would you do?

_____ 1. Take away his driving privileges for three months.
_____ 2. Cut off his allowance.
_____ 3. Restrict him to 9:00 p.m. curfew for three months.
_____ 4. Instruct him not to see the friends who were with him again.
_____ 5. Make him pay his own fine by working.
_____ 6. Force him to do extra chores around the house as an additional penalty.
_____ 7. Just discuss the situation with him without punishment.
_____ 8. Tell him it is okay if he drinks as long as he doesn't drink and drive.
_____ 9. Let him know you are disappointed in his behavior.
_____ 10. Emphasize to him that he has shamed the family name.
_____ 11. Allow him no more driving privileges with the family car(s) even after his license has been reinstated.
_____ 12. Others: _____

Another example of a case study using a different format follows:

**heart attack victim saves woman from submerged auto as 12 bystanders ignore screams for help**

Jim U. has serious heart trouble, but that didn't stop him from saving a trapped woman whose car was overturned in a murky canal—while a dozen bystanders ignored her screams for help.

Mr. U., who can't work because of three recent heart attacks, was going home from a doctor's appointment when he saw a crowd gathering by a canal.

"As I drove by, I looked in the canal and saw a car. At least a dozen people were just standing around," said Mr. U.

"I asked if anyone was still inside. There were four or five guys standing nearby with their hands in their pockets. One said: 'Yeah, there's someone inside the car.' I asked how he knew. He replied: 'Oh, we heard her screaming'."

With no thought of his illness, Mr. U. flung off his shoes and shirt and plunged into the canal. "The windows were rolled up and the doors were jammed by the muddy canal bottom," Mr. U. said. "I heard the woman scream twice, then she stopped."

"Finally I got one of the doors open a little. Water started rushing into the car. It was all black inside and I couldn't see anything." The woman lay helplessly pinned by the steering wheel after her car spun out of control, rolling over the embankment and ending on its roof in the canal.

"I leaned into the car, grabbed her legs and started pulling, but water kept rushing in so fast that we both began drowning," he said. "Finally, I dragged her out feet first. She had lost consciousness and was turning blue. At last, some guys came down and helped me pull her onto the bank. She wasn't breathing, and I gave her mouth-to-mouth resuscitation."

1. Do you think that getting involved pays?
2. Why should people "get involved" when the public has paid and assigned others (e.g., policemen, firemen, etc.) to do so?
3. Would most individuals know how to help—even if they wanted to?
4. Are you willing to help an accident victim? Do you think you are capable of helping? How could you increase your ability to assist others?
5. How would you feel if you didn't assist an accident victim who later died, but could have been saved with your assistance?

*Debate.* An excellent way of studying both sides of an issue is with a debate.

Rather than involve only a few students in a debate, the following procedure involves the whole class.

### Procedures:
1. Choose the debate topic.
2. Divide the class into two groups—one group pro and the other con.
3. Every student is to spend time researching a defense for his side—pro or con. Allow several days or a week for proper researching by the students.
4. On the day of the debate, the two groups meet separately to prepare their "offense"—questions to ask the other group opposing them. This may take 10 minutes.
5. Arrange seats so the two groups face each other.
6. Have one side ask the other a question, and let that side reply. Alternate turns asking questions.
7. Rotate the asking and answering of questions until all students (or a pre-set number) have an opportunity to participate.
8. Summarization and judging the winner can be done by one or a combination of the teacher, several students, or several parents.
9. The judging committee should:
   (a) Record arguments (questions)
   (b) Record major points arrived at by the answering group
   (c) Report to the class at the end of the period information in a and b above and declare a winner

*Demonstration.* A demonstration visually shows how some things are done. It is especially effective when teaching skills or procedures because the viewer can quickly grasp what is being done and what will result.

The instructor should practice before actually demonstrating. Credibility can be easily lost if the instructor cannot perform the intended skill in front of the class.

The following ideas may help in demonstration:

1. Will all class members be able to see the demonstration?
2. Do the steps appear in logical order?
3. Is any additional explanation needed other than showing the skill?

*Guest speaker.* A guest speaker can give valuable help. The guest speaker is one who has knowledge or skill in a specific area. Most communities have experts who are willing to assist.

Use guest speakers with these cautions: All presentations should be in harmony with acceptable safety standards and practices and what is acceptable for the class rather than what may be appropriate for another level of training. Guest speakers should not be used in the class so frequently that the technique loses its effectiveness.

*Lecture.* This is the most universally used teaching method. It consists of a verbal presentation of a body of subject matter. Because of overuse and misuse, it is sometimes questioned as an effective method of teaching. There is one-way communication with the instructor being the only one who is active.

Lecturing can be very effective if used at appropriate times. These times might be when the instructor wants to:

1. Save time.
2. Cover a lot of lesson material.
3. Present information that is difficult for the students to read because of lack of books or materials.
4. Summarize.
5. Present information to a large audience.

Criticism against lecturing includes:

1. It is often a waste of time because, being passive, the students learn little. We generally remember only about 10 percent of what we hear.
2. There is no guarantee that the student will understand the lecture's contents.
3. Unless well prepared and delivered, a lecture can become boring to the audience.

To make lecturing more effective:

1. Always use some visual aids (pictures, charts, slides, models, or chalkboard).
2. Use language which the class members can understand.
3. Express ideas and ask thought-provoking questions.
4. Vary the pitch and speed of your speech to create variety and to emphasize important points.
5. Walk around the room. Do not stand in one place and do not pace back and forth.
6. Do not read the lesson material word by word. Maintain as much eye contact as possible.
7. Whenever possible, permit questions and discussion upon a topic.

*Panel discussion.* A panel is a group of three to five class members or invited experts who are assigned to discuss a topic in front of the class.

A panel discussion can be a useful classroom variation. Class members tend to be passive learners when only the instructor is giving a lesson. When class members are used to present new material to the class, they will become more actively involved in learning. The panelists should be as well informed on the topic as possible.

For success in using a panel, ask several class members to gather information on a specific subject. When the class meets, these panelists should sit together, facing the class to discuss the subject they have researched. After each has reported, the class members may ask the panelists questions. Panelists may also be nonclass members with specialized knowledge or experience.

*Role playing.* Role playing helps students learn through involvement. In role playing, class members are assigned to act out a situation.

Tips for effective role playing include:

1.  Role play situations that relate to the lesson.
2.  Describe to the class the situation and characters that will be needed.
3.  Ask for volunteers to role play. Emphasize that the actor is to play a role and not himself.
4.  Involve the audience. Assign them tasks during the role playing, such as watching for appropriate procedures used.
5.  It takes courage to try new ideas. Allow mistakes and learn from them.
6.  Use role-playing situations that are real and important to the lesson.

*Special Report.* A special report is helpful information that is not readily available to the class. It can be research findings that will strengthen and motivate a discussion. It can be a report of an interview with an expert in a particular medical field relating to accidents and injuries.

The person making the report should have enough time to prepare properly for a presentation. Offer suggestions on content and, if necessary, where to find the information. The more specific the directions are, the more the presenter will be able to help meet the lesson objectives.

Special reports will be most effective if certain conditions are met in the presentation. Be sure the person giving the report clearly understands:

1.  The specific topic.
2.  The amount of time that will be given for reporting.
3.  That the presentation can be made more interesting through careful planning and the use of some teaching aids.
4.  Time should be allowed for questions, comments, and discussion from class members.

It is usually best not to plan a number of oral reports for one lesson.

Special reports can come either from an outside expert (similar to a guest speaker) or from class members.

*Storytelling.* This is a favorite technique among safety instructors. Stories can clarify a principle and gain and sustain attention as few other methods can.

Storytelling is the relating of experiences. It may be a personal experience or an experience of someone else.

Be cautious about too many stories. Though they might be interesting to the teller, many times students become bored with them or may even think that the teller is showing off or is bragging about his experiences. Confidentiality is important in some cases so be careful about revealing names or things which may be personal.

### Teaching Cautions

*Speculation.* One of the most common temptations is to speculate on matters about which there is very little information or knowledge. The disciplined teacher has the courage to say, "I don't know," and leave it at that. It is no discredit to intelligence or to our integrity to say, "I do not know."

*Misquoting.* The disciplined instructor will be sure of his sources and will make every effort to determine whether a statement properly represents standard policies and practices or is merely the opinion of someone.

*Special interests.* "Pet" topics where one principle or concept is stressed distort their place in the whole scheme of the safety curriculum. Overemphasis of certain topics does an injustice to the students and the curriculum. To tell a class everything you know on a subject is not always wise or necessary. It is a good idea to have something in reserve in case someone asks a question. It gets a little uncomfortable to be continually standing at the brink of your knowledge, especially since there is usually someone present who is anxious to entice you to take one more step.

*Sensational story.* Perhaps the greatest temptation of the instructor struggling to maintain the attention of a class is the use of the sensational story. A good story is always good, but soon the glimmer of such sensational reports bears a negative reaction from students. Some may even wonder about the real purposes of the teller who may seem to relish in reliving the vivid and often gory descriptions of the latest car crash victim. Soon every story sounds alike.

*Class discussion.* Such discussions can be excellent because they stimulate personal involvement, but they must have definite objectives or goals. Class discussions should not be used to kill time. Preparation is important to the success of a class discussion. Further, it should be understood that correct principles and concepts are not determined by conducting an opinion poll, which is what many class discussions amount to.

*Use of statistics.*   The field of safety is replete with figures, statistics, numbers, and rates. There is little literature available on the proper use of accident statistics. The practice of citing statistics and then requiring their memorization for an examination is all too common.

The use of statistics is not all bad. They can point out and describe problems. It is suggested that proportional data (rates or ratios) rather than numbers and figures be used. For example, rather than saying a hundred thousand accidental deaths occurred, statements similar to the following are suggested:

1. Accidents are the fourth leading cause of death in the United States.
2. There is, on the average, one person dying from an accident every five minutes in the United States.
3. Accidents cause more deaths each year than all infectious diseases combined.
4. One in four Americans is annually injured enough to require medical attention or activity restriction for at least one day.

Another pitfall is the attention drawn to catastrophes because these events make newspaper headlines. It is significant that a very small percentage of accident catastrophes occur as a result of natural disasters (e.g., floods, earthquakes, etc.) when contrasted with the number of deaths resulting from other types of unspectacular, unpublished accidents.

*Use of scare tactics.*   Perhaps we all can remember a class where a film, pictures, or stories were used of bizarre, gory accident scenes. This is a common practice in driver education and industrial safety meetings.

Experts have come to the following conclusions regarding the use of scare tactics to change or influence behavior:

1. Fear methods tend to be short term in their effectiveness.
2. If scare tactics are used too often, a person may become calloused or too accustomed to their use for any desired behavior change to occur.
3. Fear techniques can adversely affect some people by causing undue worry and anxiety and thus negatively affect behavior.
4. Scare tactics can influence behavior by preventing one from doing something dangerous.
5. There is a need for further research since the question of the effectiveness of scare tactics is not fully answered. Few studies on the use of scare tactics exist specifically in safety instruction. If used, fear techniques should be used sparingly.

*Use of rules.*   Safety rules have been used as a means to prevent accidents. Violations of safety rules usually represent the major causes of accidents and a rule was developed for the purpose of alerting people about hazards. One problem regarding rules is that a person may know the rule, but chooses not to follow the rule; the time and effort expended for safety instruction is therefore wasted. Instruction must be more than recall and memorization of facts and information.

Another problem with safety rule usage is that if all listings of rules were compiled, most people could not know or remember all safety rules. Besides, such listings would probably be incomplete.

Another problem is that if rules are made or provided to govern behavior, in many settings they then must be enforced. The enforcement can pose serious problems and difficulties.

Safety rules can be useful. However, the following should be considered:

1. The number of rules should be kept to a minimum.
2. The rule should be clear and unambiguous.
3. Rules should ordinarily be written in positive terms.
4. In certain settings (e.g., plants, schools, etc.) only those rules that will be strictly enforced should be given.

## CRITICISM AGAINST SAFETY INSTRUCTION

We now find many who say that the emphasis should be diverted from educational efforts concerned with averting accidents to those efforts which assume accidents will occur and place emphasis on prevention of further loss. Walter Kohl offers another very discerning suggestion with regard to the placement of emphasis:

> Building more reliable devices, safer cars, better highways, is all to the good, but as one observer said, "it is similar to the attempt of reducing the occurrence of crime by making it harder to steal, or to kill, rather than by improving the social climate." The attitude of people is the basic issue. This attitude cannot be managed, but only improved slowly by the individual's acceptance of a different set of values.

It would seem that through educational efforts we can truly affect attitudes. The critics of safety instructional programs do not intend to eliminate safety courses but believe these programs should rely on scientific evaluation for their justification rather than on mere "common sense." Any safety instructor should want the same.

# 23

# Legal Aspects of Accidents

Can you be sued? There is the possibility and because of it, it is wise to study those aspects of the law dealing with accidents resulting in death, injuries, and property damage. Personal harm and financial loss spark most lawsuits, but some are prompted by the lure of dollars.

Today any accident resulting in death, injury, or property damage can wind up in court. For example, there was the case of a woman who collected $50,000 damages from San Francisco with the contention that her fall against a pole in a runaway cable car transformed her into a nymphomaniac. Other examples include suing because a prize was missing from a box of Cracker Jack or a rock was found in a can of beans.

TABLE 23-1   A SAMPLING OF MULTIMILLION-DOLLAR VERDICTS

The chances of winning big stakes in a lawsuit are getting better.

The sums often are pushed up by what are called punitive damages. These awards—assessed on top of whatever is deemed to be adequate to compensate for the injury itself—are aimed at punishing the party at fault and deterring others. Many large verdicts are not paid in full, however. Sometimes, higher courts find them excessive. And because of the possibility that judges will reduce the amount, suits often are settled out of court for figures well below the verdict.

Some of the biggest money awards granted, as reported by Jury Verdict Research, Inc. include:

$128,466,280—auto gas-tank explosion. A California jury awarded the biggest verdict on record after one person was killed and another badly burned in a Ford Pinto hit from behind. Punitive damages of $125 million were reduced by a judge, but the Ford Motor Company is appealing the final $7 million judgment.

$124,000,000 structured settlement—boating accident. A 13-year-old boy was injured when a towing line broke free from a boat and struck him on the head. The cleat broke free due to an alleged defect in the cleat's attaching mechanism. Guaranteed payments to the boy, who received brain damage, total $116 million over his lifetime. The settlement has a present value of $6.6 million.

$43,000,000—truck accident. A 16-year-old boy died instantly when a thirty-ton asphalt truck that he was hired to drive went out of control on a steep highway. The boy had no license to drive and the accident occurred only two hours after he had gotten the job. Suit was brought by the parents and a brother against the company that hired the boy.

$26,500,000 structured settlement—automobile accident. Two trucks were racing on a rain-slick highway when one truck crossed the freeway median and struck a car head-on. The father suffered permanent brain damage. He is unable to care for himself and has essentially the brain of an infant. It takes $35,000 to $85,000 per year to provide full-time care. The mother was killed. A daughter and a son suffered injuries. The defendants will pay $3.5 million now, and $11 million to the two surviving children when they reach eighteen. They will also put $12 million into a trust fund. The settlement included punitive damages.

$21,766,000—plane crash. The survivors of four men killed in the crash of a two-engine private plane sued the manufacturer, claiming that the accident was caused by a fuel-system defect. The award included punitive damages. Courts later reduced the award to a total of $1.8 million.

$16,500,000—automobile crash. A man left paralyzed after a collision was awarded $16.5 million. But the total award may never be collected. The driver of the car which struck the victim's vehicle head-on has filed for bankruptcy, and Ford Motor Company settled out of court for $3.5 million. The victim is paralyzed from the neck down and must be moved at least once every fifteen minutes to avoid bed sores.

$9,341,683—seat-belt failure. A dentist became a quadriplegic when his small foreign car was hit by another car and his head smashed into the visor. He sued the other driver for negligence and the auto maker for a defective seat-belt design.

$7,000,000—swimming-pool accident. A man became a quadriplegic after landing on his head while diving into a swimming pool at a hotel. A jury upheld his claim that the diving board was too flexible and that there was not enough water in the pool. The award later was cut to $4.68 million.

$5,565,700—job accident. A construction worker went into a coma when he was struck by a power line that had been knocked down by a fellow worker. The man's wife sued the utility company claiming that the line was improperly placed.

$5,200,000—football accident. A high school athlete was paralyzed in a football game. A jury agreed with the family that the youth's helmet was not designed properly, assessing damages against the maker. The award was reduced by a settlement providing monthly payments that could total $3 million or more.

$2,500,000—explosion. An underground gasoline storage tank was left unattended at a construction site. The tank exploded when a boy dropped a match. Another boy with him suffered permanent brain damage, paralysis, hearing loss, and other damages.

$1,900,000—skiing accident. The injured had reached the end of a ski trail when a dead tree fell, hitting him on the head. The injured was in a coma, suffered brain damage, and now has partial paralysis accompanied by spasms. The jury agreed that the ski-area operators were responsible for removing the dead tree from the area near the trail.

## TORT AND CRIME

A tort is an act, or absence of an act, by which someone causes an injury to person, property, or reputation, either directly or indirectly.

A tort is never the same thing as a crime, although the two have several features in common. A criminal case is not concerned with compensation of the individual against whom the crime may be committed, and the crime victim serves as an accuser and witness against the offender. The crime victim will leave the courtroom empty-handed.

On the other hand, a tort case is started and maintained by the injured person. The purpose of such action is to obtain compensation for the damage suffered at the hands of the offender. If the injured person is successful in the court action, he or she receives a judgment for a sum of money.

## NEGLIGENCE

Today legal action for damages for personal injuries is based on the determination of negligence. Negligence is defined as acting or failing to act as a "reasonable person" would in a similar circumstance.

There is no rule of thumb for determining or predicting what constitutes negligent action in all cases. However, there are several factors which a judge or jury weighs in establishing negligence. These include:

*Proximate cause* is the direct or immediate cause of the injury, the last act prior to injury without which the injury would not have resulted. An example of negligence would be a driver hitting a pedestrian walking in a marked cross-walk. An example of not being negligent involved two players who bumped heads while playing basketball, one of them dying. The teacher was absent from the scene and was not held negligent because there was not a close causal connection with the accident since such events are normally possible in basketball.

*Contributory negligence* is when the injured person failed to act with reasonable care to safeguard himself. For example, a driver of a car hitting a pedestrian ordinarily will not be negligent when the pedestrian is illegally walking across a street. This is void in cases involving children between ages one and seven years. Contributory negligence is debated when youths between the ages of seven and twenty-one years are involved.

*Attractive nuisance.* Most of these are hazardous conditions of one kind or another. Examples include:

- Swimming pool without a fence.
- Backyard trampoline within easy access.
- Raised sprinkler heads on an athletic field.

An attractive nuisance is an object so enticing that it could reasonably be expected to attract the curiosity of one who lacks the intelligence, maturity, or experience to recognize the danger it poses.

*Assumption of risk* is voluntarily choosing to enter an activity with the realization of the risk of injury involved. In other words, assumption of risk means the acceptance of the foreseeable dangers associated with an activity. For example, athletics and sports participants assume the normal risks involved (e.g., football players receiving torn knee cartilage or a brain concussion).

*Foreseeability* is the term applied to an event that could have been anticipated and hence prevented by prudent action. An example of a negligent teacher involved moving a top-heavy piano with a broken roller. The teacher enlisted several students to help. The piano tipped over, crushing and killing one of the students. The court held that the teacher should have foreseen the potential of the piano tipping over.

## PROTECTION AGAINST LAWSUITS

In unprecedented numbers, Americans are suing each other for just about every reason imaginable. The surge of lawsuits, building for decades, shows no signs of peaking.

Any one of the following accidents could result in a huge lawsuit: The mail carrier slips on your icy steps; a guest trips over a rug; your dog attacks somebody; you are blamed for an auto accident. Chances are a lawsuit will not happen; most people go through life without being brought to court. Nevertheless, here are some protective measures to consider:

*Insurance.* Automobile and homeowners policies provide only limited protection. There is extended personal-liability insurance. A typical extended policy would pay judgments for accidents involving your home, motor vehicles, boat, and other property, and for libel or slander. Most major property and casualty insurers sell the coverage.

*Counsel.* The choice of a lawyer, should one be needed, requires great care. A good lawyer should know the available strategies if you are sued with a groundless nuisance suit.

*Safety instruction.* Everyone should learn how to recognize existing hazards in the environment. Moreover, safety instruction should also include prevention measures and ways to control injuries in the event of an accident.

*Inspections.* Regardless of the location (e.g., home, school, motor vehicle, work), periodically taking time to search for potential hazards is well worth the time and effort. Checklists are available from insurance companies and other agencies and can offer guidelines as to what to look for.

## ACTUAL COURT CASES INVOLVING ACCIDENTAL INJURIES

As an aid in understanding negligence and legal liability, actual court cases from around the United States are presented. These cases are by Bryant Berry, Jr., attorney-at-law, who wrote them for newspaper syndication.

People with specific legal problems should consult an attorney for advice relative to laws in their locality, since laws will vary from state to state.

### Teacher Liable for the Scars?

### CASE

Henry Merrick had been a science teacher at Jefferson High School for ten years. He was an excellent teacher and liked by all the students. He had earned a master's degree and was lacking only his dissertation to obtain a doctor's degree in science. But one day Henry goofed.

The experiment Henry was demonstrating to his class was to show how to put out a fire with carbon dioxide. It called for lighter fluid to be used as the source of a fire in a glass beaker. A carbon dioxide mixture was then to be poured on the fire to extinguish it. For some reason, Henry did not have cigarette lighter fluid and used alcohol instead. When the carbon dioxide mixture was poured on the alcohol fire, it did not totally extinguish the fire but instead left a nearly invisible flame. Henry then started to reconduct the experiment. When he poured new alcohol into the beaker, a flamethrower effect was created. Alice, a 17-year-old student, was standing near the beaker. The fire jumped to her neck and arms and, before it was all over, she had sustained severe burns which left her with scars for life.

A suit was brought by Alice against Henry for $150,000. Alice contended that Henry was negligent in conducting the experiment. "He should have known better than to use alcohol as a source of the fire," she told the court. "He was negligent and he should pay for these ugly scars."

Henry argued that since the injury occurred while he was performing his duties as a teacher, the school district should be the one sued—not him. Who should win the suit?

## DECISION

Alice won. The court held that a public school teacher may be held liable for injuries sustained by a student that are caused by his negligence. "Here," the court concluded, "Henry, with all of his education and experience, knew or should have known the results of using the alcohol instead of lighter fluid in his experiment."

Based on a decision of the Supreme Court of Ohio.

### Is School Liable for Student's Injury?

## CASE

Gary was fourteen years old at the time of the accident. Due to his extremely hyperactive behavior and his parents' inability to care for him, Gary had been placed in a series of schools since he was six years old. The school he attended and lived at when the injury occurred was on open land. It was unfenced, and had inadequate personnel to supervise the students. Gary had escaped from the facility many times and had been returned by passers-by or by school personnel. Relatives visiting him at the school often found him wandering on the grounds in inappropriate or no clothing.

On the evening of the accident, Gary escaped again and attempted to cross a very busy street on foot. He was struck and thrown into the air by an automobile and sustained a fractured pelvis and compound fractures of his right leg.

A lawsuit was brought on behalf of Gary by his parents against the school. They asked for $400,000 in damages and showed that Gary required numerous surgeries and medications. He was restrained several times to prevent reinjury due to his hyperactivity, was in considerable pain, and suffered permanent shortening of his right leg of two inches. The permanent injuries interfered with Gary's ability to run and swim, both activities which are important in the care of hyperactive people because they enable them to remain quiet for short periods of time after exercising.

The school argued they should not be responsible for Gary's running away and being hit by the car. "We can't keep a constant watch on all the students," they claimed. Should Gary win the lawsuit?

## DECISION

Yes. The court held the school was negligent in their care of Gary, particularly since Gary had a previous history of wandering off.

Based on a decision of the New York Court of Claims.

### Was Death of Golf Student Caused by School's Negligence?

## CASE

Tom Davis was entering his second year of high school when he decided to take golf classes offered by the school. He was inexperienced in golf and had been absent on the first day of instruction due to illness. In the second session, the regular male instructor was absent and instruction was left to a first year women's instructor who was in charge of twenty-five girls and a male substitute teacher who was in charge of thirty boys. The boys were divided into groups of six or seven and were told to stand on mats and hit wiffle balls against a far wall of the gym with golf clubs. Tom was unable to hit the ball so he asked another student to assist him. Suddenly, Tom was accidentally struck in the head with a golf club wielded by another student during the demonstration. He suffered a cranial hemorrhage and died three days later.

Tom's parents filed a lawsuit against the school district asking for $80,000 as damages for the wrongful death of their son. The school district's authorities expressed sympathy to the parents but denied they were in any way liable. "It was just an unfortunate accident," they pleaded to the court.

The parents persisted, saying the school's supervision was not adequate. Should the parents win the suit?

## DECISION

Yes. The court agreed with the parents, holding that the instructors were too few or not well-enough qualified. They felt the parents were entitled to the $80,000 asked for.

Based on a decision of a County District Court in Nebraska.

### Should School Allow Dangerous Activity?

## CASE

Howard Barnes, an 18-year-old college freshman, was really enjoying his first year of college. His grades were good and he had made many friends. The "tray-sliding" accident changed all of this. It left him paralyzed from the chest down.

"Tray sliding" was described in an orientation pamphlet distributed by the university as a "school tradition." It involved sliding down an unlighted snow-covered slope on plastic cafeteria trays. Howard fell off his tray and was struck by another student in the back. The impact broke his spine.

Howard filed a lawsuit against the college asking for $500,000 as damages for his injury. He alleged liability of the university in that it encouraged and supported the student's participation in the tray-sliding activity which it should have known was dangerous.

The university argued that Howard assumed the risk and had fallen off his tray before and had seen other people colliding on the hill. Should Howard win the lawsuit?

## DECISION

Yes. The court held in favor of Howard. They noted that the university support of the tray-sliding activity included providing trays, stationing campus security guards at the foot of the hill to close a street there, prohibiting sleds and toboggans on the slope, and placing bales of hay around trees and other obstacles on the course. The court also observed that a year after the accident the university placed lights on the slope and, after Howard's suit was filed, prohibited the activity altogether.

Based on a decision of the United States District Court.


## Was Football Coach Negligent?

### CASE

Albert had been a football player for as long as he could remember. He enjoyed the game and now, at the age of eighteen, was anticipating a football scholarship for college.

During a high school football practice, he noticed that his helmet was cracked. When he advised the coach of the crack, he was told to put adhesive tape on it and to continue playing. A few plays later, Albert was hit hard. He suffered a flexion compression fracture, resulting in permanent major paralysis of the left leg, left hand, and left arm. He now requires the use of a cane and leg brace and probably will for the rest of his life.

A suilt was filed on behalf of Albert against the school district for $1 million. Albert contended the coach should have obtained another helmet for him to use. He also contended that the tackling drill in which he was participating was unnecessarily dangerous in that it matched one ball carrier (Albert) against four tacklers.

The school district argued that they should not be held liable since football is known to be a relatively dangerous sport because of the physical contact. "Albert assumed the risks associated with the sport," they claimed, "and we should not be required to pay the $1 million." Should Albert win the suit?

## DECISION

Yes. The court concluded that the evidence showed the coach was negligent in conducting the football practice. It was also noted that the coach, in contravention of all approved first-aid methods, removed Albert's helmet after he was injured and was lying on the ground unable to move.

Based on a decision of the Los Angeles County Superior Court.

### Was Revolver Unsafe for Careless Hunter?

## CASE

Edward loved to hunt and, after many years of planning, he made his first trip to Alaska. He had taken a single action .44 caliber revolver and a shotgun with him into the woods. As he approached a roadway walking out of a wooded area, Edward breached the shotgun to unload it and as he did so the butt of the shotgun struck the hammer on the revolver causing it to discharge. The bullet passed through his right leg into his left ankle. After several unsuccessful attempts to save the right leg, it was determined that amputation below the knee was necessary. His left leg healed after approximately one year. Edward was totally disabled for a year but later received an artificial leg and was rehabilitated as a welder. He filed a lawsuit against the manufacturer of the revolver asking for $400,000 in damages. Edward claimed the revolver was negligently manufactured since it discharged without the trigger being touched.

The manufacturer argued that the injury was due to Edward's carelessness in hitting the hammer of the revolver with the shotgun. "We should not be required to pay for an injury caused by the injured party's negligence," they stated to the court. Should Edward win the lawsuit?

## DECISION

Yes. The court held that the event causing the revolver to fire was reasonably foreseeable by the manufacturer. Therefore, they should have so designed the revolver to prevent this type of accident.

Based on a decision of a United States District Court.

**Was Lawn Mower Misused?**

## CASE

Alvin was using his new rotary power lawn mower to cut the grass around his house. The rear housing of the mower was embossed with the warning, "Keep Hands and Feet From Under the Mower." The instruction booklet that accompanied the mower warned operators to mow slopes horizontally, not from top to bottom. This warning was repeated twice in the booklet in easy-to-understand language. Alvin, however, disregarded the instruction booklet advice and mowed the lawn up and down a steep slope instead of mowing the lawn horizontally. While mowing in a vertical direction, Alvin lost his balance and fell. His foot slipped under the mower housing and the mower blade severed two toes and partially severed a third toe.

Alvin sued the manufacturer of the lawn mower for $150,000 in damages, arguing that the mower was defectively designed because it lacked a rear trailing guard to shield the operator from the whirling blades.

The manufacturer denied liability, maintaining that Alvin was responsible for the accident by mowing up and down the hill, contrary to the explicit warning instructions in the booklet. Should Alvin win the suit?

## DECISION

No. The court acquitted the manufacturer noting that the warning in the instruction booklet was adequate, the design of the lawn mower was not the cause of the accident and that Alvin's misuse of the mower was the primary cause of his injuries.

Based on a decision of the Supreme Court of New Hampshire.

**Is "Hittee' or 'Hittor' Liable?**

## CASE

At the trial, William Summers testified that his car was stopped and the light was green at the time of the collision. Neck and back injuries suffered in the accident required him to be hospitalized for eight weeks.

Mrs. Bradley was the woman who ran into the back of William's car. She also suffered injuries which required hospitalization.

She testified that she was about one-half block from the intersection when she first noticed William's car stopped in her lane of traffic even though the light was green. "I let off on the accelerator to see what he was going to do—to see if he was going to go ahead," she told the jury.

"When I decided that he was not going to move forward, I applied my brakes, locked all the wheels, skidded the tires, and spent everything I had attempting to stop my car."

William sued Mrs. Bradley for $4,000 in damages and Mrs. Bradley countersued William for $3,000. "She was not keeping a proper lookout," William argued, "and since I was stopped, the accident was her fault."

Mrs. Bradley argued, "The light was green. William being stopped on a green light was negligent on his part and he should pay my damages." Who should win the lawsuit?

## DECISION

Mrs. Bradley won. The jury and the court looked at this case from the standpoint of "negligence" and "ordinary care." The evidence showed Mrs. Bradley did not discover William's perilous position in time to use all means at her command to avoid the collision.

Seeing the green light, it was normal for Mrs. Bradley to anticipate that William would proceed forward. His failure to do so constituted negligence. He failed to use ordinary care. "Mr. Summers failed to use that degree of care that would be exercised by a reasonably prudent person under the same or similar circumstances," the court concluded.

Based on a decision of the Texas Court of Civil Appeals.

### Was Danger of Wet Floor Open and Obvious?

## CASE

Walter had been a hotel night auditor for most of his working life. He had become accustomed to working all night and sleeping all day, and now at fifty years of age seemed very content with his situation in life. Most of Walter's work was done in the hotel's front office, but one night he was having some trouble balancing the restaurant receipts so he carried them into a larger rear office to spread them out. He sat down at a desk facing away from the door and completed his work. Meanwhile the custodian came in and mopped the floor around the door of this office. Walter did not see the custodian and slipped on the wet floor when he was walking out, severely injuring his back. He had dizzy spells and lost consciousness several times over the next few months. He also required several visits to hospital emergency rooms and was operated on three times. Further surgery has been recommended, but even if it is performed Walter will be in pain and unable to work for the rest of his life. He filed a lawsuit against the maintenance company that was responsible for cleaning the building asking for $300,000 in damages and contended they were negligent in not placing warning signs around the freshly mopped area.

The maintenance company argued that the wet floor was an open and obvious danger and there was therefore no duty to warn Walter of its existence.

"He should have been more careful," they claimed." The accident was due to his carelessness." Should Walter win the suit?

## DECISION

Yes. The court discounted the maintenance company's argument, pointing out that clear water placed on the floor was not such an open and obvious hazard as to eliminate the maintenance company's responsibility for providing some type of warning of the dangerous condition.

### Did Ambulance Attendants Cause Paralysis?

## CASE

The party was getting just a bit wild. Tom was one of the guests who had had too much to drink. He was intoxicated when he dove into the swimming pool and struck his head. Some other guests quickly pulled Tom out and called the ambulance. When the ambulance attendants arrived, they found Tom lying on his back. Their examination revealed no evidence of spinal injury and Tom used his arms and legs to assist himself when they placed him in a chair. In the ambulance on the way to the hospital, Tom began complaining of neck pain and leg numbness. At the hospital, damage to the spinal cord was diagnosed. Tom was rendered partially paralyzed.

Tom sued the ambulance company for $300,000 in damages. He argued that the attendants should have immobilized him and that, when they placed him in an upright position, they caused the spinal cord damage. The defendant contended that the attendants were unable to obtain information about Tom's accident because he and the crowd around him were intoxicated and belligerent. Further, the company argued that, even if the attendants were negligent, either Tom was paralyzed when he struck his head, or the initial impact produced sufficient trauma to the spinal cord that in the natural course of swelling he would have been paralyzed in any event. Should Tom win the lawsuit?

## DECISION

Yes. The court held that the attendants were negligent in their investigation of Tom's injury before moving him. The condition of the crowd is no defense and their other arguments were, at best, speculative.

Based on a decision of a California County Superior Court.

### Can Five-Year-Old Boy Appreciate Danger?

## CASE

For several years, Larry's Restaurant had distributed various promotional items in an attempt to increase their business. The current give-away was a toy rocket which was launched by a rubber band. The rocket was given to every child who ate at the restaurant. Tommy and his mother had gone to Larry's at least once a week for about four months. Tommy was five years old and always enjoyed getting the promotional items which were for children, such as candy, gum, comic books, or toys. After eating lunch at the restaurant, the mother paid the bill and the cashier gave Tommy the rocket. As soon as Tommy got home, he went into the living room and began playing with the toy. His mother, who was in the kitchen, suddenly heard him scream, "The rocket hit my eye." Tommy was rushed to the hospital where it was determined he suffered laceration of the cornea, iris, and lens, resulting in the loss of the left eye.

The mother filed a lawsuit on behalf of Tommy against the restaurant asking for $200,000 in damages and claiming they were negligent in distributing a toy so dangerous to a 5-year-old boy.

The restaurant argued they should not be held responsible and told the court, "The boy could well see how the toy worked and certainly should have appreciated the danger." Should Tommy or Larry's Restaurant win the lawsuit?

## DECISION

Tommy won. The court, after hearing the testimony of a mechanical engineer, held that the toy rocket was designed so that it was unreasonably dangerous. They also heard a psychologist testify that, in his opinion, a child of five would not appreciate the potential hazard of the toy.

Based on a decision of an Ohio County Court of Common Pleas.

### Was Ski Slope Maintained Properly?

## CASE

Walter was doing the best he could to learn how to snow ski. He had paid his fee and was on a novice trail owned and maintained by a ski resort. Walter was moving down the trail at a slow rate when his right ski became entangled in a small clump of brush. The brush was concealed by loose snow and caused Walter to fall. His injuries resulted in permanent quadriplegia. Walter filed a suit against the resort asking for damages in the amount of $1,250,000. He contended the resort negligently maintained its ski trails and failed to give notice of hidden dangers.

The resort argued that Walter assumed certain risks by engaging in the sport of snow skiing and that they should not be held responsible. They produced evidence which showed they had an excellent reputation for meticulous grooming of their ski slopes with sophisticated machinery which was used to remove everything, stumps and brush included, to achieve a fairway flatness. It was also noted that the resort had several ski patrolmen on duty, plus a trail crew, to check for hazards. Should Walter win the lawsuit?

## DECISION

Yes. Walter was awarded the $1,250,000. The court held that the clump of brush, covered by snow, on a novice trail was not part of the inherent risk of the sport of skiing. Walter did not assume this type of risk. "While skiers fall, as a matter of common knowledge," the court concluded, "that does not make every fall a danger inherent in the sport."

Based on a decision of the Vermont Supreme Court.

## Was Chughole County's Responsibility?

### CASE

Mr. and Mrs. Stewart had picked up another couple and were on their way to a Saturday afternoon football game. Suddenly Mr. Stewart, who was doing the driving, hit a chughole. The wheels started shaking and the car flipped over. Mr. Stewart broke two ribs and his wife broke her collar bone. The other woman had broken glass all over her face and nearly lost an ear. Her husband sustained a knee injury and was on crutches for three weeks.

The foursome filed a lawsuit against the county, which was responsible for maintenance of the road. They asked for $50,000 in damages contending the county was responsible for the six-to-ten-inch deep hole spanning ninety percent of the road's width.

The county argued that they should not be held liable for several reasons. First, they said they were unaware of the road damage before the wreck. Second, the county claimed it was unreasonable to assume every highway problem could be solved immediately since that was beyond the resources of mortal man; and third, they felt Mr. Stewart was negligent in not seeing the hole. Should the county win the lawsuit?

## DECISION

No. The county was ordered by the court to pay the $50,000 in damages. The court held the abnormally large hole was a special defect and the county should have at least put up warning signs. They noted that the evidence showed the hole had reached the proportions of a ditch across the highway and although a driver could see the hole from two hundred feet away, he could not tell its depth from that distance.

Based on a decision of the Supreme Court of Texas.

### Is Hotel Liable for Loose Carpet?

## CASE

The company Christmas party was going well. Betty, a 42-year-old telephone operator for the company, was walking across the room when she tripped over a loose, removable carpet that had been installed a short time before the accident. The fall caused a severe injury to Betty's left hip. This incident occurred at a local hotel where Betty's employer had arranged to have the party. She was rushed to a nearby hospital where she was put in traction. Ten days later, Betty was allowed to go home and nine months later she returned to her job as a telephone operator. However, due to the increasing pain and an inability to sit or stand for normal lengths of time, Betty was forced to retire after six months. The pins that had been placed in the hip were removed in an attempt to relieve the pain.

Betty sued the hotel for $1,400,000. She contended the hotel should have taped the carpet to the floor with plastic tape so as to not create a toe or heel trap. She argued that the $1,400,000 was not excessive considering that she could not now work, and that she had experienced so much pain in the past and would have more in the future.

The hotel claimed, and had a witness so testify, that Betty was bumped into by someone at the party and that was what caused her to trip over the carpet. "We should not be held liable for the negligent actions of other people," the hotel's lawyer stated to the court. Should Betty win the suit?

## DECISION

Yes. The court held that the hotel was responsible for taking reasonable precautions to protect the guests at the party. The evidence indicated they failed to do so and must therefore pay Betty the $1,400,000.

Based on a decision of the New York County Supreme Court.

### Was Electric Company Negligent?

## CASE

Albert Evans was enthusiastic about his father's day gift of a large CB antenna. He had expressed his desire for this type of antenna several months before but had never anticipated that his children would get him one. It was so large that Albert had two of his neighbors over to assist him in the installation. While moving the antenna, it crossed underneath the electric company's uninsulated, seventy-five thousand volt power lines. It was never known whether the antenna actually touched the lines, but a surge of electricity from the lines to the antenna caused Albert's instant death and severe injuries to his friends who were handling the antenna at the time.

A lawsuit was filed by Albert's wife against the electric company wherein she asked for damages of $600,000. She argued and presented evidence at the trial which showed that the electric company knew of other antenna contact accidents within its service area, including one on the same distribution line three blocks away from Albert's home. She also showed that the company was aware of the changing character of the neighborhood and that insulation should have been placed on such lines since they were located in a residential area.

The electric company contended they should not be held responsible for Albert's death since their power lines were in the company's right-of-way and were at least thirty feet in the air. Should Albert's wife be awarded the $600,000?

## DECISION

Yes. The court concluded that there had been a conscious disregard by the electric company of the public safety and consequences of not implementing known safety procedures and programs. They therefore should pay the $600,000.

Based on a decision of a County District Court of Nevada.

# Index